FEMALE INFERTILITY

CORE PRINCIPLES AND CLINICAL MANAGEMENT

FEMALE INFERTILITY

CORE PRINCIPLES AND CLINICAL MANAGEMENT

Bryan Woodward PhD FRCPath
Consultant Reproductive Scientist
X & Y Fertility Ltd
Leicester, UK

Jayant Mehta PhD DipRCPath
Sub-Fertility Laboratory Director
Quality Control Manager
Barking, Havering and Redbridge NHS University Trust
Romford, UK

JP medical publishers

London • New Delhi

Published by Jaypee Brothers Medical Publishers,
4838/24 Ansari Road, New Delhi, India

Tel: +91 (011) 43574357 Fax: +91 (011)43574390

Email: info@jpmedpub.com, jaypee@jaypeebrothers.com
Web: www.jpmedpub.com, www.jaypeebrothers.com

JPM is the imprint of Jaypee Brothers Medical Publishers.

ISBN: 978-1-909836-50-1

British Library Cataloguing in Publication Data
A catalogue record for this book is available from the British Library

Library of Congress Cataloging in Publication Data
A catalog record for this book is available from the Library of Congress

Development Editor: Harsha Madan
Editorial Assistant: Keshav Kumar
Cover Design: Rakesh Kumar

Preface

Pregnancy outcomes are highly dependent on oocyte quality. Although sperm quality influences fertilization, embryo development and implantation, it is the oocyte that orchestrates these processes to produce a successful pregnancy and a healthy baby. The birth of Louise Brown in 1978 marked the beginning of our journey towards an understanding of the dynamics of assisted female reproduction. Today, four decades later, our efforts to expand and improve on this knowledge are greater than ever.

The purpose of *Female Infertility: Core Principles and Clinical Management* is to provide a comprehensive understanding of various aspects of female reproduction in order to overcome infertility with appropriate treatments.

The book opens with an introduction to the basic anatomy and physiology and concludes with a chapter on fertility preservation for future treatment. Chapters in between cover a broad range of topics: those dedicated to investigative techniques describe how to establish the physiologically normal functionality of the ovaries, the measurement of ovarian reserves, stimulation protocols and the process of oogenesis and oocyte collection.

Conditions such as polycystic ovarian syndrome and endometriosis influence the quality of oocytes and implantation. Dedicated chapters therefore address the underlying causes of these diseases and how to treat them to achieve successful pregnancies. The preservation of oocytes offers women facing chemo- or radiotherapy the opportunity to realize their reproductive potential: relevant techniques and concepts are described in chapters on cryo-banking and oncology. Concluding chapters address future technologies, including deriving oocytes from stem cells. Correcting mitochondrial disease by application of the three-parent child concept is also discussed. The dynamic journey of describing female reproduction ends with a chapter on transplantation of cryopreserved ovaries.

Female Infertility: Core Principles and Clinical Management is richly illustrated throughout and we hope it will serve as an essential resource for all clinicians, nurses and clinical scientists specialising in reproductive medicine, gynecology, oncology, infertility and embryology.

Bryan Woodward
Jayant Mehta
March 2019

Contents

Contributors

Masoud Afnan MB BS FRCOG
Chief Medical Officer
Tianjin United Family Hospital
Tianjin
China

Fidelis Akagbosu BSc(Hons) MBChB MMedSc(ART) FWACS FRCOG FACOG
Obstetrician, Gynecologist, Reproductive Endocrinology and Infertility Specialist
Kaiser Center for Reproductive Health
Fremont
California
USA

Montserrat Barragán PhD
Researcher
Eugin Clinic
Barcelona
Spain

Kate Brian
Chair of the RCOG Women's Network
Royal College of Obstetricians & Gynaecologists
London
UK

Melanie Brown MSc
Nutritionist
Melanie Brown Nutrition
London
UK

Neelke De Munck PhD
Clinical Embryologist
UZ Brussel
Centre for Reproductive Medicine,
Brussels
Belgium

Michel De Vos MD PhD
Clinical Professor of Reproductive Medicine
UZ Brussel
Centre for Reproductive Medicine,
Brussels
Belgium

Simone Ferrero MD PhD
Associate Professor of Obstetrics and Gynaecology
Academic Unit of Obstetrics and Gynaecology
IRCCS Ospedale Policlinico San Martino
Genova
Italy

Tony Gordon PhD
Vice President Business Development
CooperGenomics
London
UK

Juan José Guillén MD
Specialist in Assisted Reproduction
Eugin Clinic
Barcelona
Spain

Corinne Hargreaves MBChB MRCOG
Consultant Obstetrician and Gynaecologist
Department of Obstetrics and Gynaecology
Queen's Hospital
Romford
UK

Roy Homburg FRCOG
Professor of Reproductive Medicine
Homerton Fertility Centre
Homerton University Hospital
London
UK

Louise Hyslop BSc, PhD
Principal Embryologist
Newcastle Fertility Centre
International Centre For Life
Newcastle upon Tyne
UK

Stamatina Iliodromiti PhD MD MSc MRCOG
Senior Lecturer in Obstetrics and Gynaecology
School of Medicine
University of Glasgow
Glasgow
UK

Benjamin P Jones MRCOG BSc(Hons)
Clinical Research Fellow in Fertility Preservation and Restoration
Department of Surgery & Cancer,
Imperial College London
London
UK

Semra Kahraman MD
Professor in Obstetrics and Gynecology Fertility Specialist
ART&Reproductive Genetics Unit
İstanbul Memorial Hospital
Istanbul
Turkey

Mohan S Kamath MS DNB
Reproductive Medicine Consultant
Department of Reproductive Medicine
Christian Medical College
Vellore
India

William Ledger MA DPhil (Oxon) MB ChB FRCOG FRANZCOG CREI
Professor of Obstetrics and Gynaecology
School of Women's and Children's Health
University of New South Wales
Sydney
Australia

Maria Jesus López MD
Specialist in Assisted Reproduction
Eugin Clinic
Barcelona
Spain

Umberto Leone Roberti Maggiore MD, PhD
Gynaecologist
Academic Unit of Obstetrics and Gynaecology
IRCCS Ospedale Policlinico San Martino
Genova
Italy

Mariano Mascarenhas MS(OG) DNB MRCOG
Clinical Fellow
Leeds Teaching Hospitals NHS Trust
Leeds
UK

Scott M Nelson BSc PhD MRCOG
Muirhead Chair in Obstetrics & Gynaecology
University of Glasgow
Glasgow Royal Infirmary
Glasgow
UK

Wendy Norton RCN BSc(Hons) MSc PhD
Senior Lecturer
The Leicester School of Nursing and Midwifery
De Montfort University
Leicester
UK

Caroline Pirkevi MSc PhD
Assisted Reproductive Technologies and Reproductive Genetics
Centerl stanbul Memorial Hospital
Istanbul
Turkey

Annalisa Racca MD
Gynaecologist
Academic Unit of Obstetrics and Gynaecology
IRCCS Ospedale Policlinico San Martino
Genova
Italy

Amelia Rodríguez Aranda MD PhD
Medical Director
Eugin Clinic
Barcelona
Spain

Sara Rodríguez López RN
Fertility Service Coordinator
Braunschweig
Germany

Kathryn Sanders BSc(Hons)
Genetics PhD Student
CooperGenomics
University of Kent
Canterbury
UK

Srdjan Saso MRCOG BSc PhD
Subspecialty Trainee in Gynaecologic Oncology
West London Gynaecology Cancer Centre
Hammersmith Hospital
London
UK

Susan Seenan
Chief Executive
Fertility Network UK
London
UK

Ingrid Segers PhD
Senior Clinical Embryologist
Centre for Reproductive Medicine
UZ-Brussel, Vrije Universiteit Brussel
Brussels
Belgium

J Richard Smith FRCOG MD
Consultant Gynaecology Oncologist
West London Gynaecology Cancer Centre
Hammersmith Hospital,
London
UK

Karen Sohan MBBS(UWI) FRCOG
Consultant Obstetrician
Diagnostic (Mother & Baby) Ltd.
Chaguanas
Trinidad and Tobago

Dominic Stoop MD PhD
Professor of Reproductive Medicine
Centre for Reproductive Medicine
UZ Brussel
Brussels
Belgium

Sesh Kamal Sunkara MBBS MD MRCOG
Consultant Gynaecologist and Subspecialist in Reproductive Medicine
Queen's Hospital
Barking Havering and Redbridge University Hospitals NHS Trust
Essex
UK

Gustavo Tiscornia PhD
Researcher
Eugin Clinic
Barcelona
Spain

Rita Vassena DVM PhD
Scientific Director
Eugin Clinic
Barcelona
Spain

Greta Verheyen PhD
Head, ART Laboratory
Centre for Reproductive Medicine
UZ Brussel
Brussels
Belgium

Kieren Wilson MBBS MRMed MWomHMed FRANZCOG
Consultant Obsterician & Gynaecologist
Royal Australian and New Zealand College of Obstetricians and Gynaecologists
Melbourne
Australia

Chapter 1 Anatomy and physiology

Fidelis T Akagbosu

ANATOMY OF THE FEMALE REPRODUCTIVE SYSTEM

The human female reproductive system is composed of anatomical structures that must interact with hormones within a defined time-frame in order for conception, pregnancy, and birth to occur. The primary sex organs are the ovaries which produce oocytes and hormones, mainly estrogen and progesterone. The secondary sex organs are the external genitalia, vagina, uterus and fallopian tubes. Their function is to receive sperm, and to provide sites for fertilization, implantation and development of the embryo to term and parturition. The mammary glands provide nourishment for the young and may be considered accessory reproductive organs.

External genitalia

The vulva (or pudendum) is the collective term for all the visible external genital organs in the female. It consists of the mons pubis, labia majora, labia minora, hymen, clitoris, vestibule, urethra and Skene's and Bartholin's glands (see **Figure 1.1**).

The mons pubis is the subcutaneous fat pad overlying the symphysis pubis. The labia majora are two folds of fat pad and skin that have hair and sweat glands. The labia majora are homologous to the scrotum in the male. They act together with the labia minora as the gatekeeper into the vagina. The vulva is covered by keratinized stratified squamous epithelium. The labia minora are two folds of hairless skin with sweat glands that merge anteriorly to form the prepuce (covering of the clitoris) and serve to protect the vaginal and urethral openings. The labia minora are homologous to the penile urethra and part of the skin of the penis in males. The clitoris is a small cylindrical erectile body, situated in the most anterior part of the vulva. It is homologous to the penis in the male but it differs in being entirely separate from the urethra. It is attached to the under surface of the symphysis pubis by the suspensory ligament.

The vestibule is the triangular space bounded anteriorly by the clitoris, posteriorly by the fourchette and on either side by labia minora. The four openings into the vestibule are the urethral opening, the vaginal orifice and hymen, the opening of Bartholin's ducts, and the Skene's ducts openings in the vestibule on either side of the external urethral meatus. The vestibular bulbs are bilateral elongated masses of erectile tissues situated beneath the mucus membrane of the vestibule. Each bulb lies on either side of the vaginal orifice in front of the Bartholin's gland and is incorporated with the bulbocavernosus muscle. They are homologous to the bulb of the penis and corpus spongiosum in the male.

The external genitalia develop in the region of the cranial aspect of ectodermal cloacal fossa and form by the end of the 12th week of fetal development. The clitoris develops from the genital tubercle, the labia minora from the genital folds, the labia majora from the labioscrotal swelling and the vestibule from the urogenital sinus.

Internal genitalia

The internal genital organs are located in the lower abdominal/pelvic cavity and include the vagina, uterus, fallopian tubes and ovaries (**Figure 1.2**).

Vagina

The vagina is a flattened but distensible musculomembranous canal that links the uterine cavity with the exterior at the vulva. It is the excretory channel for uterine secretions and menstrual blood, the organ

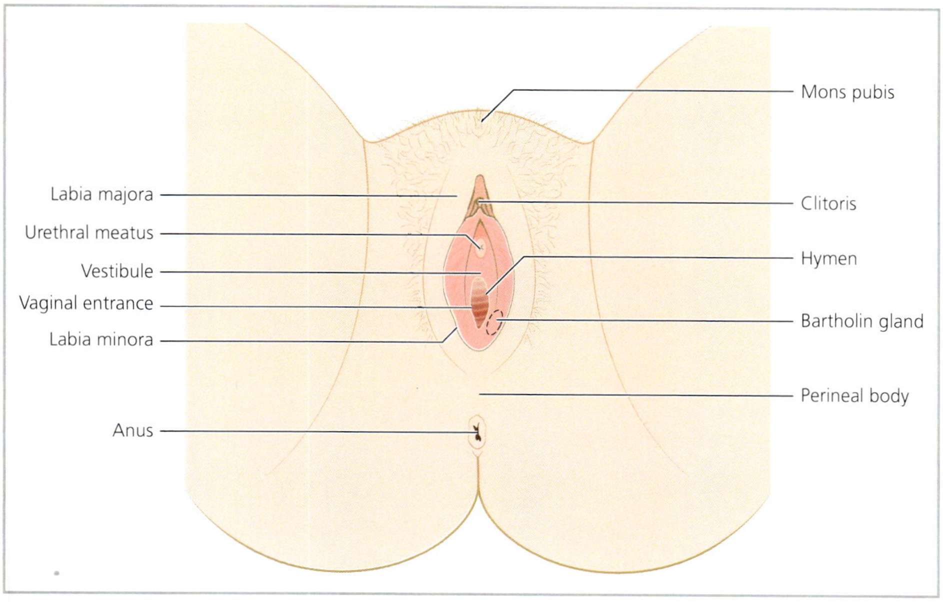

Figure 1.1 The external structure of the female reproductive system. The vulva is the collective term for all the visible external genital organs in the female. This includes of the mons pubis, labia majora, labia minora, hymen, clitoris, vestibule, urethra and Skene's and Bartholin's glands and mons pubis. The labia minora and majora protect the clitoris, urethral meatus and vaginal entrance.

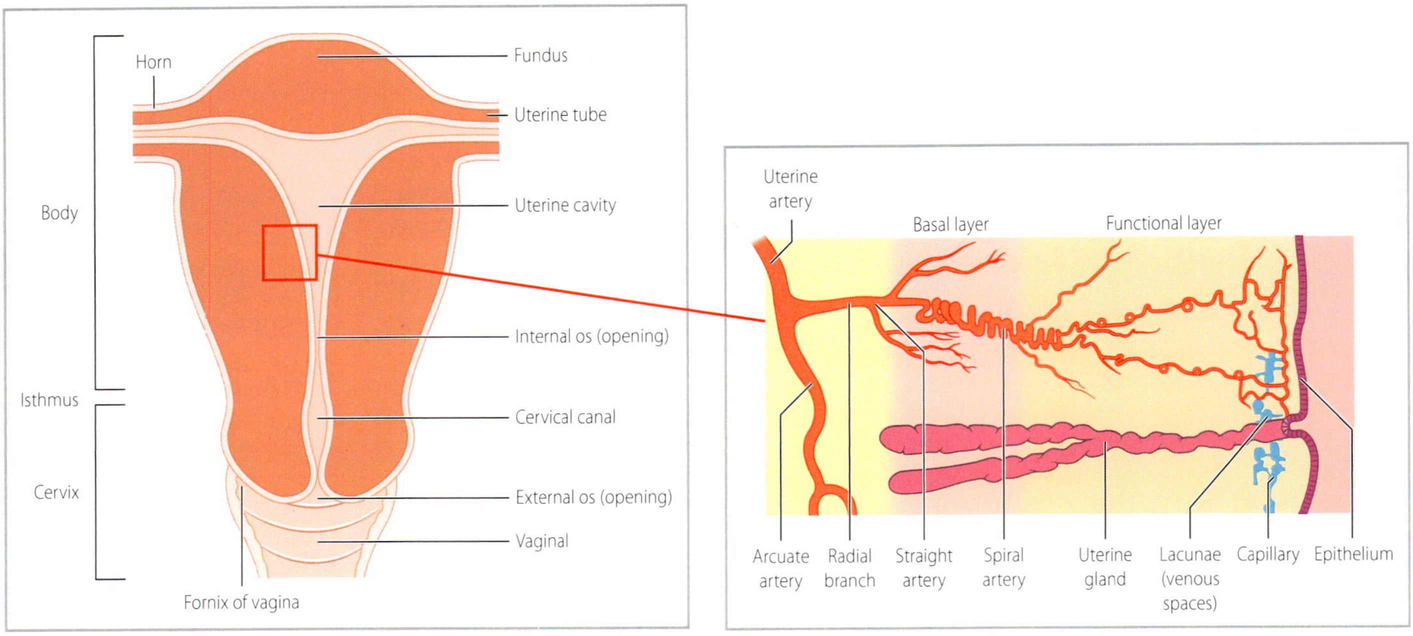

Figure 1.2 The internal structures of the female reproductive system. The female internal genital organs are located in the lower abdominal/pelvic cavity and include the vagina, cervix uterus, fallopian tubes and ovaries. The uterine wall has three layers: the perimetrium is the outer serosal layer; the myometrium is the middle muscular layer; and the endometrium is the inner mucosal lining. The endometrium consists of a functional layer, which contains secretory glands and is shed during menses, and a basal layer, which is highly vascularized and regenerates the functional layer.

of copulation and forms the birth canal of parturition. The canal is directed upwards and backwards forming an angle of about 45° with the horizontal in erect posture. The length of the anterior wall is about 7 cm and that of the posterior wall is about 9 cm (Dutta 2015). The vaginal walls are separated where the uterine cervix projects into the vaginal cavity. The space which exists between the intravaginal part of the cervix and the vaginal wall is divided into anterior, lateral and posterior fornices.

The vagina has three layers: an inner mucosal layer that is comprised of non-keratinized stratified squamous epithelium; a muscularis layer made of smooth muscle; and a fibrous layer that covers the vagina and attaches it to the surrounding pelvic organs. The vaginal pH, from puberty to menopause, is acidic because of the presence of Doderlein's bacilli which are large gram-positive bacteria that produce lactic acid from the glycogen present in the exfoliated cells (**Figure 1.3**).

The mucus membrane of the upper four-fifth of the vagina, above the hymen, is derived from endoderm of the canalized sinovaginal bulbs, while the musculature is developed from the mesoderm of two fused paramesonephric (Müllerian) ducts. The lower one-fifth, below the hymen, is developed from the endoderm of the urogenital sinus. The external vaginal orifice is formed from the genital fold ectoderm after rupture of the urogenital membrane (Dutta 2015).

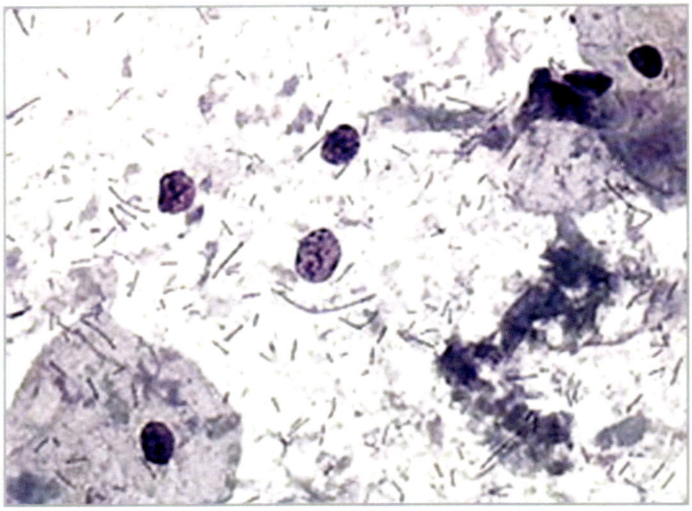

Figure 1.3 Doderlein's bacilli are large rod-shaped gram-positive bacteria that produce lactic acid from the substrate glycogen present in exfoliated cells. Vaginal pH is acidic because of the presence of these bacteria, and this environment prevents the growth of other pathogens. They are detectable in the vagina 3–4 days after birth, and then at puberty; however, they are no longer detectable postmenopause. They most likely originate from the intestine and their presence is dependent on estrogen.

Uterus

The uterus is a pear-shaped muscular organ that is intermediate in position between the bladder, rectum and broad ligaments. After puberty, the normal length is about 7.6 cm and width is 4.5 cm. The normal uterus weighs about 60 g but can weigh up to 200 g when associated with various pathologies. The uterus is developed from the fused vertical part of the two Müllerian ducts.

The uterus is composed of three regions: the bulging upper section called the fundus; the body which is the usual site of implantation; and the narrow lower section called the cervix. The cervix is about 2.5 cm long and is divided into supravaginal and intravaginal portions. The inner walls of the cervix contain nabothian follicles, small sacs that, in response to rising estradiol levels, secrete an alkaline mucus which protects sperm from the acidity of the vaginal secretions. These follicles are also known as nabothian cysts, which may appear as harmless bumps on the surface on the cervix.

The uterus is supported by four paired ligaments. The broad ligament attaches the pelvis walls and floor to the uterus; the uterosacral ligament attaches the lateral pelvic wall to the uterus; the cardinal ligament runs laterally from the cervix and vagina to the walls of the pelvis; and the round ligament extends from the lateral border of the uterus below the uterine tube to the lateral pelvic wall.

The uterine wall has three layers:

1. The perimetrium is the outer serosal layer
2. The middle muscular layer is called the myometrium
3. The endometrium is the inner mucosal lining. The endometrium consists of a functional layer, which contains secretory glands and is shed during menses, and a basal layer, which is highly vascularized and regenerates the functional layer (see **Figure 1.2**).

The uterus is capable of undergoing major changes during a woman's reproductive life. From puberty to menopause, the inner lining of the uterus (the endometrium) provides a suitable environment for embryo implantation and development during pregnancy. The endometrial lining in response to hormones released from the ovaries, thickens during the proliferative phase of the menstrual cycle, and then forms secretory glands in the second half of the menstrual cycle. If implantation does not occur, the endometrium is shed and excreted from the body via the vagina during menstruation (see **Figure 1.4**).

Fallopian tubes

The fallopian tubes, or oviducts, are paired structures approximately 10 cm long that lead from the uterus and end in finger-like projections called fimbriae. The fimbriae are suspended over the ovaries, and during ovulation receive the mature oocyte that is released from an ovarian follicle.

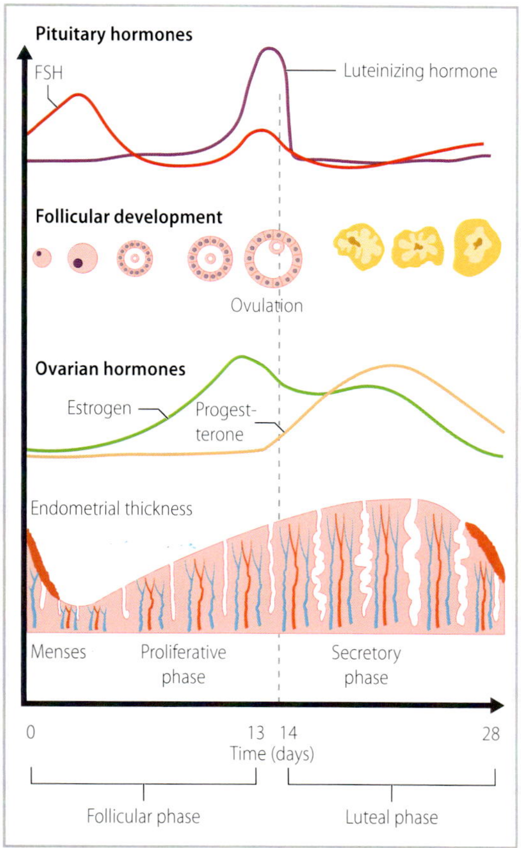

Figure 1.4 The menstrual cycle. The uterus undergoes major changes during the menstrual cycle. The inner lining of the uterus (the endometrium) provides a suitable environment for embryo implantation. The endometrial lining responds to hormonal signals from the ovaries, thickening during the proliferative phase and then forming secretory glands in the second half of the cycle. If implantation does not occur, the endometrium is shed and excreted from the body via the vagina during menstruation.

The fallopian tube has four subdivisions; the interstitial part is the short portion that begins at the upper angle of the uterine cavity with which it connects by a minute ostium; the isthmus is the medial 2.5 cm; the ampulla is the widest and longest subdivision of the tube; and the infundibulum is funnel-shaped leading from the ampulla, which contains the fimbriae.

After release from the follicle, the oocyte remains in the fallopian tube for about 3 days, with fertilization normally taking place at the distal end. The resulting embryo is propelled through the fallopian tube by a combination of rhythmic contractions of the muscular layer and the action of tiny hair-like projections, called cilia, toward the uterus. Pregnancy may be established via implantation of the embryo into the uterine lining 5 or 6 days following fertilization.

The fallopian tube has three layers (see **Figure 1.5**):

1. A serous layer (serosa) has peritoneum on all sides except along the line of attachment of mesosalpinx
2. A muscular layer (smooth muscle) has an outer longitudinal and inner circular layer
3. A mucus membrane layer (mucosa). Columnar ciliated epithelial cells line the mucus membrane layer and are predominant near the ovarian end of the tube, whilst secretory columnar cells are present at the isthmic segment, with peg cells found in between

The fallopian tube is developed from the upper vertical part of the corresponding Müllerian duct at about 6–10th week of pregnancy.

Ovaries

The ovaries are paired sex glands in the female, located on either side of the uterus. Each ovary is a pinkish/white ovoid structure which resembles a large almond in size and shape. A normal adult healthy ovary measures about 3 cm long × 1.5 cm wide × 1 cm thick.

The ovary lies near the lateral wall of the pelvic cavity in a slight depression between the ureter posterior medially, the external iliac artery being lateral and the uterine tube in the free margin of the broad ligament anteriorly. The extremity of the uterine tube curves around the lateral end of the ovary and is attached to it by one of its fimbriae. The ovary is attached to the superior surface of the broad ligament by a short peritoneal fold (mesovarium), through which the ovarian vessels enter its hilus. The medial extremity of the ovary is attached to the uterus by the ligament of the ovary.

The ovary consists of four layers. The germinal epithelium is the outermost layer and is made up of simple cuboidal epithelium. Next is the tunica albuginea, a collagenous layer, then the outer cortex and inner medulla layers. Throughout the cortex and medulla is a

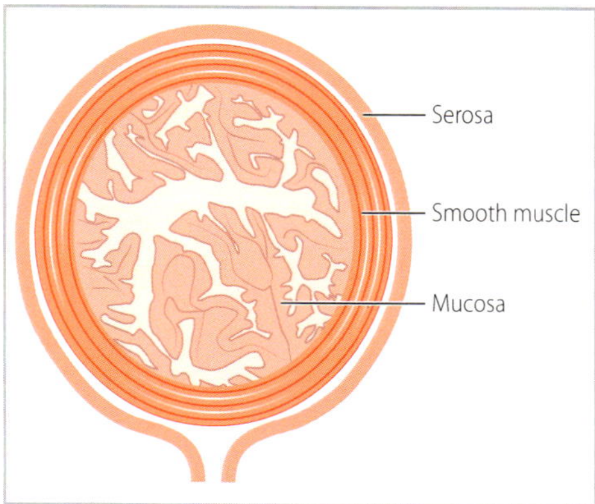

Figure 1.5 A cross-section of a fallopian tube, showing the three layers: the serosa layer has peritoneum on all sides except along the line of attachment of mesosalpinx; the smooth muscle layer has outer longitudinal and inner circular layers; and the mucosa layer is lined with columnar ciliated epithelial cells, predominantly near the ovarian end of the tube, whilst secretory columnar cells are present at the isthmic segment, with peg cells found in between.

connective tissue matrix known as stroma. The stromal tissue has the ability to respond to luteinizing hormone (LH) or human chorionic gonadotropin (hCG) with androgen production (Speroff & Fritz 2005). Embedded in the stroma are blood vessels and thousands of microscopic structures called ovarian follicles. Each follicle contains an oocyte. The rete ovarii (the hilum) is the point of attachment of the ovary to the mesovarium. It contains nerves, blood vessels, and hilus cells, which have the potential to become active in steroidogenesis or to form tumors. The ovary is developed from the cortex of the undifferentiated genital ridges by about 9th week of gestation.

BLOOD SUPPLY AND INNERVATION OF THE FEMALE SEX ORGANS

External genitalia

The arterial blood supply to the external genitalia is via:

- Branches of internal pudendal artery – the labial, transverse perineal, artery to the vestibular bulb and deep and dorsal arteries to the clitoris
- Branches of femoral artery – superficial and deep external pudendal. Venous drainage of the external genitalia is via venous plexuses that drain into the internal pudendal vein, the vesical or vaginal venous plexus and the long saphenous vein

Innervation of the external genitalia is through bilateral spinal somatic nerves. The anterosuperior part is supplied by the cutaneous branches from the ilio-inguinal and genital branch of genitofemoral nerve (L1 and L2) and the posterior-inferior part by the pudendal branches from the posterior cutaneous nerve of thigh (S1.2.3). The vulva is also supplied by the labial and perineal branches of the pudendal nerve (S2.3.4).

Internal genitalia

Vagina

Arterial blood supply to the vagina is via:

- The cervicovaginal branch of the uterine artery
- The vaginal artery – branch of anterior division of internal iliac
- The middle rectal artery
- The internal pudendal artery

These anastomose with one another and form two azygos arteries – anterior and posterior. The veins drain into internal iliac veins and internal pudendal veins.

Nerve supply of the vagina is via sympathetic and parasympathetic fibers from the pelvic plexus. The lower part of the vagina is supplied by the pudendal nerve.

Uterus

Blood supply to the uterus is from the uterine artery, one on each side. The artery arises directly from the anterior division of the internal iliac. Other sources are ovarian and vaginal arteries with which the uterine arteries anastomose. The venous channels correspond to the arterial course and drain into the internal iliac veins (see **Figure 1.6**).

The nerve supply of the uterus is derived principally from the sympathetic system and partly from the parasympathetic system. Sympathetic components are from T5 and T6 (motor) and T10 to L1 spinal segments (sensory). The somatic distribution of uterine pain is that area of the abdomen supplied by T10 to L8. The parasympathetic system is represented on either side by the pelvic nerve which consists of both motor and sensory fibers from S2, S3, S4 and ends in the ganglia of Frankenhauser.

Fallopian tubes

Arterial supply to the fallopian tubes is from the uterine and ovarian arteries. Venous drainage is through the pampiniform plexus into the ovarian veins. The nerve supply is derived from the uterine and ovarian nerves.

Ovaries

Arterial supply to the ovary is from the ovarian artery, a branch of the abdominal aorta. The ovarian artery sends branches through the mesovarium to the ovary, continues medially in the broad ligament, gives branches to the uterus and anastomoses with the uterine artery. Venous drainage is through the pampiniform plexus, to form the ovarian veins, which drain into the inferior vena cava on the right side and the left renal vein on the left side. Sympathetic innervation of the ovary is from T10 segment (Dutta 2015).

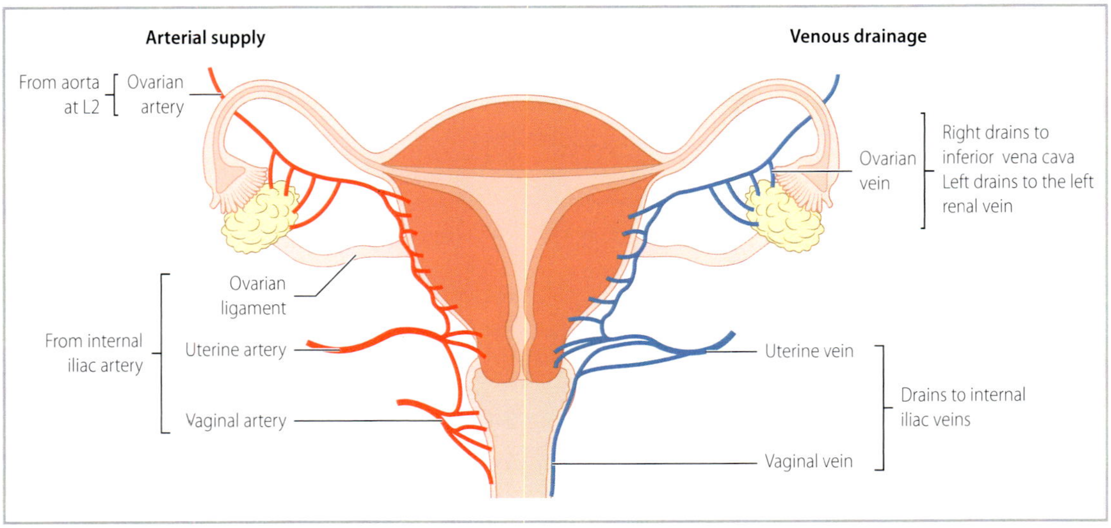

Figure 1.6 The blood supply to the uterus is from the uterine artery. This artery arises directly from the anterior division of the internal iliac. The venous channels correspond to the arterial course and drain into the internal iliac veins.

NOMENCLATURE OF FEMALE ANATOMY AND PHYSIOLOGY

- Skene's gland is also known as the periurethral, paraurethral, lesser vestibular gland or the female prostate. Anatomically, Skene's gland is positioned on the upper wall of the vagina, at the lower end of the urethra. Skene's gland was named after British gynecologist Alexander Skene (1837–1900).
- Bartholin's glands are also called the major vestibular glands. They are two compound glands, approximately the size of two peas, located slightly posterior and to the left and right of the opening of the vagina. They secrete mucus to lubricate the vagina. Bartholin's glands were named after Dutch anatomist Caspar Bartholin (1655–1738).
- Doderlein bacteria were named after Albert Döderlein (1860–1941), a German gynecologist who first described vaginal flora or microbiota.
- Nabothian follicles, also known as nabothian cysts, are mucinous retention cysts that can appear as firm bumps on the surface of the cervix. They were named after the German anatomist Martin Naboth (1675–1721).
- Fallopian tubes are the tubes that lead from the ovaries to the uterus. They are named after the Italian anatomist Gabriele Falloppio (1523–1562).
- Frankenhäuser ganglia is derived from the inferior hypogastric plexus. These gangia are the autonomic plexus located either side of the cervix, and were named after the German gynecologist Ferdinand Frankenhäuser (1832–1894).

OOGENESIS AND PRODUCTION OF OOCYTES

Early development of the ovary

During fetal life, the development of the ovary can be traced through three stages:

1. Indifferent gonad stage
2. Ovarian differentiation, oogonal multiplication and oocyte formation
3. Follicle formation

Indifferent gonad stage

At approximately 5 weeks of gestation, the paired gonads are structurally consolidated coelomic prominences overlying the mesonephros forming the genital ridge. This indifferent gonad stage lasts approximately 7 days. The primordial germ cells originate within the primitive ectoderm and are first identified at the end of the 3rd week after fertilization. They 'migrate' from the yolk sac around the hindgut to their gonadal sites between 4–6 weeks of gestation. The germ cells are the direct precursors of sperm and oocytes and, by the 6th week of gestation, on completion of the indifferent stage, have multiplied by mitosis to an estimated 10,000 (Speroff & Fritz 2005).

Ovarian differentiation, oogonal multiplication and oocyte formation

Oogenesis refers to the sequence of events by which oogonia (primordial oocytes) are transformed into primary oocytes. The process begins during the fetal period but is not completed until after puberty. At 6–8 weeks of development, the first signs of ovarian differentiation are reflected in the rapid mitotic multiplication of germ cells, reaching 6–7 million oogonia by 16–20 weeks of development (Baker 1963, Gordon et al. 1971). This is the maximal oogonal content of the gonad. At 11–12 weeks of development, the oogonia are transformed into primary oocytes as they enter the first meiotic division and arrest in the diplotene stage of prophase I. It is estimated that two-thirds of all primordial oocytes undergo programmed cell death. This 'quality control' mechanism occurs via an intrinsic apoptosis pathway and has been named the 'apoptotic wave' (De Felici et al. 2005).

At 18–20 weeks, the newly formed oogonia begin to be surrounded by the pregranulosa cells to become primordial follicles. As soon as the oocyte is surrounded by the rosette of pregranulosa cells, the entire follicle has the potential to undergo variable degrees of maturation.

At birth, the ovaries contain about 2 million primordial follicles with germinal vesicles and stay at this stage of development until puberty. Atresia of the primordial follicles persists and at puberty there are approximately 3-400,000 primordial follicles left. During reproductive life, 400–500 are selected to ovulate if there are regular menstrual cycles. The primary follicles will eventually be depleted to a point at menopause, when only a few hundred remain (Richardson et al. 1987).

Follicular growth

The time that elapses in progressing from a primary follicle to ovulation is approximately 85 days (Gougeon 1996). The number of follicles that mature is dependent on the amount of follicle stimulating hormone (FSH) available to the gonad and the sensitivity of the follicles to the gonadotropins. FSH receptor expression is greatest in granulosa cells, but significant expression can be detected in ovarian surface epithelium and fallopian tube epithelium. FSH acts on the growing cohort of follicles and causes an increase in size of the primary oocyte and the follicle.

On the first day of the menstrual cycle, about 5–10 growing follicles in the ovaries are available for recruitment. The increasing concentration of FSH causes selection of usually one follicle to grow, with proliferating granulosa cells. The follicle forms an antrum and the granulosa cells now make estrogen. The tertiary follicle is the last stage of the folliculogenesis before ovulation, growing to 16–19 mm in diameter (as assessed by ultrasonography). Granulosa cells give rise to all the cells of the follicle - the theca (interna and externa), the coronal radiata directly adjacent to zona pellucida (ZP) and the cumulus oophorus (**Figure 1.7**).

The rising estradiol level just before ovulation triggers a surge of LH, and informs the oocyte to resume its division via gap junction communication. The primary oocyte completes the first meiotic division (meiosis I) just before ovulation. At ovulation, the secondary oocyte begins meiosis II, but progresses only to the metaphase II stage, where the cell cycle is temporarily arrested. If the secondary oocyte is fertilized by a sperm, meiosis II is completed and a second polar body is formed. At this stage, the secondary oocyte is large, being just visible to the unaided eye (see Chapter 9 for a detailed description of the oocyte).

ESTROGEN

Estrogen is primarily synthesized by the granulosa cells of the ovarian follicles and the corpora lutea. However, some estrogens are also produced in smaller amounts by other tissues such as the liver, adrenal glands, breasts and fat cells. These secondary sources of estrogens are especially important in postmenopausal women.

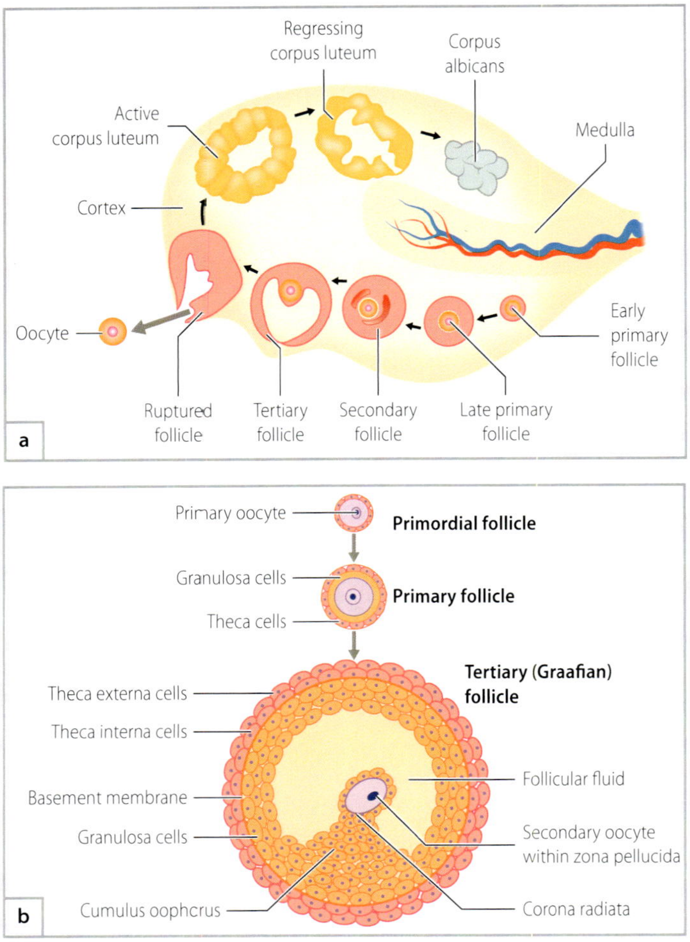

Figure 1.7 (a) Structure of the ovary and (b) oocyte. The ovary consists of the cortex which contains developing follicles and a vascular central core, the medulla. On the first day of the menstrual cycle, about 5–10 growing follicles are available for recruitment. As follicle-stimulating hormone (FSH) levels rise, usually one follicle is selected to grow. The follicle forms an antrum and makes estrogen via granulosa cells. The tertiary follicle is the last stage of the follicle before ovulation, growing to 16–19 mm in diameter. After ovulation, the empty follicle forms the corpus luteum.

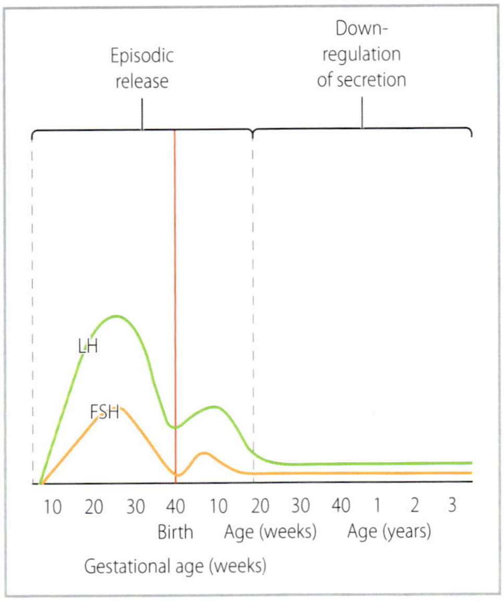

Figure 1.8 Levels of follicle-stimulating hormone (FSH) and luteinizing hormone (LH) during gestation, childhood and adulthood. There is a postnatal rise in FSH and LH. Between the ages of 2 and 11 there is very low amplitude and episodic release of both FSH and LH. By the ages of 11-13 secretion and episodic release of FSH and LH both rise - FSH to a higher level than LH - and then level out between the ages of 14 and 17 with amplitude and frequency of release dependent on the phase of cycle.

HORMONE RECEPTOR EXPRESSION (ABILITY OF THE OVARY TO RESPOND TO ENDOCRINE SIGNALS)

The anterior pituitary gland begins development between 4 and 5 weeks of gestation and the hypothalamic-pituitary portal circulation is functional by the 12th week. Pituitary levels of FSH peak at 20–23 weeks, and circulating levels peak at 28 weeks. Ovaries in anencephalic fetuses, which lack gonadotropin-releasing hormone (GnRH) and gonadotropin secretion, lack antral follicles and are smaller at term; progression through meiosis and development of primordial follicles occur, indicating that this process is independent on gonadotropins (Rabinovici 1990). The ovary develops gonadotropin receptors only in the second trimester. There is a postnatal rise in FSH with levels greater than the levels reached during a normal adult menstrual cycle, decreasing to low levels usually by 1 year of age, but sometimes later (Burger et al. 1991). LH levels are in the range of lower adult levels (**Figure 1.8**).

Ovarian-derived sex steroid hormones dictate the menstrual cycle in humans and are essential for the establishment and maintenance of pregnancy. The steroid receptors are part of the family of nuclear receptors and consist of estrogen, progesterone, androgen and glucocorticoid receptors. The functions of the sex steroids and their cognate receptors in ovarian function are multifaceted. Progesterone, testosterone and estradiol are all synthesized in the ovary during folliculogenesis and act via both extraovarian (i.e. endocrine) and intraovarian (i.e. paracrine/autocrine) pathways to influence all aspects of ovarian function. The endocrine actions of the sex steroids in the hypothalamic-pituitary axis are critical to the regulation of gonadotropin secretion and the ovarian cycle (Binder et al. 2015).

High-affinity estradiol binding sites in normal human ovaries have been described. Estrogen receptor beta (ER beta) is the predominant estrogen receptor form and is most often exclusively localized to granulosa cells of follicles from the primary to pre-ovulatory stage. Although FSH is the primary stimulus for both granulosa cell proliferation and differentiation, both FSH and estrogen are required for full antrum formation in pre-ovulatory follicles (Binder et al. 2015). Acquisition of aromatase activity and estradiol synthesis is a hallmark of healthy pre-ovulatory follicles and 90% of the circulating estrogen is estimated to originate from the dominant follicle in the ovary. Unlike thecal cells, granulosa cells express LH only in follicles in the late pre-ovulatory stage. This limited expression of LH receptors in the granulosa cells of healthy pre-ovulatory follicles provides for an intraovarian mechanism that ensures only those follicles that are suitable for ovulation acquire the capacity to respond to the LH surge (Binder et al. 2015).

Like granulosa cells, follicular thecal cells also undergo a process of differentiation during progression from a pre-antral to pre-ovulatory follicle. The two-cell, two gonadotropin paradigm of steroidogenesis in maturing follicles is that thecal cells exclusively possess the 17-β hydroxylase: C17-20-lyase activity necessary for synthesizing androgens, forcing the granulosa cell layer to be dependent on the theca as a source of aromatizable precursors (see **Figure 1.9**).

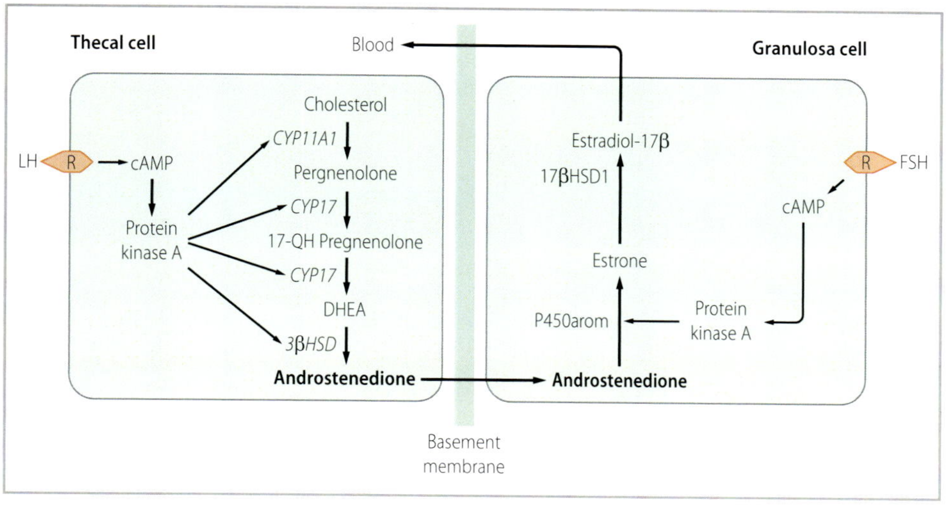

Figure 1.9 The two-cell, two-gonadotropin theory of steroidogenesis in maturing follicles. Thecal cells possess the 17-β hydroxylase: C17-20-lyase activity necessary for synthesizing androgens, forcing the granulosa cell layer to be dependent on the theca as a source of aromatizable precursors.

Androgens are necessary and serve as both a stimulus of and substrate for aromatase activity in granulosa cells. An intraovarian mechanism exists to negatively modulate thecal cell androgen synthesis so that levels do not surpass the aromatase capacity of the granulosa cell layer. Defects in this intraovarian mechanism are postulated to be an underlying cause of the excess thecal cell androgen synthesis that is a hallmark of polycystic ovarian syndrome in women (Binder et al. 2015).

Progesterone receptor (PR) expression has been primarily localized to the theca of large pre-ovulatory follicles, the surface epithelium, and ovarian stroma. The dramatic increase in PR expression in the granulosa cells of ovulatory follicles is absolutely essential to follicle rupture (Conneely et al. 2002).

The hypothalamic feedback mechanism and ovulation

The hormonal interactions that regulate the female reproductive cycle are initiated and maintained by a feedback mechanism that originates in the hypothalamus. The hypothalamus influences the anterior pituitary gland's secretion of FSH and LH by transmitting gonadotropin releasing hormone (GnRH) in a pulsatile fashion. In normal menstrual cycles, the hypothalamus releases GnRH at 60–120 minute intervals in the follicular phase. The FSH and LH stimulate follicular development in the ovary, resulting in the production of estradiol. Rising levels of estradiol in the bloodstream provide the 'feedback' to the hypothalamus for further regulation of FSH and LH. Shortly following ovulation, the high levels of progesterone and estradiol promote a negative feedback mechanism causing the pituitary gland to taper off the release of FSH and LH. As a result, concentrations of estrogen and progesterone decrease until levels are low enough to trigger menstruation and start the next menstrual cycle (**Figure 1.4**). In anovulatory cycles, the endometrium remains in the proliferative phase until menstruation begins.

Fertilization, implantation and initiation of pregnancy

Fertilization occurs when the mature oocyte is penetrated by one of the few sperm that survives the journey to enter the fallopian tube. If the oocyte is fertilized, a cortical reaction within the ooplasm changes the oolemma and causes structural changes in the protective ZP. This prevents other sperm from entering. Unfertilized oocytes are expelled during menstruation.

The fertilized oocyte, now termed a zygote, migrates down the fallopian tube, propelled by the action of cilia lining the tubal lumen. The early preimplantation embryo divides several times during this period to form a morula on day 4 and then a blastocyst on day 5. Approximately 5–6 days following fertilization, the blastocyst reaches the uterus where it implants itself in the endometrium. Implantation is dependent on several factors, such as adequate formation of the corpus luteum and an adequately developed endometrial lining. If implantation is not successful, the blastocyst is expelled from the uterus with menstruation. Pregnancy can only ensue following successful implantation.

Implantation signals the pituitary gland to release additional LH. This hormone supports the granulosa cells in their critical role of maintaining early pregnancy, by continuing to release an increasing amount of progesterone. Progesterone is vital to maintaining the endometrium during this phase. The corpus luteum continues to produce progesterone until the placenta is able to produce a sufficient supply of its own progesterone, typically at about the 9th or 10th week of pregnancy.

During the assisted conception cycle, additional supplies of progesterone are usually provided to the female once oocytes have been released, either via ovulation induction or egg collection for in-vitro fertilization (IVF) treatment. This is known as 'luteal phase progesterone' and the hormone is usually supplemented in the form of vaginal pessaries or gel, which needs to be continued on a daily basis.

Just before implantation, the developing blastocyst starts to produce hCG from the outer cell's layer, known at the trophectoderm. The rise in secretion of hCG is exponential, as the blastocyst implants and the trophectoderm cells continue to divide and grow.

The hCG is the hormone tested to determine pregnancy; hCG can be detected in urine or via a blood test. At the end of a successful pregnancy, the uterus undergoes powerful, rhythmic contractions during labor, resulting in the delivery of the fetus at birth.

REFERENCES

Baker G. A quantitative and cytological study of germ cells in human ovaries. Proc Roy Soc Lond 1963; 158:417–433.

Binder AK, Winuthayanon W, Hewitt SC. Steroid receptors in the uterus and ovary. In: Plant TM, Zeleznik AJ (eds), Knobil and Neill's Physiology of Reproduction, (4th edn). New York, NY: Elsevier, 2015.

Burger HG, Famada Y, Bangah MI, et al. Serum gonadotropin, sex steroid, and immunoreactive inhibin levels in the first two years of life. J Clin Endocrinol Metab 1991; 72:682.

Conneely OM, Mulac-Jericevic B, DeMayo F, et al. Reproductive functions of progesterone receptors. Recent Prog Horm Res 2002; 57:339–355.

De Felici M, Klinger FG, Farini D, et al. Establishment of oocyte population in the fetal ovary: primordial germ cell proliferation and oocyte programmed cell death. Reproductive BioMedicine Online 2005; 10:182–191.

Dutta DC. Anatomy of female reproductive organs. Dutta's Textbook of Obstetrics, 7th edn. Konar H (Ed). New Delhi: Jaypee Brothers Medical Publishers 2015.

Gordon B, Bhiraleus, P, Hobel C. Ultrastructural observations on germ cells in human fetal ovaries. Am T Obstet Gynecol 1971; 110:644–652.

Gougeon A. Regulation of ovarian follicular development in primates: facts and hypothesis. Endoc Rev 1996; 17:121–125.

Rabinovici J, Jaffe RB. Development and regulation of growth and differentiated function of human and subhuman primate fetal gonads. Endocr Rev 1990; 11:532–557.

Richardson SJ, Senikas V, Nelson JF. Follicular depletion during the menopausal transition: Evidence for accelerated loss and ultimate exhaustion. J Clin Endocrinol Metab 1987; 65:1231.

Speroff L, Marc A, Fritz MA. The Ovary – Embryology and Development. Clinical Gynecologic Endocrinology and Infertility (7th edn). Philadelphia, PA: Lippincott, Williams & Wilkins, 2005.

Chapter 2 Investigation of female infertility in primary care

Corinne Hargreaves, Jayant Mehta

INTRODUCTION

Infertility is a common condition in primary care. Fertility problems are estimated to affect one in six heterosexual couples in the UK. Most couples (about 84 out of every 100) having regular unprotected sexual intercourse (i.e. every 2–3 days) conceive within a year. About 92 out of 100 couples who are trying to conceive will do so within 2 years (HFEA 2013).

Infertility is defined as the inability to conceive after regular unprotected intercourse. In the absence of any known cause of infertility, a woman who has been trying to conceive for more than 1 year if <36 years old or for more than 6 months if >36 years old should be advised to have investigations to determine whether there are any treatable causes for the inability to conceive (NICE, 2013).

Initial investigations should be performed in primary care. This chapter aims to describe those investigations and discuss the rationale behind them, with explanations of the ramifications of abnormal results.

PRECONCEPTION COUNSELING

The initial consultation with the woman in primary care is an opportunity to determine whether or not there are factors related to her health or lifestyle that need to be adjusted or managed prior to pregnancy.

Obesity

A woman with a body mass index (BMI) >30 is less likely to conceive than a woman with a BMI in the normal range (20–25); and fertility treatments are also less likely to be successful (Friedler et al. 2017). In the UK, many National Health Service commissioners do not fund fertility treatment for women with a BMI >30. Pregnancy outcomes are also suboptimal for these women, with an increased risk of stillbirth, miscarriage and fetal abnormality. The risks of pre-eclampsia, gestational diabetes and operative delivery are all increased. The BMI should be recorded at the first visit and advice given around how to lose weight when it is found to be high (see Chapter 4).

Increasingly, women are turning to surgical solutions for their weight problems. Gastric banding and bypass procedures have been shown to be effective techniques for inducing weight loss. There is no evidence that having a surgical procedure to treat obesity increases a woman's chances of conception, but it is hoped that the weight loss will improve the outcome of any future pregnancies. Women who have bariatric surgery are advised to avoid pregnancy for at least 12 months in order for any complications of surgery to be dealt with, such as malabsorption, which can lead to growth retardation in the fetus. Future pregnancies require careful monitoring with regular growth scans and assessment for gestational diabetes (Cornthwaite et al. 2016).

A low BMI can also be detrimental to reproductive health. Too little body fat can cause ovulation to cease and render the woman amenorrhoeic. Furthermore, inducing ovulation in these women can be difficult. Some women with a low BMI have complications during pregnancy such as a low birth weight baby.

Anemia

Anemia may result from deficiency of hematinics (also known as hematics, hematinics are used to promote red blood cell production and the amount of circulating hemoglobin), e.g. due to dietary insufficiency, or from chronic blood loss as would be seen if the woman has heavy menstruation. There is no good evidence that vitamin B_{12}, folate and iron deficiencies can cause infertility, but, if an anemic woman becomes pregnant, there are risks to her and her baby. She is more likely to succumb to infection and is more likely to have a postpartum hemorrhage. There is also an increased risk of low birthweight and prematurity (Jagadish Kumar et al. 2013). If the woman has iron deficiency anemia, her baby may be born with low iron stores and this has been shown to have an adverse effect on neurodevelopment (Georgieff, 2008). It is therefore important that anemia is investigated and appropriately managed prior to pregnancy.

Rubella infection

Despite active international programs to eliminate rubella, if this viral infection is contracted in pregnancy it can be a major concern (Hübschen et al. 2017). If maternal infection occurs in the first trimester, fetal infection rates are up to 50%, reducing to <1% after 12 weeks (Silasi et al. 2015).

It is therefore very important that women of reproductive age are immunized against rubella infection. In the UK, a single dose of rubella vaccine was originally given to females at around the age of 14 years for this purpose. In 1988, the measles, mumps and rubella (MMR) vaccination program replaced the single dose rubella vaccine. However, in 1998, a study was published in *The Lancet* medical journal that suggested that administration of the MMR vaccine to children was associated with the development of inflammatory bowel disease and autism. This paper has since been retracted (see Godlee et al. 2011), but for a time it resulted in fewer women of reproductive age in the UK being immune to rubella. Nowadays, the MMR vaccination program has been re-accepted in the UK and the present incidence of rubella susceptibility amongst women of reproductive age is so low that routine testing of rubella immunity in the pregnant population is no longer needed (Public Health England, 2016) (see **Figure 2.1**).

Women who have not had access to such immunization programs continue to be susceptible to rubella infection. In order to eliminate this risk in the pregnant population, when a woman consults her general practitioner (GP) about fertility concerns, the rubella IgG level should be measured to assess her immunity. If the woman is nonimmune then she is recommended to receive two doses of MMR vaccine, 4 weeks apart. As this is an attenuated live vaccine, the woman should be advised that she should avoid trying to conceive until 4 weeks after the second dose, when the rubella IgG level should then be measured

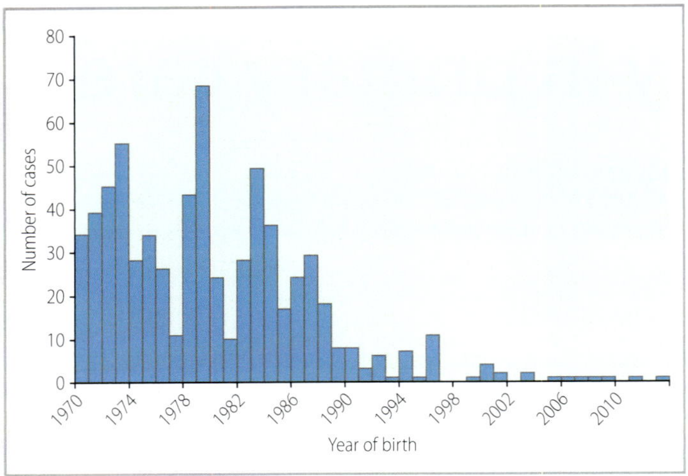

Figure 2.1 Congenital rubella cases in the UK: 1970–2014. There is a decline in the frequency of congenital rubella in the last half century due to the MMR vaccination program.

again. If the woman fails to seroconvert, it is important to check that the full schedules of two doses of MMR were given. Over 95% of women will become immune to rubella after the first dose of MMR (Plotkin & Orenstein 2004). Most cases of 'failure' of sero-conversion are due to the fact that the woman didn't attend to have the vaccination. If there is any uncertainty about a woman's immunity to rubella, it is safer to assume nonimmunity. There is no evidence that repeated doses of MMR cause any harm to the woman (Public Health England, 2016).

Hemoglobinopathies

Hemoglobinopathies are inherited single-gene disorders that result in an abnormal structure of one of the globin chains of the hemoglobin molecule. A hemoglobinopathy screen is an essential part of the investigation of all women with infertility. If the woman is found to be a carrier of one of the conditions, there is then the opportunity for her partner to be tested (see Chapter 15). Formal genetic counseling can be offered as necessary. Affected couples will be able to consider their options prior to conception, rather than finding out that there may be a problem when they are already pregnant.

Sexually transmitted infections

The initial consultation is an opportunity to screen for sexually transmitted infections (STIs). Where possible, nucleic acid amplification tests (NAT) should be used (Nwokolo et al. 2016) via a self-taken vaginal swab, or a cervical swab if a vaginal examination is necessary for another reason. The swab will pick up >90% of chlamydial and gonococcal infections with almost 99% specificity (Papp et al. 2014). If undetected and untreated, these infections may cause tubal disease and infertility in the future, in addition to neonatal conjunctivitis and maternal sepsis postpartum, in the event of a pregnancy.

Screening at this point in the woman's investigations may save time if she is referred to secondary or tertiary care. Screening is advised if a woman is to have tests of tubal patency and many fertility clinics insist on an up-to-date chlamydial and gonococcal screen prior to performing any assisted reproductive technology (ART).

The human immunodeficiency virus (HIV) and hepatitis infections in the woman are not a bar to receiving fertility treatments. However, by definition, attempting to conceive requires unprotected intercourse which increases the risk that the woman's partner may contract the infection. If a woman is found to be positive for blood-borne viruses, she should be advised of the risk to her partner from unprotected intercourse. If a woman tests positive for the hepatitis B virus and the male partner tests negative, he can be appropriately vaccinated. However, if the woman tests positive for either the hepatitis C virus or HIV, and the male partner tests negative, then the couple should consider assisted conception, to reduce the risk of the male partner contracting the disease.

Cervical cytology

We have found that 3–4% of women attending our fertility clinic have either never had a cervical smear, or have not attended for a repeat smear in the last 3 years. Women need to be informed of the problems they may encounter if they become pregnant and are then found to have cervical cytology abnormalities. It is the responsibility of the primary care physician to ensure that women are up-to-date with their smear tests and that the results are normal, before considering referral to secondary care for further investigation of infertility.

Folate

Spina bifida affects around 1 in 1000 babies in the UK. Folate supplementation is proven to reduce the risk of this condition occurring in the fetus. Folate is naturally found in leafy green vegetables, citrus fruits and lentils, but it cannot be assumed that all women are replete in their folate stores (see Chapter 4).

It is advised that all women of reproductive age who plan conceptions should take 400 μg of folate daily and continue with this until 12 weeks' gestation. This dose can be purchased without prescription and is present in many of the multivitamin supplements marketed to women hoping to become pregnant. A GP should ensure that the woman understands why she is being asked to take folate. Many women are unaware of why they are asked to take folate and may take it because they think that it will help them to become pregnant. If they don't become pregnant, they stop taking the folate because they think that it doesn't work!

Since women with diabetes and epilepsy are at increased risk of spina bifida, they need to take a higher dose of 5 mg daily, which requires a prescription.

Alcohol

Studies have shown that self-reported high alcohol consumption in women is associated with lower fertility rates compared to moderate or low alcohol consumption (Mikkelsen et al. 2016). The main concern about alcohol and fertility relates to those women who may drink alcohol in the early stages of pregnancy, before their pregnancy has been confirmed.

Due to this, the UK's Chief Medical Officer issued advice that: "if you are pregnant or planning a pregnancy, the safest option is not to drink alcohol at all, to keep risks to your baby to a minimum."

The guidance goes on to say that heavy drinking in pregnancy can cause fetal alcohol syndrome and that drinking lesser amounts can also be associated with behavioral problems or learning difficulties in the baby.

Tobacco

Smoking has been shown to cause premature aging in a variety of tissues including the ovary (Morita 2007). Although there is limited evidence that smoking cessation improves pregnancy rates, the UK's National Institute for Health and Care Excellence (NICE) states in their fertility guidelines that women who smoke should be informed that both active and passing smoking may reduce their fertility (NICE, 2013).

The main concern with regard to cigarette smoking is its strong known association with a poor pregnancy outcome if smoking continues during pregnancy. It is important to ask female patients about their tobacco intake and to offer support to help stop smoking. There is no evidence regarding the safety of using nicotine replacement in pregnancy and women should be advised about this.

Caffeine

There is no evidence that consumption of caffeine in drinks or foodstuffs influences the chances of conception (see Chapter 4).

FEMALE MENSTRUAL CYCLE

Hormonal changes

From puberty onwards, the hypothalamus secretes gonadotrophin releasing hormone (GnRH) in a pulsatile fashion; in response to this, luteinizing hormone (LH) and follicle stimulating hormone (FSH) are secreted by the anterior pituitary gland. LH mainly stimulates the production of hormones by the ovary, whilst FSH mainly stimulates development of the germ cells (**Figure 2.2**). Each developing ovarian follicle consists of an immature egg (oocyte) surrounded by granulosa and theca cells. The theca cells produce androgens (testosterone and androstenedione) which are then converted into estrogens (mainly estradiol) in the granulosa cells (see Figure 1.9).

Three types of estrogen are found in the plasma. Estradiol is the physiologically most important form. Ovarian and adrenal androgens are also converted in the liver and subcutaneous fat to another form of estrogen, known as estrone. This is a less physiologically active form of estrogen than estradiol, but still has significant clinical effects. This explains why women with extra subcutaneous fat may suffer less with symptoms of estrogen withdrawal at the time of menopause than do thin women. Finally, both estradiol and estrone are metabolized to the least active form of estrogen, known as estriol.

In order for a woman to menstruate spontaneously, a number of prerequisites need to be in place. Most importantly, the woman must be 'well-estrogenized', meaning she must have a threshold level of estrogen. Toward the end of a woman's menstrual cycle, estrogen (estradiol) levels are low. As a result, FSH is produced in the first part of the next menstrual cycle. The rising FSH stimulates the ovary to recruit a number of immature primordial follicles which then produce estradiol, as described above.

The majority of these follicles remain small and their only function is to produce estradiol. After a few days, in response to the increasing estradiol levels, one of the follicles will continue to grow and become the dominant follicle for the cycle. This is the follicle that will hopefully release the oocyte. The increasing estradiol levels in the first part of the menstrual cycle also cause release of LH, which is acute and occurs over 1–2 days. In a 28-day cycle, the LH surge occurs at around day 13 (mid-cycle) and triggers ovulation (see Figure 1.4).

Following the release of the oocyte, the empty follicle develops into a corpus luteum. This gland secretes progesterone, with levels starting to rise during this luteal phase. The peak progesterone level occurs around 7 days after ovulation. If there is no pregnancy, progesterone falls gradually to almost undetectable levels over the course of the next 7 days (see Figure 1.4).

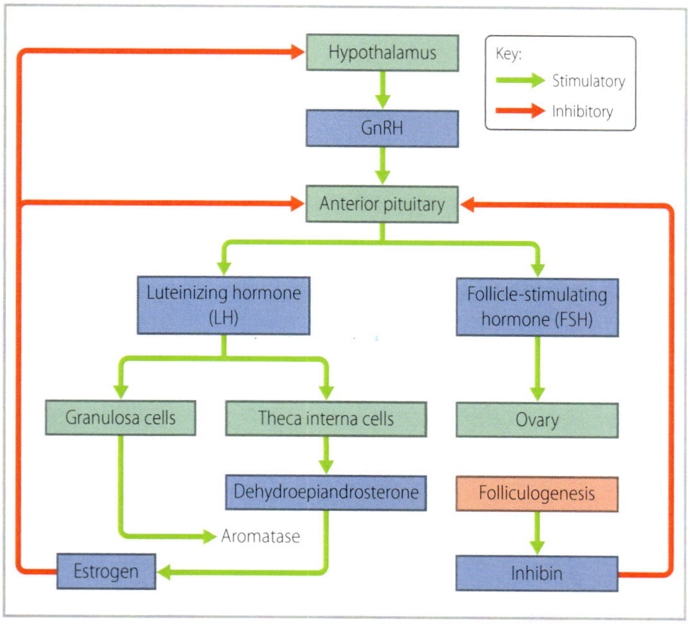

Figure 2.2 The hypothalamic–pituitary–ovarian axis. The hypothalamus, pituitary and ovaries secrete hormones that regulate their own production and secretion. Together, they control the function of the female reproductive system.

Hormonal effects on the endometrium

The increasing estrogen level, at the end of menstruation and the beginning of the next menstrual cycle, causes the endometrium to proliferate. If an ultrasound scan of the endometrium is performed, it is evident that the endometrial thickness has increased (**Figure 2.3**). Histologically, the endometrial stroma proliferates and becomes more vascular. The endometrial glands become enlarged and, later in the cycle, become coiled (**Figure 2.4**).

When the corpus luteum forms and progesterone levels rise, the endometrium becomes secretory. Histologically, the endometrial glands dilate and produce mucus, as the stroma becomes edematous and fragmented.

Menstruation usually results from the withdrawal of progesterone that occurs if there is no pregnancy. Importantly, if the endometrium has not proliferated under the influence of estrogen, then it will not respond to the progesterone produced by the corpus luteum. In these cases, even if the woman ovulates, she will not have a menstrual bleed. Progesterone can be supplemented to promote a withdrawal bleed in a woman with amenorrhea. When the woman is hypoestrogenic, e.g. due to menopause, hyperprolactinemia or hypothalamic hypogonadism, she will not have a withdrawal bleed in response to any additional progesterone that has been administered.

Women who persistently fail to ovulate, but have normal serum estrogen levels, may still have periods although the cycle length is usually very long. The menstrual flow is usually in response to breakdown of the endometrium after a long episode of estrogen exposure. This may occur in patients with polycystic ovarian syndrome (PCOS, see Chapter 6).

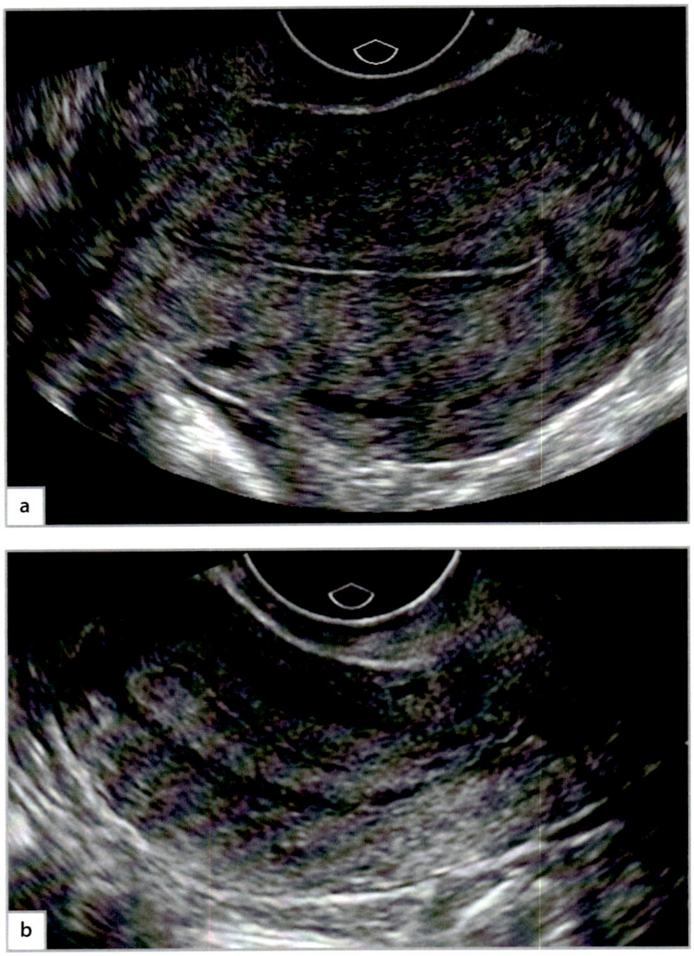

Figure 2.3 Ultrasound scans showing (a) the increasing endometrial thickness at the beginning of the menstrual cycle and (b) the loss of endometrial thickness at the end of the menstrual cycle (menses).

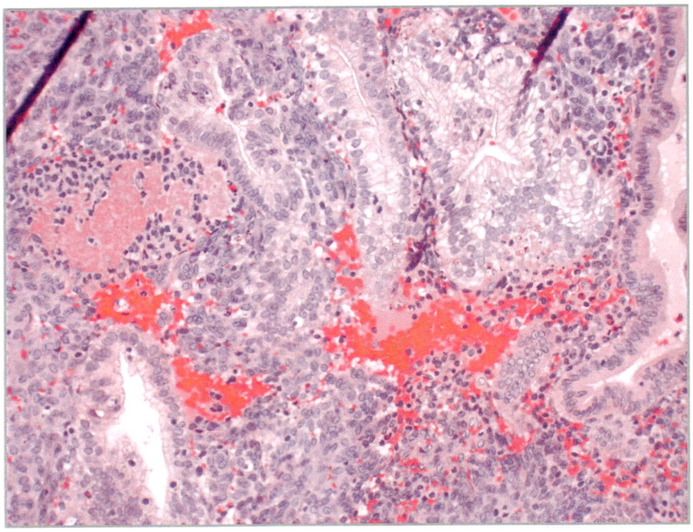

Figure 2.4 Proliferative endometrium showing the more vascular stroma and enlarged endometrial glands.

HISTORY

Duration of infertility

The duration of infertility is a prognostic marker for the success of any fertility treatment. The longer a couple have been trying to conceive unsuccessfully, the lower the likelihood that any fertility treatment will be successful, particularly if no obvious abnormality can be found after investigation.

It can take up to 2 years for a couple to achieve a pregnancy spontaneously and they should be reassured about this. However, it has been recommended that investigations should begin if a couple has been trying to conceive for >12 months (NICE, 2013). This period can be shortened to 6 months if the woman is >36 years.

Frequency of intercourse

It is not uncommon to find that couples with infertility are not having regular intercourse, which is defined as taking place every 2–3 days. There may be a variety of reasons for this, e.g. some couples may attempt to time intercourse to the day when they think that the woman is most fertile. However, a Cochrane review found no good evidence that 'timed intercourse' improves pregnancy rates (Manders et al. 2015). This study also found that attempting to predict the fertile period may have adverse effects on quality of life, risk of depression and levels of stress.

Another reason for decreased frequency of intercourse may be that the woman may have pain on intercourse or her partner may have erection difficulties. It is important to ask about difficulties with intercourse as this not only affects the chances of fertility, but can also be the cause of relationship breakdown. Effective management of these conditions at this stage may mean that no further investigation or treatment is necessary for the couple's inability to conceive.

Menstrual history

It is essential to enquire about a woman's history of amenorrhea, which may be primary (the woman has never had a period), or secondary (no periods after menarche has occurred). There are a number of causes of amenorrhea and some of these are listed in **Table 2.1**.

When asking about the menstrual history, the average length of the woman's menstrual cycle should be determined. The endometrium prepares for pregnancy in the proliferative phase of the menstrual cycle and extends through the luteal phase. In a 28-day cycle, the follicular phase usually lasts for 14 days and the luteal phase for a further 14 days. However, it is estimated that only 10–15% of women will have a 28-day menstrual cycle (Vollman 1977). It is assumed that most of these cycles will be ovulatory and this allows for around 12 attempts at conception each year. A cycle length of >35 days may suggest that a woman is not ovulating regularly, but even if she does ovulate, her chance of conception is less than a woman who ovulates every 28 days.

A short cycle length (<28 days) may also be problematic. This may be because ovulation takes place early in the cycle (a short follicular phase with a normal 12–16 day luteal phase), or because ovulation takes place around day 14, but there is a short luteal phase. The short follicular phase was previously thought to lead to a suboptimal secretory phase in the endometrium, with reduced pregnancy rates, but pregnancy rates have been shown to be similar whether there is early or late ovulation (Wilcox et al. 2000). A short luteal phase might be expected to be associated with reduced pregnancy rates because the endometrium sheds before the blastocyst has the opportunity to implant.

Table 2.1 Causes of amenorrhea

Type of hypogonadism	Primary amenorrhea	Secondary amenorrhea
Hypergonadotrophic hypogonadism	Chromosomal (e.g. Turner's syndrome)	Menopause
Hypogonadotrophic hypogonadism	Isolated GnRH deficiency Kallman's syndrome Systemic illness Eating disorder Hypopituitarism	Hyperproctinemia Low BMI/eating disorder Hypopituitarism Nonspecific hypothalamic (e.g. stress)
Eugonadotrophic hypogonadism	Rokitansky–Mayer–Kuster–Hauser syndrome (RMKH) Congenital adrenal hyperplasia (CAH)	Asherman's syndrome PCOS

The amount of bleeding reported during menstruation varies greatly between women. Most women lose between 35–40 mL of blood during their period, with 90% losing no more than 80 mL. However, the amount of blood loss is objectively difficult to assess and women may under- or over-estimate this. Very heavy menstruation may indicate the presence of endometrial pathology, such as submucous fibroids, whilst very light periods may indicate a hypo-estrogenic state.

Pain experienced during periods (dysmenorrhea) may indicate pathology, but many women, even with severe dysmenorrhea, have no gynecological pathology to account for this. Possible causes include endometriosis, adenomyosis and pelvic adhesions.

Past obstetric history

All previous pregnancies including miscarriages, terminations and ectopic pregnancies should be documented. Any complications in the management of these pregnancies should be enquired about, such as infections. For pregnancies resulting in live births, the mode of delivery should be documented and any complications related to the birth and postnatal period are important to note. There is no evidence to suggest that fertility rates following uncomplicated cesarean section are reduced (Evers et al. 2014).

Some women may have a history of recurrent miscarriage (three or more consecutive pregnancy losses) and this should be investigated prior to attempting any fertility treatment. At the time of the third miscarriage, products of conception should have been sent to a cytogenetics laboratory for karyotyping to identify if there might be a chromosomal cause for the miscarriage. If this is the case, the parents should be karyotyped to see if one of them has a balanced translocation. Genetic counseling can then be offered (see Chapter 15 for further details).

If there is no obvious genetic basis for the miscarriages, the woman should have a blood test for anticardiolipin antibodies and lupus anticoagulant. If either of these antibodies are raised, aspirin and low molecular weight heparin can be considered for future pregnancies.

Past medical and surgical history

Enquiries should be made about pre-existing and past medical problems. Conditions such as diabetes and hypertension should be optimally managed before any attempt at conception. In some conditions, such as epilepsy and depression, medications may carry a risk for the developing fetus. In these cases, the maternal condition must always take priority when considering whether to stop or change current medication.

Previous abdominal surgery may have implications for future fertility. The risk of tubal damage and subsequent infertility in women with a previous uncomplicated appendectomy is minimal. However, whilst appendectomy is significantly associated with an increased risk of ectopic pregnancy, this is not significantly associated with future infertility in women (Elraiyah et al. 2014).

Ovarian surgery, particularly if performed laparoscopically with diathermy, can destroy healthy ovarian tissue, and potentially, reduce ovarian reserve. A number of studies have shown that ovarian reserve is reduced when ovarian diathermy is carried out to treat polycystic ovaries (Kandil et al. 2005) (**Figure 2.5**).

Previous abdominal surgery may carry risks for the woman if she needs to have a diagnostic laparoscopy as part of her fertility investigations in secondary care and this should be discussed with her.

Family history

If there is a significant history of a hereditary condition such as a hemoglobinopathy or cystic fibrosis, then the couple should receive genetic counseling before embarking on a pregnancy. Many teaching hospitals have a genetics department and the primary care physician can ask for advice about how to refer (see Chapter 15).

Medication

If a woman is taking regular medication for an ongoing medical problem, it is important to establish whether the medication is known to be

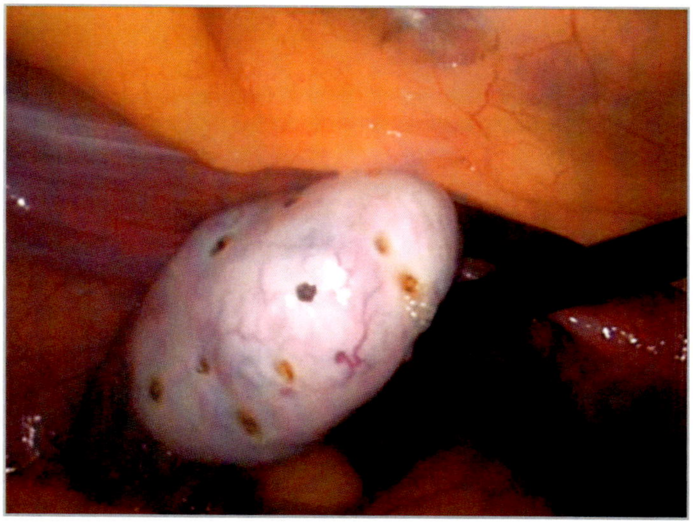

Figure 2.5 Ovarian drilling. This may be helpful for women with polycystic ovarian syndrome, to promote ovulation in future cycles.

safe in pregnancy or not. The general advice is to stop any medication that is not absolutely necessary. If the medication needs to be continued, this should be at the lowest possible dose. If the medication is known not to be safe in pregnancy, if at all possible, it should be substituted for a drug with a safer profile.

EXAMINATION

General

The woman's height, weight and BMI should be documented. Features of PCOS, such as hirsutism, acne and acanthosis nigricans should be noted. If there is amenorrhea, the breasts should be examined for evidence of galactorrhea. The abdomen should be examined for evidence of a pelvic mass and for scars indicating previous surgery.

Gynecological examination

A speculum examination should be performed to assess the vulva, vagina and cervix. Local conditions of the vulva such as lichen simplex or vulvar intraepithelial neoplasia may be present and result in painful intercourse. More rarely, there may be congenital anatomical abnormalities that are preventing conception. For example, in Mayer-Rokitansky-Küster-Hauser syndrome, there is absence of the uterus and cervix with a blind ending vagina.

A bimanual pelvic examination may reveal the presence of uterine enlargement due to fibroids or painful thickening behind the uterus that might indicate the possibility of endometriosis.

NON-NEOPLASTIC EPITHELIAL DISORDERS OF VULVA AND MUCOSA

Lichen simplex

Lichen simplex chronicus (LSC) is a skin disorder, whereby a localized area of skin has thickened via a process of 'lichenification', as a result of persistent abrasion and rubbing. It can occur on normal skin of individuals as well as people with psoriasis, atopic, seborrheic or contact dermatitis. Common sites for LSC are the sides of the neck, ankles, vulva, pubis, scrotum, and extensor sides of the forearms. This condition is also classified as neurodermatitis. LSC frequently seen in women than men, and is more common between ages of 35 and 50 years. LSC is also classified as neurodermatitis.

Vulvar intraepithelial neoplasia

Vulvar intraepithelial neoplasia (VIN) is localized to the skin that covers the vulva. VIN is an intraepithelial lesion of the vulva, whereby cells of the skin of part, or several parts, of the vulva become abnormal and change in their appearance. Many cases of VIN are linked to human papillomavirus, passed on by having sex with an infected person. VIN may disappear without treatment, but more commonly surgery or ablation is required. If the changes to the vulva become more severe, there is a chance that cancer might develop after many years, and so it is referred to as a precancerous condition.

ASSESSMENT OF REPRODUCTIVE FUNCTION

Assessment of ovulation

Ovulation results in corpus luteum formation, which secretes progesterone. Progesterone is a thermogenic hormone that causes a rise in basal body temperature (BBT) in around 25% of women if ovulation has already occurred. BBT is taken when the woman wakes up, before any activity. However, measuring BBT has significant limitations, but remains simple, noninvasive, and cheap, so many women download BBT charts from the internet in an attempt to help them to time intercourse (Wark et al. 2015) (**Figure 2.6**).

Women will often tell the primary care practitioner that they have been using ovulation predictor kits, which can be bought in a pharmacy. LH, which is released 24–48 hours prior to ovulation, can be detected in urine at this time, and studies have shown that there is a 90% correlation between the urine LH surge and ultrasound evidence of ovulation (Behre et al. 2000).

However, some national guidelines do not recommend use of such kits (NICE, 2013). Women may find it difficult to know when they should start to look for the LH surge and as a result they may spend an unnecessarily large amount of money before the surge is detected. Also, women with PCOS may have a naturally high LH level during the menstrual cycle such that an LH peak may not be detected. As previously discussed, ovulation predictor kits encourage couples to practice timed intercourse, which has not been shown to be helpful in increasing pregnancy rates.

A more accurate way to check if ovulation is taking place is to measure serum progesterone levels in the luteal phase. Progesterone peaks at around 7 days after ovulation, so a blood test is taken 7 days before the next period is due. To do this, it is important to ask the woman

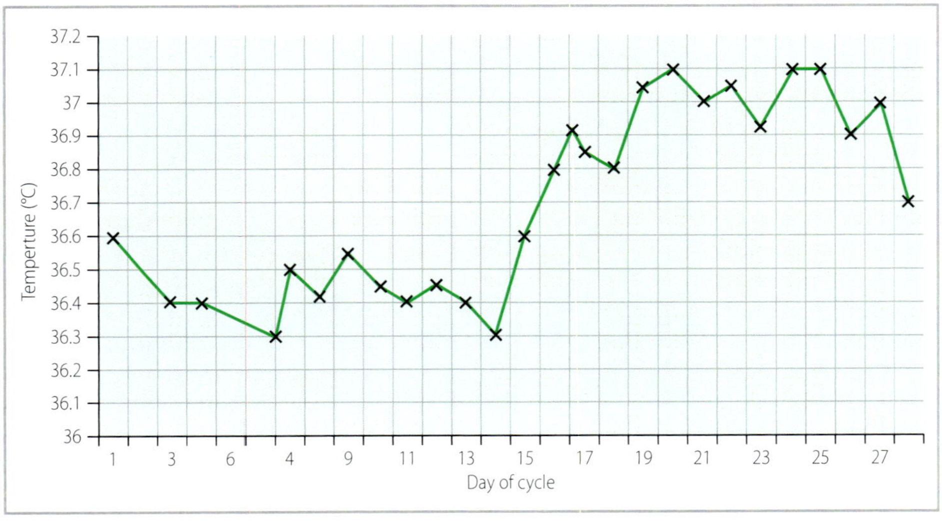

Figure 2.6 An example basal body temperature (BBT) chart.

about the length of her menstrual cycles, where menstrual cycle length is calculated from the first day of menstruation to the next first day of menstruation. If the menstrual cycle length is 28 days, the blood test should take place on day 21 of the cycle; and if it is 35 days, the blood test should take place on day 28 of the cycle. For women whose menstrual cycle varies, e.g. from 21–35 days, a series of progesterone levels can be obtained, e.g. on days 17, 23 and 28.

A progesterone level >16 nmol/L indicates ovulation (NICE, 2013). The test needs to be repeated if ovulation was not confirmed (<16 nmol/L) and the timing of the test was not optimal.

If a woman has infrequent menstrual cycles (e.g. a cycle length of >56 days) then she is not ovulating on a regular basis and a progesterone test will not be useful. In this case, further investigations will be required and treatment to induce ovulation may be needed.

Ovarian reserve testing

A woman is born with her full complement of oocytes. Since oocyte quality reduces with advancing age, it is important to explain the risk of delaying conception, and also to try to estimate the 'ovarian reserve'.

Measurement of serum anti-Müllerian hormone

Anti-Müllerian hormone (AMH) is produced by the ovarian granulosa cells. As women age, the functional capability of granulosa cells falls and, consequently, the level of serum AMH falls (Tatone et al. 2008). Thus, the serum AMH level can be used to try to predict ovarian reserve (see Chapter 5).

Woman's age and serum follicle stimulating hormone

The age of a woman when she is trying to conceive can provide a broad estimate of her chances of conception (see **Table 2.2**).

As a woman nears menopause, the number of oocytes declines and higher levels of FSH are required to stimulate ovulation. Thus, the FSH level in the early follicular phase of the menstrual cycle (day 2–4) can be predictive of ovarian reserve, where an FSH <8.9 IU/L is considered normal. There is some evidence to suggest that an FSH >8.9 IU/L predicts a poor response to ovarian stimulation regimes in in-vitro fertilization (IVF) treatment (NICE, 2013). However, FSH levels can fluctuate significantly from month to month and the results should be interpreted with caution to avoid creating unnecessary distress for the woman.

Antral follicle count

An antral follicle count (AFC) can be performed via a transvaginal ultrasound scan performed in the first few days of the menstrual cycle. The number of follicles measuring <10 mm in each ovary is then counted (**Figure 2.7**). A low AFC (<4 follicles) indicates a poor ovarian reserve and a poor response to ovarian stimulation in IVF.

Table 2.2 The relationship of a woman's age to the chances of conception after 1 or 2 years. (Adapted from NICE Clinical Guideline, 2013)

Age (years)	% pregnant after 1 year	% pregnant after 2 years
19–26	92	98
27–29	87	95
30–34	86	94
35–39	82	90

Assessment of cervical mucus

Cervical mucus is produced by the cells of the endocervix (see Chapter 1). Cervical mucus production varies throughout the menstrual cycle and is greatest mid-cycle. During the proliferative phase of the menstrual cycle, under the influence of estrogen, cervical mucus is thin and watery. At the time of ovulation, it becomes very stretchy, and is likened to egg white, with a water content is about 98%, compared to 90% at other times of the cycle (Sharif 2006).

The postcoital test (PCT) assesses mucus quality, as this may affect sperm transport. A specimen of mid-cycle mucus is collected around 24 hours after coitus. If the mucus is 'stretchy' and contains motile sperm (as assessed by microscopy), this is considered a good result. However, despite many years as an assessment tool, due to lack of efficacy, very few clinics still perform PCTs (Hessel et al. 2014).

Assessment of the endometrium

In order for pregnancy to occur the endometrium must be receptive to the fertilized oocyte. A number of biochemical factors such as cytokines and interleukin 1 appear to be involved in the process of endometrial receptivity, but there are currently no reliable tests to investigate this.

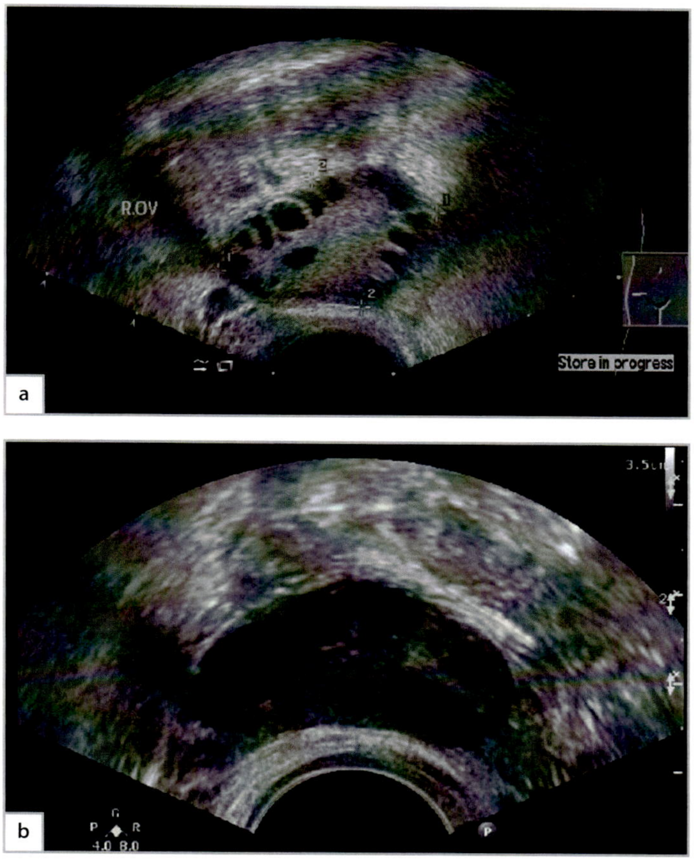

Figure 2.7 (a) A PCOS ovary with a high antral follicle count. (b) A normal ovary with a normal antral follicle count.

In cases where there is a history of amenorrhea, the primary care physician can perform a simple progesterone challenge test to assess whether the endometrium has been exposed to estrogen. A progesterone preparation, e.g. Provera 10 mg daily, can be given for 7 days and in the well-estrogenized woman there will be menstrual bleeding (a progesterone withdrawal bleed) 3–4 days later. If no bleed occurs, this is indicative of hypogonadotrophic hypogonadism.

Ultrasound assessment of the pelvis

It is reasonable for the GP to organize a pelvic scan as part of the primary care investigations. This may demonstrate the presence of fibroids or adenomyosis within the uterus (**Figure 2.8**). Intramural and subserous fibroids, and adenomyosis, are not known to be a cause of infertility, whilst submucous fibroids may need to be removed prior to attempting ART.

A pelvic scan may also detect the presence of endometriosis. Mild endometriosis is not proven to cause infertility, but moderate to severe cases can reduce the chances of natural conception (see Chapter 7).

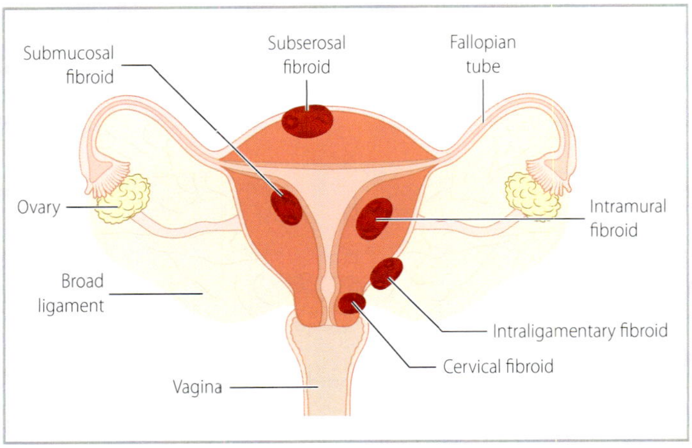

Figure 2.8 Types of fibroids occurring within the uterus.

OTHER ENDOCRINE INVESTIGATIONS

Serum prolactin

Prolactin is produced by the anterior pituitary gland. It has a wide range of effects in the female, but its main function is to stimulate the breast to produce milk after delivery of the baby. Outside of pregnancy, a high serum prolactin (>500 IU/L) may suppress ovarian function, causing failure of ovulation, amenorrhea and infertility. High prolactin levels may also cause the breast to produce milk inappropriately (galactorrhea). A serum prolactin is usually reserved for women with amenorrhea, anovulation or galactorrhea.

Hyperprolactinemia (raised prolactin) may be due to a microprolactinoma in the pituitary gland; a side-effect of some drugs, e.g. antidepressants and antipsychotics (La Torre 2007); or hypothyroidism.

Before investigating a raised serum prolactin, a repeat blood test is recommended to exclude the presence of macroprolactin. This is an isomer of biologically active prolactin which is bound to an anti-prolactin immunoglobulin. This molecule has very little biological activity and when present requires no investigation or treatment (Vaishya et al. 2010). If macroprolactinemia can be excluded, then a woman with a raised prolactin needs further investigations of her endocrine system, especially the hypothalamus and pituitary gland.

Serum insulin

Insulin resistance is most common in women with PCOS and overweight women (Tsilchorozidou et al. 2004). The condition can be diagnosed by measuring fasting insulin levels, but can be suspected by searching for clinical clues such as obesity, acanthosis nigricans (hyperpigmentation of the skin) and raised serum triglycerides (see Chapter 6 for more details).

CONCLUSION

Infertility is a problem that is commonly seen in primary care. The GP is perfectly placed to ensure that pre-conception issues are addressed. Careful history taking, appropriate examination of the female and an understanding of the underlying science behind female reproduction will help to guide the doctor toward prompt and efficient investigation.

REFERENCES

Morita A. Tobacco smoke causes premature skin ageing. J Dermatol Sci 2007; 48:167–175.
Api M. Is ovarian reserve diminished after laparoscopic ovarian drilling? Gynae Endocrinol 2009; 25:159–165.
Behre HM, Kuhlage J, Gassner C, et al. Prediction of ovulation by urinary hormone measurements with the home use ClearPlan® Fertility Monitor: comparison with transvaginal ultrasound scans and serum hormone measurements. Hum Reprod 2000; 15:2478–2482.
Cornthwaite K, Jefferys A, Lenguerrand E, et al. Pregnancy after weight loss surgery. BJOG 2016; 123:165–170.
Department of Health. UK Chief Medical Officers' Alcohol Guidelines Review (online only). London: Department of Health, 2016.
Eggert J, Theobald H, Engfeldt P. Effects of alcohol consumption on female fertility during an 18-year period. Fertil Steril 2004; 81:379–383.
Evers EC, McDermott KC, Blomquist JL, Handa VL. Mode of delivery and subsequent fertility. Hum Reprod 2014; 29:2569–2574.
Elraiyah T, Hashim Y, Elamin M, Erwin PJ, Zarroug AE. The effect of appendectomy in future tubal infertility and ectopic pregnancy: a systematic review and meta-analysis. J Surg Res 2014; 192:368–374.
Faddy MJ, Gosden RG. A model conforming the decline in follicle numbers to the age of menopause in women. Hum Reprod 1996; 11:1484–1486.
Faddy MJ, Gosden RG, Gougeon A, Richardson SJ, Nelson JF. Accelerated disappearance of ovarian follicles in mid-life – implications for forecasting menopause. Hum Reprod 1992; 7:1342–1346.
Friedler S, Cohen O, Liberty G, et al. Should high BMI be a reason for IVF treatment denial? Gynecol Endocrinol 2017; 20:1–4.
Georgieff MK. The role of iron in neurodevelopment: fetal iron deficiency and the developing Hippocampus. Biochem Soc Trans 2008; 36:1267–1271.

Godlee F, Smith J, Marcovitch H. Wakefield's article linking MMR vaccine and autism was fraudulent. BMJ 2011; 342:c7452.

Hessel M, Brandes M, de Bruin JP, et al. Long-term ongoing pregnancy rate and mode of conception after a positive and negative post-coital test. Acta Obstet Gynecol Scand 2014; 93:913–920.

Hübschen JM, Bork SM, Brown KE, et al. Challenges of measles and rubella laboratory diagnostic in the era of elimination. Clin Microbiol Infect 2017; 23:511–515.

Human Fertilisation and Embryology Authority (HFEA). HFEA fertility trends 2013 (online only, last updated 2018). London: HFEA, 2013.

Jagadish Kumar K, Asha N, Srinivasa Murthy D, et al. Maternal anaemia in various trimesters and its effects on Newborn Weight and Maturity: An Observational Study. Int J Prev Med 2013; 4:193–199.

Kandil M, Bork SM, Brown KE, et al. Hormonal and sonographic assessment of ovarian reserve before and after laparoscopic ovarian drilling in polycystic ovary syndrome. BJOG 2005; 112:1427–1430.

La Torre D, Falorni A. Pharmacological causes of hyperprolactinaemia. Ther Clin Risk Manag 2007; 3:929–951.

Manders, McLindon L, Schulze B, et al. Timed intercourse for couples trying to conceive. Cochrane Database Syst Rev 2015:CD011345.

Mikkelsen EM, Riis AH, Wise LA, et al. Alcohol consumption and fecundability: prospective Danish cohort study. BMJ 2016; 354:i4262.

National Institute for Health and Care Excellence (NICE). Clinical guideline GC156. Fertility problems: assessment and treatment London: NICE, 2013.

Nwokolo NC, Dragovic B, Patel S, et al. 2015 UK national guideline for the management of infection with Chlamydia trachomatis. Int J STD AIDS 2016; 27:251-267.

Papp JR, Schachter J, Gaydos C, Van Der Pol B. Centers for disease control and prevention. Recommendations for the laboratory-based detection of Chlamydia trachomati and Neisseria gonorrhoeae, 2014.

Pepling ME. From primordial germ cell to primordial follicle: mammalian female germ cell development. Genesis 2006; 44:622–632.

Plotkin SA, Orenstein W. Vaccines, 4th edn. Philadelphia: WB Saunders Company, 2004.

Public Health England. Rubella susceptibility screening in pregnancy to end in England. Press Release. London: UK Gov/Public Health England, January 2016.

Sharif K, Olufowobi O. The structure, chemistry and physics of human cervical mucus. In: Jordan J, Singer A, Jones H, Shafi M (Eds), The Cervix (2nd edn) 2006:155–168.

Silasi M, Cardenas I, Kwon JY, et al. Viral infections during pregnancy. Am J Reprod Immunol 2015; 73:199–213.

Tang T, Lord JM, Norman RJ, Yasmin E, Balen AH. Insulin-sensitizing drugs (metformin, rosiglitazone, piogliatazone, D-chiro-inositol) for women with polycystic ovary syndrome, oligo-amenorrhoea and subfertility. Cochrane Gynaecology and Fertility Group 2012.

Tatone C, Amicarelli F, Carbone MC, et al. Cellular and molecular Aspects of ovarian follicle ageing. Hum Reprod Update 2008; 14:131–142.

te Velde ER, Eijkemans R, Habbema HDF. Variation in couple fecundity and time to pregnancy, an essential concept in human reproduction. Lancet 2000; 355:1928–1929.

Tsilchorozidou T, Overton C, Conway GS. The Pathophysiology of PCOS. Clin Endocrinol 2004; 60:1–17.

Vaishya R, Gupta R, Arora S. Macroprolactin: a frequent cause of misdiagnosed hyperprolactinaemia in clinical practice. J Reprod Infertil 2010; 11:161–167.

Vollman RF. The menstrual cycle. Philadelphia: WB Saunders, 1977.

Wark JD, Henningham L, Gorelik A, et al. Basal Temperature Measurement Using a Multi-Sensor Armband in Australian Young Women: A Comparative Observational Study. JMIR Mhealth Uhealth 2015; 3:e94.

Wilcox AJ, Dunson D, Baird DD. The timing of the "fertile window" in the menstrual cycle: day specific estimates from a prospective study. BMJ 2000; 321:1259–1262.

Chapter 3 Investigations in secondary care

Sara Rodríguez López, Masoud Afnan

INTRODUCTION

An estimated 1 in 7 couples seek medical advice for difficulties conceiving.[1]

The aim of investigations in secondary care is to quickly and accurately categorize patients into the correct diagnosis group. The clinician can then provide clear guidance on the chances of conceiving and on treatment options available, with the risks and benefits of each one made clear. Only then can an informed decision be made about how to proceed.

Many people will seek medical advice early on in their quest for a child. Consequently, background pregnancy rates are reasonably high, even in patients waiting for procedures such as in vitro fertilization (IVF). Furthermore, up to 40% of couples will not proceed with any additional treatment after the female has undergone hysterosalpingogram (HSG). It is therefore important to consider the costs and invasiveness (in terms of risks) of the initial investigations.[2]

Whilst this book focuses on female infertility for heterosexual couples it is important to consider the couple as a whole obtaining semen analysis results early on will often guide the diagnostic and therapeutic plan. For example, if the man has severe oligozoospermia, an option for the couple is intracytoplasmic sperm injection (ICSI), and the investigations will be geared to optimizing outcomes from that treatment.

Even if a cause is clearly identified in one partner, there may be a problem with the fertility of the other partner too. This is because approximately a quarter of couples will have borderline problems in both partners (odds multiply, so significantly decreasing the chances of pregnancy). Of the remaining three quarters, it is estimated that one quarter of couples will have male factor, one quarter female factor and one quarter unexplained infertility, with no obvious cause.

In the case of the female partner, basic investigations in secondary infertility care will involve three major areas: tubal patency, uterine cavity and ovulation. In the past, fertility specialists looked for cervical factors, for example by doing a postcoital test, or did repeated follicle tracking or performed tests on the semen, such as antisperm antibodies. However, questions have been raised regarding the reliability and cost-effectiveness of these tests, and whether the results alter management. They have therefore fallen out of favor and are no longer routinely carried out.

CHECKING THE FALLOPIAN TUBES

Tubal disease accounts for 20–25% of all female infertility, with pelvic inflammatory disease (PID) the most common cause (**Table 3.1**). PID is often asymptomatic, and a common cause is due to a sexually transmitted infection (STI) such as *Chlamydia trachomatis* infection.[3,4] Another important infection to consider is gonorrhea

Table 3.1 Sexually transmitted infections that can cause pelvic inflammatory disease (PID) and tubal blockage

Disease	Examples	Organism	Prevalence	Treatment
Chlamydia	*Chlamydia trachomatis*	Bacteria	>20% in sexually active men and women aged <24 years	Azithromycin: 1 g orally in a single dose or doxycycline: 100 mg orally twice a day for 7 days
Gonorrhea	*Neisseria gonorrhoeae*	Bacteria	0.6% per 100,000 men and women between the ages of 20–24 in the USA (2016)	Centre for Disease Control (USA) recommends dual therapy, or using two drugs, to treat gonorrhea – a single dose of 250 mg of intramuscular ceftriaxone and 1 g of oral azithromycin
Syphilis	*Treponema pallidum*	Bacteria	9.5 cases per 100,000 population in the USA (2017). Men account for most cases of syphilis, with the majority of cases occurring among men who have sex with men (MSM)	A single intramuscular injection of long-acting benzathine penicillin G (2.4 million units administered intramuscularly) will cure a person who has primary, secondary or early latent syphilis. Three doses of long-acting benzathine penicillin G (2.4 million units administered intramuscularly) at weekly intervals is recommended for individuals with late latent syphilis or latent syphilis of unknown duration. Treatment will kill the syphilis bacterium and prevent further damage, but it will not repair damage already done
Mycoplasma	*Ureaplasma urealyticum* *Mycoplasma genitalium*	Mycoplasma	10–30% in women with clinical cervicitis	1 g single dose of azithromycin is significantly more effective against *Mycoplasma genitalium*
Tuberculosis	*Mycobacterium tuberculosis*	Bacteria	2.8 cases per 100,000 population in the USA (2017). Tuberculosis (TB) can cause latent TB infection and TB disease. If not adequately treated, TB disease can be fatal	Anti-tuberculous therapy, dependent on extent and area of infection

(*Neisseria gonorrhoeae*), with the reported incidence of this condition increasing.[5] The significance of mycoplasma (*Ureaplasma urealyticum*) is unclear. In developing countries tuberculosis must also be considered.

The other main cause for tubal infertility is previous pelvic pathology (e.g. peritonitis from a burst appendix), and pelvic surgery (e.g. ovarian cystectomy or tubal surgery for an ectopic pregnancy). Previous sterilization is also a significant cause, though less so nowadays, as there are many reliable, reversible methods of contraception on the market. A less common cause for tubal disease is endometriosis, which can cause scarring in the tubal wall (see Chapter 7).

Distal tubal blockage is the most common form of tubal disease, and is usually caused by PID or previous surgery. It is important to identify and treat distal tubal disease which has resulted in a hydrosalpinx (either with occlusion or salpingostomy), prior to IVF, as this untreated condition can halve pregnancy rates.[6]

Approximately 10-15% of the cases of tubal disease are due to proximal tubal blockage from different etiologies such as salpingitis isthmica nodosa (SIN), intraluminal fibrosis or endometriotic scarring in the muscle of the tube. Mucus plugs or spasm of the tube may also be responsible for apparent obstruction when assessing tubal patency.

There are three main techniques to assess tubal patency: hysterosalpingography (HSG), laparoscopy and ultrasound assessment using specially designed contrast agents.

Investigations for tubal patency

Hysterosalpingography

Hysterosalpingography is the most widely used procedure to check tubal patency, primarily because it is minimally invasive, and easily carried out in the outpatient setting (**Figure 3.1**). It is the preferred investigation for those patients without a known risk factor, such as known endometriosis, history of PID or previous ectopic pregnancy. A contrast medium is injected through the cervix into the uterine cavity to assess radiologically, the uterine cavity and the patency of fallopian tubes.

The HSG is a reliable test to exclude tubal disease, with a negative predictive value of 98%.[7,8] It has a positive predictive value of 54%, best when assessing proximal occlusion substantial for distal obstruction and hydrosalpinx and moderate to poor for adhesions.[7,8]

Hysterosalpingo sonography: contrast versus foam (HyCoSy versus HyFoSy)

Like HSG, HyCoSy and HyFoSy are minimally invasive procedures that allow the evaluation of the uterine cavity and tubal patency. Again like HSG, in HyCoSy a contrast saline-based medium is injected through the cervix to assess, in this case by ultrasound, the uterine cavity and the fallopian tubes. For HyFoSy, a hyperechogenic foam is used rather than a medium. HSG, HyCoSy and HyFoSy have comparable positive and negative predictive value, although many physicians prefer HSG on the grounds that it provides more details about the state of the fallopian tubes, such as mucosal patterns. Conversely, HyCoSy and HyFoSy are considered to have some advantages over HSG, as they have greater sensitivity and specificity for the detection of intrauterine pathologies, such as fibromas, polyps and synechiae in subfertile populations. At the same time they allow for assessment of the ovaries and myometrium.[9,10] Some consider that HyFoSY offers enhanced contrast visualization and enables clearer delineation of tubal anatomy. This may enhance confidence in the diagnosis of tubal patency, reduce false occlusion results, and improve the diagnostic yield of the test.[11]

Many clinics routinely performing an HSG may also offer a separate pelvic ultrasound.

In practice, the decision as to whether to do HSG or HyCoSy as a first-line uterine and tubal assessment will depend mainly on the expertise of and the facilities available to the physician.

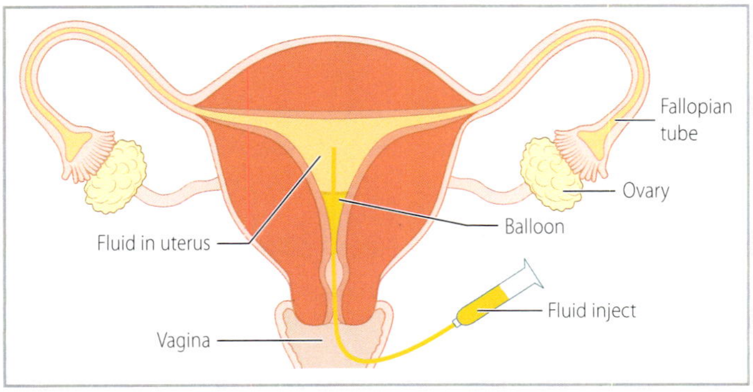

Figure 3.1 Hysterosalpingography.

Management of patients with abnormal HSG or HyCoSy

Laparoscopy and hydrotubation

Laparoscopy and hydrotubation require a general anesthetic and carry a risk of visceral injury so are not usually considered as first-line investigation for patients without a risk factor. The risk of serious complications is estimated 1 in 1,000. Furthermore, both HSG and HyCoSy/HyFoSY have a good negative predictive value. Laparoscopy is therefore only recommended for patients with suspected tubal disease in order to gain a more accurate diagnosis to guide management.[12]

Patient management is only changed in about 5% of the patients who receive a normal HSG result.[13]

Tubal disease

There are different treatment options for tubal disease management, depending on: the type of disease; whether there is complete occlusion; the patient's age; and other fertility parameters (e.g. duration of trying for a baby). Tubal disease can be treated via salpingectomy or IVF. Nowadays, however, IVF is the most commonly used fertility treatment if there is a tubal pathology, and consequently surgical expertise in tubal surgery has declined.

This is to be lamented, as in the right hands, and with good patient selection, excellent pregnancy rates can be achieved, and of course successive pregnancies can be safely and cheaply obtained, without further intervention.[14]

For apparent proximal tubal disease, selective salpingography is an excellent and simple outpatient diagnostic procedure, and if true blockage is identified, a guidewire and catheter are used to unblock the tube radiologically at the same time (Figure 3.2). The procedure can also be carried out hysteroscopically. Both treatments increase the chances of pregnancy depending on the extent of the underlying tubal damage.

Patients with distal tubal occlusion can either be treated via IVF or tubal surgery. In the case of unilateral hydrosalpinx, treatment of hydrosalpinx is recommended to maximise the chances of conceiving with a contralateral tube (**Figure 3.3**). With bilateral hydrosalpinges, both tubes should be treated before proceeding to IVF. If the tubes are too damaged, treatment should be via salpingectomy or tubal

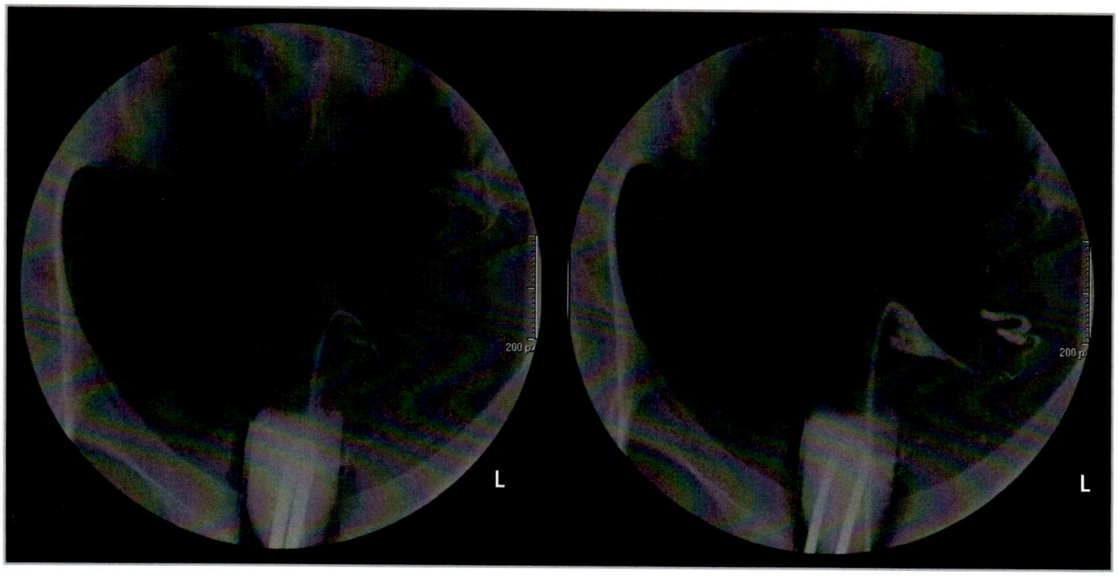

Figure 3.2 X-ray plate images during selective salpingography.

clipping, since there is good evidence that not doing so can halve the background pregnancy rates. This may be due to fluid from the hydrosalpinx draining back into the uterine cavity, which can make the environment toxic to embryo development and implantation.

A recent systematic review of salpingostomy, reported cumulative clinical pregnancy rates of 20% at 12 months after salpingostomy to treat hydrosalpinx.[15] However, there is a high risk of re-occlusion, so it is important to carefully evaluate the hydrosalpinx before undertaking salpingostomy. The risk of ectopic pregnancy following salpingostomy is also higher compared with IVF. If after 6–12 months of surgery pregnancy does not occur, IVF is indicated.

CHECKING THE UTERUS

The uterine cavity can be assessed as described above by HSG or HyCoSy/HyFoSy. In the absence of any significant clinical history of intrauterine procedures which might cause uterine synechiae, a plain transvaginal ultrasound to determine endometrial thickness and the absence of distortion of the endometrial lining can offer a satisfactory check. If a laparoscopy is being performed, then it is reasonable to simultaneously perform a diagnostic hysteroscopy to assess the cavity by direct visualization.

A pelvic ultrasound can often be used to detect uterine conditions such as the presence of fibroids; calcification in the myometrium which would indicate adenomyosis; and whether the patient has uterine malformations such as an arcuate uterus, a uterine septum, unicornuate or bicornuate uterus. Depending on the pathology, subsequent investigations to consider include a hysterosonogram (to check for submucosal fibroids) (**Figure 3.4**), an MRI (to determine the size and location of fibroids, and adenomyosis), or a laparoscopy and hysteroscopy. The latter provides a complete assessment of congenital anomalies, and in particular can be used to differentiate between a septate uterus and a bicornuate uterus. If intrauterine synechaie are suspected, then a diagnostic hysteroscopy can be performed, with the possibility to proceed at the same sitting to a hysteroscopic adhesiolysis.

Treatment of uterine fibroids, intrauterine synechiae or a significant uterine septum is generally via surgery. Arcuate uterus, bicornuate and unicornuate uterus do not usually benefit from treatment. There is no currently available therapy for adenomyosis.

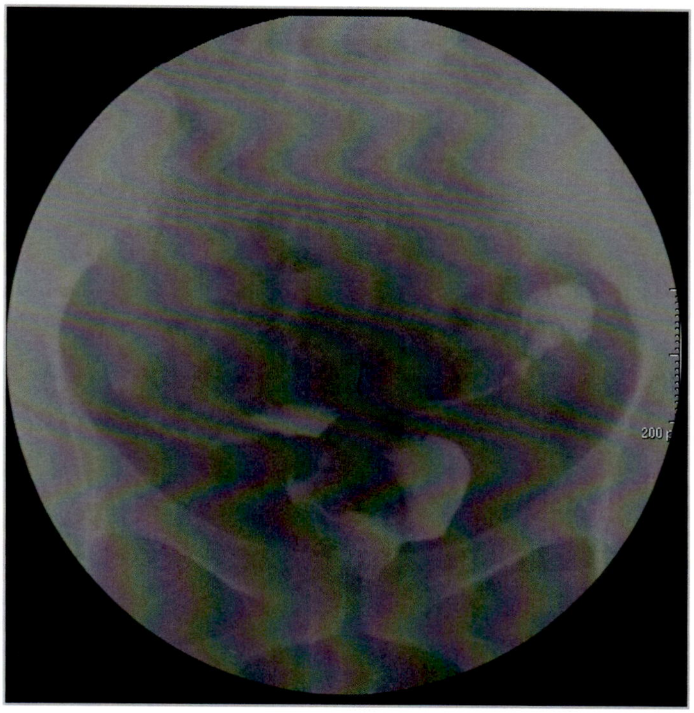

Figure 3.3 A hydrosalpinx.

Endometrial polyps are common, and may often resolve spontaneously as the endometrium is shed each month. In some cases they can persist, and if they measure over 2 cm in diameter may significantly affect the chances of conception. Between 1–2 cm in diameter, the impact is less certain, but it is reasonable to remove them if they persist. Polyps less than 1 cm in diameter are probably of little clinical significance. However, there remains a lack of clarity regarding the clinical significance of endometrial polyps. For example, endometrial polyps are highly prevalent in all types of abnormal uterine bleeding (AUB), yet they are also commonly found in women without AUB.[16]

It is important to consider the endometrial hyperplasia in patients with anovulation, and who have heavy frequent periods, which are

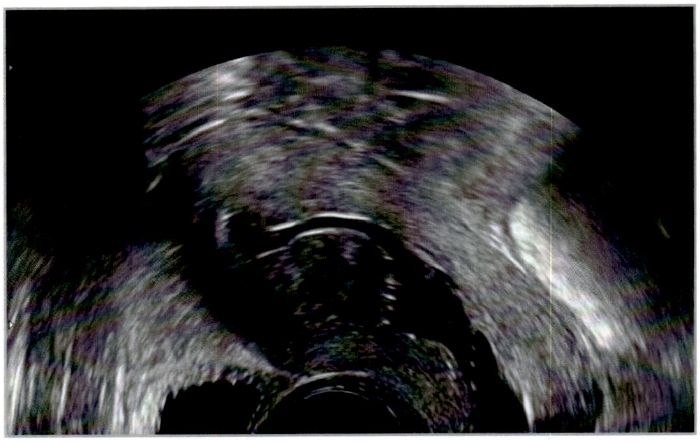

Figure 3.4 Evidence of submucosal fibroid on hysterosonogram.

indicative of high, unopposed estrogen stimulation of the endometrium. A proportion of women will have endometrial hyperplasia with atypia, which if left unchecked may progress to endometrial cancer.[17] Diagnosis is made by taking a sample of the endometrium using an endometrial sampler in the outpatient clinic.

Uterine malformations

Uterine malformations occur in about 4% of the population, with approximately the same prevalence amongst infertile women, though it is higher (10–20%) among women with recurrent miscarriage.[18] They occur either as a result of failure of fusion during fetal development (bicornuate or unicornuate uterus) or resorption (arcuate or septate uterus) of the Müllerian ducts (**Figure 3.5**). Consequences of uterine malformations may include altered vascularity; abnormal intrauterine pressure; decreased ability of the uterus to expand; cervical incompetence; and altered endometrial receptivity.

The commonest type of abnormality is the septate or arcuate uterus. Patients with these abnormalities have a higher (double) miscarriage rate, which appears to revert back to normal rates after hysteroscopic excision.[19] Unicornuate or bicornuate uterus may cause intrauterine growth retardation, fetal malposition and malpresentation later in the pregnancy. There is no useful treatment for these types of uterus. Neither type of abnormality is said to affect the chances of conception.

CHECKING THE CERVIX

The cervix is best assessed by physical examination, though occasionally cervical polyps can be observed on ultrasound and not visualized directly (**Figure 3.6**). The most common finding is a cervical ectropion, which is a physiological distal shifting of the squamocolumnar junction under estrogenic influence. This condition does not need to be treated, and does not affect chances of conception. Small cervical polyps will normally resolve on their own. Persistent polyps may be avulsed in the outpatient clinic. Cervical intraepithelial neoplasia should be treated prior to fertility treatment, and if excision cone biopsies are performed, may result if large or repeated, in cervical incompetence. Cervical treatment (such as excision, cautery, or laser) for premalignant cells on the cervix may also result in abnormal (reduced) cervical mucus, which might affect future fertility.

The 'tight' cervix will not cause infertility, but may make it difficult to pass a catheter for procedures such as HSG or embryo transfer.

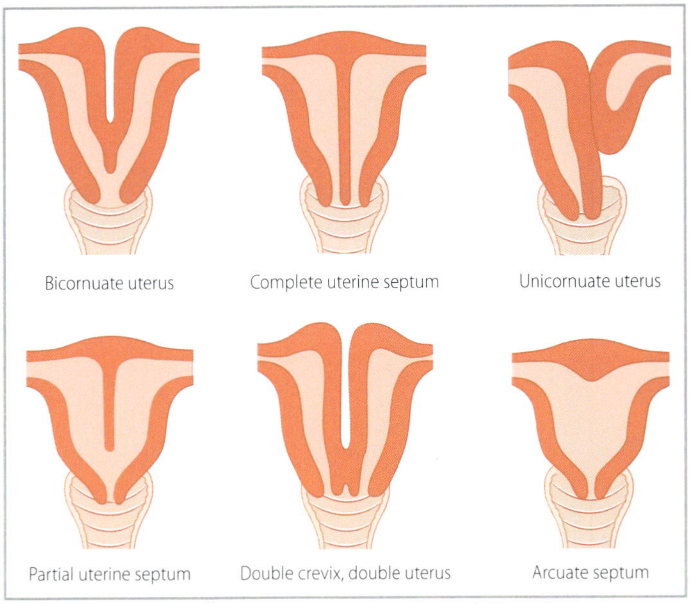

Figure 3.5 Failure of fusion of the Müllerian ducts.

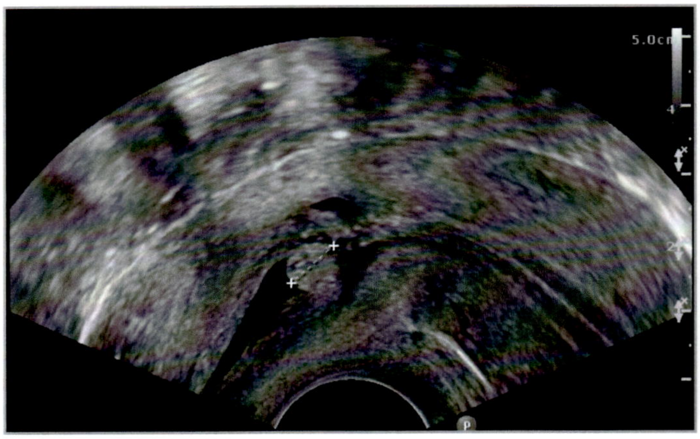

Figure 3.6 Cervical polyp seen on transvaginal ultrasound.

Evaluation of the cervix can be performed before embarking on IVF treatment if a difficult embryo transfer is anticipated.

Consideration should be given to STIs, such as chlamydia and gonorrhea, which are harbored in the cervix in high risk women (under the age of 25 years), as instrumentation of the cervix may cause further spread of the infection. Such patients should either be screened or given prophylactic antibiotics.

Finally, the role of post-coital testing is controversial, with professional societies from different countries giving different assessments of its utility. This may be because of inconsistencies in how the post-coital test is performed, and the management of the patient with cervical factor and 'unexplained' infertility is the same (IUI or IVF).

CHECKING THE OVARIES

The ovaries are the primary organs of the female reproductive system. The importance of the ovary is not only as a gonad responsible for the production of oocytes, but also as a gland responsible for the secretion of hormones such as estrogen and progesterone that have an essential role in the menstrual cycle.

The ovaries are whitish-colored organs laying on the ovarian fossa of the female pelvis on both side of the uterus; each ovary is connected to the uterus through the ovarian ligament and attached to the fallopian tubes (for a detailed description of the anatomy and physiology, see Chapter 1).

Checking morphology

Transvaginal ultrasound is the most common procedure to check ovarian morphology (see Figure 2.7), and to monitor follicular development through the menstrual cycle. As a follicle enlarges, it becomes more vascular; ovulation is followed by collapse of the follicle, and formation of the echogenic corpus hemorrhagicum and subsequently corpus luteum.

Ultrasound scans can help to identify abnormal cysts (**Table 3.2**), which can be functional (essentially, a follicle that has not developed normally, and which will normally resolve over time), to persistent cysts, which can be benign or malignant. One type of cyst is an ovarian endometrioma, which appears as an opaque cyst because it is filled with old blood.

Ultrasound can also identify the number of small antral follicles present in each ovary, which gives a measure of the ovarian reserve, and in the case of polycystic ovaries is increased (see Figure 2.7).

Luteal phase deficiency

Luteal phase deficiency (LPD) is a condition in which not enough progesterone is secreted, resulting in failure to develop normal secretory endometrium for embryo implantation and growth, whereby the luteal phase is shortened. However, a short luteal phase can occur in up to 5% of healthy fertile women, and there is no significant increase seen among sub-fertile women.[20]

Abnormal luteal function may occur as a result of underlying abnormal thyroid function, so women with a short luteal phase should be investigated for this. As women near the menopause, the luteal phase often becomes shorter. Obesity and anorexia have also been implicated.

Repeated luteal progesterone level tests and endometrial biopsies have been used to diagnose LPD, however, the validity of these tests has been questioned.

While progesterone is important for implantation and maintenance of early pregnancy, no treatment for luteal phase insufficiency has been shown to improve pregnancy outcomes in natural, unstimulated cycles. The treatment options for patients with suspected LPD are the same as for those patients with unexplained infertility, therefore efforts to diagnose LPD are not currently justified.[21,22]

ANOVULATION

Ovulatory disorders (anovulation or infrequent ovulation) are responsible for approximately 20–25% of female infertility. A normal menstrual cycle relies upon normal ovarian cycle, with a coordinated shedding of the endometrium at the end of the luteal phase. In the absence of normal ovulation, the patient will have irregular cycles. The pattern of bleeding will reflect the patient's baseline estrogen levels.

If the patient has no periods, her estrogen level will be very low whereas infrequent periods (oligomenorrhea) are usually associated with slightly higher estrogen level that tend to oscillate: if the level is above the threshold, this causes some proliferative changes in the endometrium. If the level is below the threshold, this causes a withdrawal bleed. Heavy, frequent periods reflect high estrogen levels which act unopposed (by progesterone) on the endometrium, causing endometrial proliferation until the point when it cannot maintain its own architecture and the endometrium breaks down in an uncoordinated way.

As well as considering fertility implications, it is important to consider other health-related issues such as consequences of prolonged hypoestrogenism on the cardiovascular and skeletal symptoms; the effect of prolonged, unopposed hyperestrogenism and the risk of developing endometrial cancer and anemia from heavy frequent periods.

Types of anovulation

The World Health Organization (WHO) classifies anovulation into 3 groups (**Table 3.3**):

WHO I hypogonadotropic-hypogonadism

This group accounts for 10% of anovulatory disorders. Selective failure of the pituitary gland affects the production of luteinizing hormone (LH) and follicle-stimulating hormone (FSH). The most common cause is hypothalamic amenorrhea due to anorexia nervosa or excessive exercise. Other causes include pituitary microadenoma or prolactinoma, as prolactin suppresses the secretion of gonadotropin-releasing hormone (GnRH) from the hypothalamus. These patients may experience other symptoms such as galactorrhea, headaches and visual field disturbances.

Rare causes include infarction of the anterior pituitary, such as Sheehan's syndrome, or congenital conditions causing hypopituitarism

Table 3.2 Types of ovarian cysts

Cyst	Cause
Corpus luteum cysts	Post-ovulation, the corpus luteum closes prematurely causing fluid to accumulate
Hemorrhagic cyst	Blood fills the follicle/corpus luteum, possibly causing pain
Follicular cysts	If the luteinizing hormone surge does not cause ovulation, the follicle retains clear fluid
Cystadenomas	An epithelium-lined cyst derived from ovarian tissue containing secretory material. Can be either serous (containing clear fluid) or mucinous (usually benign, with mucin-containing cavities)
Dermoid cysts	Develops from totipotent germ cells which proliferate, forming different types of tissue and structures, e.g. hair and teeth. Large cysts may cause ovarian torsion. Require surgical removal
Endometrioma / 'chocolate cysts'	Endometriotic tissue inside the ovary causes blood-filled cysts, which become viscous and brown. Cyst rupture causes pelvic pain and induce adhesions
Multiple cysts – polycystic ovaries	Polycystic ovary syndrome causes many small cysts to form on the periphery of the ovary

Table 3.3 Anovulation. The World Health Organization (WHO) provides a practical classification of anovulatory states into three groups (I, II and II) based on gonadotropin secretion

Hormone	WHO I Hypothalamic – pituitary failure	WHO I Hyper-prolactinemia	WHO II PCOS	WHO II Ovulatory dysfunction	WHO III Ovarian failure
Follicle-stimulating hormone	Very low	Normal or low	Normal	Normal	Very high
Luteinizing hormone	Very low	Normal or low	High	Normal	Very high
Prolactin	Normal	High	Normal	Normal	Normal
Thyroid-stimulating hormone	Normal	Normal or high	Normal	Normal	Normal
Testosterone	Normal	Normal	High	Normal	Normal
Anti-Müllerian hormone	Normal	Normal	High	Normal	Very low

including Kallmann's, Prader-Willi and Laurence-Moon-Biedl syndromes. These patients have estrogen levels in the postmenopausal range, with normal to low FSH levels and normal prolactin levels.

WHO II normogonadotropic, normogonadism

This group accounts for 85% of ovulatory disorders and includes patients with polycystic ovary syndrome (PCOS). Approximately 80% of oligomenorrheic and 30% of those with amenorrhea have polycystic ovaries.[23]

The primary anomaly is failure of small antral follicles to respond to normal concentrations of FSH, and therefore follicle recruitment and ovulation rarely take place. This results in a large number of small antral androgen-dominated follicles. In addition to irregular periods, PCOS patients may present with signs of androgen excess, such as hirsutism and acne. In addition, at least a third will be overweight.

PCOS is an endocrine disorder that affects 15–20% of women of fertile age. It is the commonest cause of amenorrhea and oligomenorrhea.

The symptoms are variable but some of the most common clinical manifestations are irregular or absent cycles, hirsutism, acne, insulin resistance, obesity and infertility. 80–90% of women presenting with oligomenorrhea have PCOS; on the other hand, 30% of PCOS patient will have normal cycles.[24]

According to the European Society of Human Reproduction and Embryology (ESHRE) and American Society for Reproductive Medicine (ASRM), to diagnose PCOS, two out of three criteria should be present:

- Oligo- and/or anovulation (cycle >35 days)
- Clinical and/or biochemical signs of hyperandrogenism
- Polycystic ovary morphology (12 or more follicles and/or ovarian volume of >10 mL) in at least one ovary[25]

More recent studies suggest that the threshold of 12 follicles is insufficient to distinguish PCOS patients from healthy women and propose a substantially higher threshold of 26 follicles.[26]

WHO III hypergonadotropic hypogonadism

This group accounts for 5% of anovulatory disorders and includes patients with premature ovarian failure. These patients present with elevated FSH and LH and postmenopausal levels of estrogen. Many cases are of unknown origin, but some will have sex chromosome abnormalities such as Turner syndrome, metabolic disorders such as hypergalactosemia, or be autoimmune in origin.

Women are born with a predetermined number of primordial follicles; this number reaches a peak before the birth, at 20 weeks of gestation, and starts decreasing from then. At the time women reach puberty only around 5% of primordial follicles remain; menopause occurs when all the follicles are exhausted.

Premature ovarian insufficiency (POI), is defined by the presence of oligoamenorrhea for at least 4 months and two determinations of FSH in the menopausal range (at least 1 month apart) in women younger than 40 years.

POI can be caused by follicle depletion or dysfunction (also known as resistant ovary syndrome) when even though there are follicles, they do not function normally. The cause is often unknown (90%), but may be due to ovarian autoimmunity, G protein mutation, enzyme deficiency or a defect on the signal receptor of FSH or LH.[27]

Genetic testing such as a karyotype analysis or testing for an *FMR1* premutation, which is responsible for fragile X syndrome (FXS), may be helpful to identify a cause, but usually does not alter management. It is reasonable to screen for autoimmune conditions in other endocrine glands such as the thyroid or adrenal, in order to check for early disease.

Treatment options

Women with amenorrhea (absence of periods), or oligomenorrhea (irregular cycles/ >35 days cycles) should be fully investigated to understand which type of anovulation they are suffering from in order to better recommend treatment options.

WHO anovulation group 1

The appropriate treatment to achieve ovulation for patients with anovulatory disorders will depend on the etiology of anovulation. For WHO I group patients, normalisation of weight or decreasing exercise may help women to resume periods. Alternatively, treatment with pulsatile administration of GnRH can be considered if the pituitary is intact, or gonadotropins can be used directly. Both LH and FSH stimulation is necessary for normal steroidogenesis.

For women with hyperprolactinemia, medical treatment with dopamine agonists, such as bromocriptine, cabergoline or quinagolide restores ovulation.

WHO anovulation group 2

In those PCOS patients presenting with obesity, weight loss should be recommended before starting treatment, not only because weight loss improves fertility and obstetric outcomes but also because obese women require more stimulation to achieve ovulation.[28]

The first-line of treatment for PCOS is oral ovulation induction (OI). Clomiphene citrate (CC) has for many years been the initial of treatment for PCOS. CC is an antiestrogen which binds to estrogen receptors, blocking the negative feedback to the hypothalamus, and therefore increasing the production of gonadotropins, particularly FSH, leading to follicle recruitment and ovulation (see Figure 6.1).

Recently, letrozole has been shown to produce better outcomes, with higher ovulation and pregnancy rates. Letrozole is an aromatase inhibitor that reduces oestradiol production by diminishing the androgen conversion to estradiol in the granulosa cell. Consequently, there is less negative feedback on the hypothalamic-pituitary axis, so FSH stimulation of the follicle is increased. Legro and colleagues reported cumulative live birth rates of 27.5% in patients with letrozole compared with 19.1% in those patients on CC.[29] It is hypothesized that letrozole has better results because of the negative effect of CC on the endometrium and cervical mucus.

For those who do ovulate with OI but fail to achieve a pregnancy after 6 months of treatment, OI and IUI may be offered.

For those who fail to ovulate with oral OI, injectable gonadotropin (hMG or FSH) can be used to stimulate follicular development. This requires close follicle monitoring as it carries a high risk (16%) of multiple births and a 1% risk of ovarian hyperstimulation syndrome.[30]

Ovarian drilling is a procedure performed by laparoscopy that involves the creation of small holes with diathermy, which appears to trigger ovulation. For those patients that fail to ovulate on CC or letrozole, diathermy ovarian drilling may be offered as a treatment option. Ovulation rates of up to 80% have been reported, with the effect lasting up to 2 years. Of significance, as there is no external ovulation induction, these are usually single ovulatory cycles.

Finally, IVF is an option for patients who do not conceive with the treatment strategies outlined above.

WHO anovulation group 3

For anovulatory women due to a premature ovarian failure or who are perimenopausal, OI is not recommended and the most appropriate treatment is donor oocytes.

As well as the emotional impact for women diagnosed with POI, there are many other health issues to consider such as low bone density and higher risk of heart disease because of the prolonged estradiol deficiency. Therefore, hormone replacement therapy (HRT) should be offer to women suffering POI.

Unexpected pregnancies have been reported in 5–10% of patients diagnosed with POI.[27] For patients who actively wish to achieve conception, oocyte donation is the only treatment option that should be offered.

CONCLUSION

Management of the infertile couple has been revolutionized in the last 25 years by the advent of IVF and ART. In place of extensive, detailed, repeated diagnostic assessments, we are now able to offer rapid diagnostic assessment within a single menstrual cycle to categorize patients into a diagnostic group and subsequently offer effective treatment. Simpler, more cost-effective treatment options should be offered where possible, resorting to IVF treatment as an effective final step. Much of the focus in infertility investigation research therefore has been to ensure the effectiveness of the diagnostic process, reduce waste and reduce costs. This has largely been achieved. Future work will be directed to the social trend of delayed childbearing, and the implications for the chances of conception.

At every step of the diagnostic process, the competent physician should be able to discuss with their patients the increased likelihood of conceiving, in percentage terms. This patient-centerd, patient-informed approach will do much to ensure only appropriate investigations are conducted.

REFERENCES

1. Leaver RB. Male infertility: an overview of causes and treatment options. Br J Nurs 2016; 25:S35–S40.
2. Duthie EA, Cooper A, Davis JB, et al. A conceptual framework for patient-centered fertility treatment. Reprod Health 2017; 14:114
3. Rogstad K. Complications in the female and their management. In: Moss T (Ed.) International handbook of Chlamydia, 3rd edn. Alden Press, Haslemere, UK 2008:111–121.
4. Peipert JF. Clinical practice. Genital chlamydial infections. N Engl J Med 2003; 349:2424–2430.
5. Suay-García B, Pérez-Gracia MT. Drug-resistant Neisseria gonorrhoeae: latest developments. Eur J Clin Microbiol Infect Dis 2017; 36:1065–1071.
6. Strandell A, Lindhard A, Waldenstrom U, Thorburn J. Hydrosalpinx and IVF outcome: cumulative results after salpingectomy in a randomized controlled trial. Hum Reprod 2001; 16:2403–2410.
7. Berker B, Şükür YE, Aytaç R, et al. Infertility work-up: To what degree does laparoscopy change the management strategy based on hysterosalpingography findings? J Obstet Gynaecol Res 2015; 41:1785–1790.
8. Papaioannou S, Bourdrez P, Varma R. Tubal evaluation in the investigation of subfertility: A structured comparison of test. BJOG 2004; 111:1313–1321
9. Papaioannou S, Bourdrez P, Varma R, et al. Tubal evaluation in the investigation of subfertility: a structured comparison of tests. BJOG 2004; 111:1313-1321.
10. Saunders RD, Shwayder JM, Nakajima ST. Current methods of tubal patency assessment. Fertil Steril 2011; 95:2171–2179.
11. Rajesh H, Lim SL, Yu SL. Hysterosalpingo-foam sonography: patient selection and perspectives. Int J Womens Health 2016; 9:23–32.
12. National Institute for Health and Care Excellence (NICE). Fertility problems: assessment and treatment. London: NICE, 2013.
13. Lavy Y, Lev-Sagie A, Holtzer H, Revel A, Hurwitz A. Should laparoscopy be a mandatory component of the infertility evaluation in infertile women with normal hysterosalpingogram or suspected unilateral distal tubal pathology? Eur J Obstet Gynecol Reprod Biol 2004;114:64-68.
14. Johnson N, van Voorst S, Sowter MC, Strandell A, Mol BW. Surgical treatment for tubal disease in women due to undergo in vitro fertilisation. Cochrane Database Syst Rev 2010:CD002125.
15. Chu J, Harb HM, Gallos ID, et al. Salpingostomy in the treatment of hydrosalpinx: a systematic review and meta-analysis. Hum Reprod 2015; 30:1882–1895.
16. Clark TJ, Stevenson H. Endometrial polyps and abnormal uterine bleeding (AUB-P): What is the relationship, how are they diagnosed and how are they treated? Best Pract Res Clin Obstet Gynaecol 2016; 40:89–104.
17. Royal College of Obstetricians and Gynaecologists. Long-term Consequences of polycystic ovary syndrome. Green-top Guideline No. 33. London: RCOG; 2014.
18. Prior M, Richardson A, Asif S, et al. Outcome of assisted reproduction in women with congenital uterine anomalies: a prospective observational study. Ultrasound Obstet Gynecol 2018; 51:110-117.
19. Sugiura-Ogasawara M, Ozaki Y, Suzumori N. Müllerian anomalies and recurrent miscarriage. Curr Opin Obstet Gynecol 2013; 25:293–298.
20. Lenton EA, Landgren BM, Sexton L. Normal variation in the length of the luteal phase of the menstrual cycle: identification of the short luteal phase. Br J Obstet Gynaecol 1984; 91:685–689.
21. Practice Committee of the American Society for Reproductive Medicine. The clinical relevance of luteal phase deficiency: a committee opinion. Fertil Steril 2012; 98:1112–1117.
22. Bukulmez O, Aric A. Luteal phase defect: myth or reality. Obstet Gynecol Clin North Am 2004; 31:727–744.

23. Vander Borght M, Wyns C. Fertility and infertility: Definition and epidemiology. Clin Biochem 2018. pii: S0009-9120(18)30220-0.
24. Sirmans SM, Pate KA. Epidemiology, diagnosis and management of polycystic ovary syndrome. Clin Epidemiol 2014:6 1–13
25. Rotterdam ESHRE/ASRM-Sponsored PCOS consensus workshop group. Revised 2003 consensus on diagnostic criteria and long- term health risks related to polycystic ovary syndrome (PCOS). Hum Reprod 2004; 19:41–47.
26. Lujan ME, Jarrett BY, Brooks ED, et al. Updated ultrasound criteria for polycystic ovary syndrome: reliable thresholds for elevated follicle population and ovarian volume. Hum Reprod 2013; 28:1361–1368.
27. Nelson LM. Primary ovarian insufficiency. N Engl J Med 2009; 360:606–614.
28. Balen AH, Platteau P, Andersen AN, et al. The influence of body weight on response to ovulation induction with gonadotrophins in 335 women with World Health Organization group II anovulatory infertility. BJOG 2006; 113:1195–1202.
29. Legro RS, Brzyski RG, Diamond MP, et al. Letrozole versus clomiphene for infertility in the polycystic ovary syndrome. N Engl J Med 2014; 371:119–129.
30. Legro RS. Ovulation induction in polycystic ovary syndrome: current options. Best Pract Res Clin Obstet Gynaecol 2016; 37:152-159.

Chapter 4 Pre-conceptual nutrition and health

Melanie Brown

INTRODUCTION

A woman's preconception health and nutritional status are important predictors of fertility, maternal and fetal health and pregnancy outcome. Moreover, poor diet and lifestyle habits may contribute to infertility, so addressing these may help to restore natural fertility. If a positive dietary change is made, it introduces a 'locus of control' for women (and men) who might otherwise feel overwhelmed by their infertility (Cobb-Clark et al. 2014, Omani Samani et al. 2017).

A woman's nutritional status before pregnancy affects oocyte development, which has repercussions during early pregnancy and also for the health of offspring years later (De-Regil et al. 2016, Gluckman et al. 2008). Research in rural West Africa showed that adults who were conceived during the rainy season, when availability of folate-rich vegetables was high, enjoyed better health and longevity compared to those who conceived during the dry season, when green vegetables were scarce and the staple diet was rice (Waterland et al. 2007).

Historically, the link between nourishment and fertility is well recognized. In 17th century France, the birth rate fell when the price of wheat was high (Meuvret 1946). Furthermore, the famine caused by the Nazi blockade of Holland in 1945 clearly demonstrated the relationship between substantial food shortage and infertility, with a dramatic fall in conception during this time, followed by an increase in pregnancies upon allied liberation and food restoration (Lumey et al. 2007).

However, even in the absence of hardship, diet may be suboptimal. For example, in the UK, the National Diet and Nutrition Survey (NDNS) frequently reports women having nutrient deficiencies relating to fertility, e.g. vitamin A, iron, iodine, vitamin D, riboflavin, folate, magnesium and selenium (Food Standards Agency, 2014). Moreover, both malnutrition and obesity can have an adverse impact on fertility.

This chapter reviews various aspects of diet and lifestyle that affect female fertility and related aspects of maternal health.

THE MEDITERRANEAN DIET

The Mediterranean diet is considered by many to be the optimal preconception diet, given its high levels of B vitamins, omega three fatty acids (ω-3 FAs) and antioxidants (see **Figure 4.1**). The diet has been linked to longevity and low levels of chronic disease, and has even been shown to benefit in vitro fertilization (IVF) patients (Dinu et al. 2017).

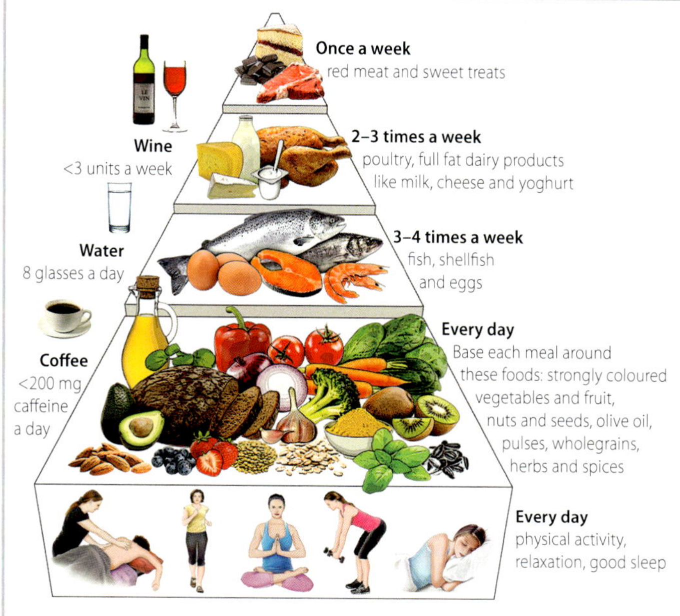

Once a week
red meat and sweet treats
Wine
<3 units a week
2–3 times a week
poultry, full fat dairy products like milk, cheese and yoghurt
Water
8 glasses a day
3–4 times a week
fish, shellfish and eggs
Coffee
<200 mg caffeine a day
Every day
Base each meal around these foods: strongly coloured vegetables and fruit, nuts and seeds, olive oil, pulses, wholegrains, herbs and spices
Every day
physical activity, relaxation, good sleep

Figure 4.1 The Mediterranean diet for optimum fertility. This diet typically comprises high monounsaturated (olive oil)/low saturated fat ratio; moderate levels of red wine; low levels of refined sugars; high consumption of whole grains, fruits and vegetables; low levels of meat products; increased levels of fish; and moderate consumption of milk and dairy products.

MACRONUTRIENTS

According to the Barker hypothesis, macronutrient deficiencies during critical periods of fetal development may have serious implications for susceptibility to adult disease (Barker 1990). Both under- and overnutrition of macronutrients can influence all stages of female reproduction, whilst ovulation is primarily affected by glucose metabolism, micronutrients and fiber content.

THE BARKER HYPOTHESIS

The Barker hypothesis was proposed by the British epidemiologist David Barker in 1990. He suggested that fetal growth retardation, premature birth and low birth weight may be linked to adult diseases such as hypertension, coronary heart disease, and noninsulin-dependent diabetes. The hypothesis originated from a study that revealed a link between the occurrence of these diseases in middle age and premature birth or low birth weight.

Carbohydrates

Carbohydrates with a high glycemic load, (i.e. quickly raise blood glucose) are associated with poor ovulatory function (Chavarro et al. 2009). Sharp rises in glucose affect insulin sensitivity, and women with polycystic ovarian syndrome (PCOS) are particularly susceptible, as this can raise luteinizing hormone (LH) and androgen levels. By contrast, unrefined whole-grain carbohydrates and soluble fibers (e.g. oat bran) facilitate the growth of colonic bacteria to slow down digestion, improving insulin sensitivity (Anderson et al. 2009). Wholegrains also contain B vitamins, selenium, magnesium and manganese, which enhance the nutrient content of the diet.

Protein

For women with PCOS having IVF treatment, a high dietary protein content has been shown to improve menstrual function and reduce androgen levels (Stamets et al. 2004). However, whilst replacing carbohydrates with protein may improve glucose metabolism and insulin sensitivity, there is little evidence (beyond weight loss) that this approach improves fertility outcomes. Furthermore, evidence from a large cohort study (18,000 women from the Nurses' Health Study, see Box below) showed that consumption of animal protein (particularly red meat and chicken) rather than vegetable or fish sources, actually increased ovulatory dysfunction (Chavarro et al. 2008).

THE NURSES' HEALTH STUDY

The Nurses' Health Study II was a prospective cohort study designed to investigate the role of diet and other lifestyle factors in common chronic diseases.

The study took place at the Brigham and Women's Hospital, Boston, USA in 1989. 116, 671 female registered nurses ages 24–42 years were enrolled in the study and have been followed every 2 years since then with mailed questionnaires.

In cattle which are fed a high protein diet, elevated plasma urea concentrations have been shown to adversely affect the bovine uterine environment (Boland et al. 2001). Furthermore, consumption of such meat may adversely influence ovulatory function in humans (Chavarro et al. 2015). To reduce related concerns, women contemplating pregnancy may benefit from a diet with adequate protein preferentially sourced from vegetables, e.g. beans, lentils, mycoproteins (e.g. Quorn), some soya and protein-rich grains like quinoa.

Fat

There are few studies examining dietary fats and human fertility. The effects of different fatty acids on health and fertility are summarized in **Table 4.1**.

MICRONUTRIENTS

Women planning pregnancy should focus primarily on a healthy diet that includes a wide variety of different foods. However, specific micronutrient deficiencies may require supplementation.

Folate

Folate is a water-soluble B-vitamin that plays a critical role in DNA methylation and cell division. Deficiency can result in ovarian malfunction, decreased ovulation or anovulation, irregular cycle length and decreased ovarian hormone production (Gaskins et al. 2012). However, the main role of this essential micronutrient relates to fetal development, since folate deficiency is strongly linked to fetal neurological malformations such as anencephaly and spina bifida.

Folate is supplemented as synthetic folic acid which requires the enzyme methylenetetrahydrofolate reductase (MTHFR) to metabolise it to its active form methyltetrahydrofolate (MTHF). A supplement of 400 µg folic acid and a folate-rich diet (e.g. dark green leafy vegetables and pulses) are recommended if planning to conceive (British Dietetic Association, 2010). Since obesity leads to an increased folic acid requirement, obese women may require a higher dose of folic acid with vitamin B_{12} and vitamin B6 which act as co-factors in the methylation cycle (see **Figure 4.2**). This increased demand is also relevant to women with MTHFR mutations.

Vitamin D

Vitamin D is a steroid hormone synthesized in response to sunlight. In the UK, the NDNS regularly shows that up to 40% of women aged between 25-34 years have low vitamin D levels. This is more so for women from ethnic minorities who 'cover up' outdoors (Henderson et al. 2003).

Furthermore, the re-emergence of rickets in the Americas, Europe and parts of the Middle East has once again focused attention on vitamin D requirements when planning pregnancy (Creo et al. 2016). It has also been reported that the vitamin D receptor (VDR) located in

Table 4.1 Dietary fatty acids, their sources and actions. Different fatty acids (FAs) have different effects on health and fertility. Unsaturated fats tend to be more unstable it is with regard to heating and oxidation (Santos et al. 2008, Scaramuzzi et al. 2010, Missmer 2010)

Fatty acid	Food source	Action
Saturated fatty acids (SFAs)	Animal fats in meat Dairy products Palm and coconut oils	SFAs regulate cell membrane integrity and may increase the risk of cardiovascular disease High levels of follicular SFAs impair oocyte quality in cattle
Monounsaturated fatty acids (MUFAs)	Oils (olive, rape seed, peanut, sesame seed)	Improvement in insulin sensitivity for women with PCOS
Polyunsaturated fatty acids (PUFAs) omega-6 (ω-6 EFAs) omega-3 (ω-3 PUFAs)	Vegetable oils and margarines (corn, soya bean, sunflower) Flax seeds, walnuts, dark green leafy vegetables	In cattle: • high levels of follicular PUFAs improved ovarian function and progesterone production. • PUFA supplementation improved granulosa cell function • ω-3 PUFA supplementation increased follicle number and the size of the pre-ovulatory dominant follicle For endometriosis, ω-3 PUFA: • decreased inflammatory cytokine and pro-coagulant thromboxane • improved insulin sensitivity and endocrine function in women with PCOS
Very long chain polyunsaturated fatty acids (VLCPUFAs) ω-3	Algae, oily fish; salmon, mackerel	Highly anti-inflammatory, decreased inflammatory cytokine and pro-coagulant thromboxane for women with endometriosis
Trans Artificial Natural	 Partially hydrogenated vegetable oils in margarines, baked and deep-fried foods. Ruminant derived meat and milk products	High intake is linked to insulin resistance, poor ovulatory function and increased risk of endometriosis

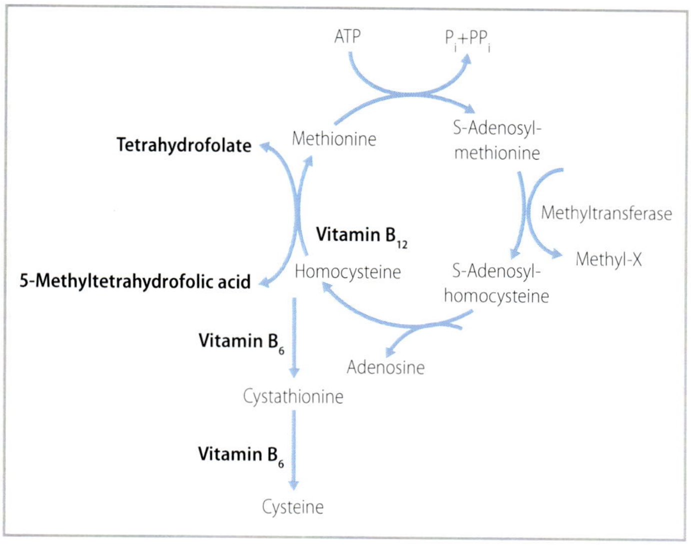

Figure 4.2 Folate synthesis. Vitamin B_{12} and vitamin B_6 act as co-factors in the methylation of folic acid to its active derivatives tetrahydrofolate and 5-methyltetrahydrofolate (MTHF).

female reproductive ovarian and endometrial tissue and VDR knock-out mice has significant reproductive abnormalities (Lerchbaum & Obermayer-Pietsch 2012).

Obesity, PCOS and certain medications (e.g. antiplatelet and corticosteroids) may further decrease vitamin D levels (Wortsman et al. 2000). Whilst there is no UK Reference Nutrient Intake (RNI) for vitamin D in adults, it may be advisable to test vitamin D levels in women presenting with infertility, particularly in women from vulnerable groups where vitamin D deficiency is common.

Iodine

Iodine is an essential trace element, critical for thyroid function, fertility and pregnancy. Requirements are greatly increased in pregnancy and fetal neuro-development is particularly sensitive to even small variances in thyroid hormones. At this stage, an iodine deficiency can lead to mental impairment (Zimmermann et al. 2009).

The RNI for iodine is 150 µg/day for women, with no increment for pregnancy, although the World Health Organization recommends an increase to 250 µg/day to cover fetal needs and extrarenal clearance (WHO Secretariat et al. 2007). Younger women often have low mean daily intakes, such that 68% of UK schoolgirls have been shown to be iodine-deficient (Vanderpump et al. 2011). The risk of iodine deficiency far outweighs the relatively small risk of excess (Zimmermann et al. 2009), so women who want to conceive are recommended to eat iodine-rich food and possibly supplement via pre-natal vitamins that usually contain 150 µg of iodine.

Iodine is found in fish and shellfish, with 100 g whitefish containing about 115 µg. A large proportion of iodine in the Western diet comes from non-organic dairy products, since iodine is used as a disinfectant in the dairy industry (iodophor disinfectants are used for cleaning dairy equipment leaving an iodine residue in milk). For example, 200 mL milk contains 50–80 µg, whereas organic milk contains 30–65 µg.

Iodine absorption may be inhibited by raw cruciferous vegetables (e.g. kale, broccoli, soya, cassava) and cigarette smoking. For women with a high consumption of these, and for vegetarians and vegans whose diet puts them at risk of deficiency, switching to iodized salt may be an appropriate recommendation.

Iron

Anemia of pregnancy affects almost 50% of pregnant women and is considered to be a global health problem due to the risk to fetal and maternal morbidity (Achebe & Gafter-Gvili 2017). Iron deficiency anemia causes maternal fatigue, compromised immunity, alopecia, and fetal organ dysfunction, low birth weight and long-term neurodevelopmental impairment (Rao & Georgieff 2007). Vulnerable women include vegetarians and vegans, those with dysmenorrhea (e.g. from endometriosis or fibroids) and coeliac disease. Prior to pregnancy, such women should have their levels of iron and ferritin measured (iron storage protein), and be given supplements accordingly.

However, excessive iron intake should also be avoided, as this increases levels of reactive oxygen species (ROS) and lipid peroxidation (Milman 2006). Moreover, approximately 10% of the population suffer from the genetic iron overload condition hemochromotosis (Bender 2008).

Iron also has a role in follicular growth and development, since iron-transport proteins and receptors are found in granulosa cells and oocytes (Chavarro 2006).

REACTIVE OXYGEN SPECIES AND ANTIOXIDANTS

ROS are naturally required for metabolism and immunity via phagocytosis, inflammation and cell signalling. Examples include the hydroxyl, superoxide and hydrogen peroxide radicals.

However, ROS are unstable molecules formed in the presence of oxygen. These free oxygen radicals cause oxidative stress by oxidizing lipids, causing cell membrane damage and DNA mutation, resulting in tissue damage and disease. As a defence, the body produces antioxidants to stabilize ROS and de-activate potential damage. Antioxidants include superoxide dismutase (SOD), glutathione and catalase. These substances are formed in vivo from dietary antioxidants such as vitamins C and E, selenium, zinc, copper and N-acetylcysteine. A balance of ROS and antioxidants is needed for conception to take place. However, if ROS levels exceed antioxidant defences, oxidative stress results, which can adversely impact infertility.

Excess ROS are generated by several factors including inflammation or infection, smoking, exposure to UV radiation, obesity, a poor diet and aging. High oxidative stress parameters in follicular fluid can adversely impact on the fertility outcomes (Bedaiwy et al. 2012). Elevated ROS levels detected in the granulosa cells of PCOS patients have also been linked to lower IVF success rates (Karuputhula et al. 2013).

Antioxidant rich diets, such as the Mediterranean diet, are recommended to mitigate ROS damage. Such diets can be supplemented with a pre-natal multivitamin if necessary.

FOOD SOURCES OF ANTIOXIDANTS

- Blueberries, strawberries, raspberries, blackberries, cherries
- Turmeric
- Kidney beans
- Broccoli, spinach, watercress, kale, Brussels sprouts
- Tomatoes and peppers
- Brazil nuts, walnuts
- Black and green tea
- Sunflower, pumpkin, chia seeds, wheat-germ, buckwheat
- Dark chocolate
- Olive oil
- Red onions, red cabbage
- Apples
- Red and black grapes, red wine

WEIGHT, BODY MASS INDEX AND BODY FAT

A woman's weight, and in particular her body fat percentage, is an important factor in pre-conception care (see Chapter 2; **Figure 4.3**).

Many weight-related metabolic and endocrine factors can reduce fertility, e.g. altered steroid hormone metabolism, dysregulated insulin secretion, nutrient deficiencies, and inflammation. These factors can increase ovulatory dysfunction such that exogenous gonadotropins may be needed for ovarian stimulation (Fedorcsák et al. 2004).

In pregnancy weight issues can be exacerbated due to nausea and vomiting, changing dietary habits and cravings and aversions which all dictate food intake. Therefore, preconception weight management is essential for both fertility and pregnancy.

Overweight

A high body mass index (BMI) can decrease fecundity, primarily due to high adipose tissue levels which are associated with ovulation disorders (Rich-Edwards 2002). Adipose tissue acts as a repository of estrogen, such that it behaves as an 'extragonadal estrogen source' (Frisch 1978). Aromatization of androgens to form estrogens occurs within adipocytes, and this process can disrupt the hypothalamic-pituitary axis.

However, the risk of metabolic problems seems to depend on how the adipose tissue is distributed. Vague (1947) hypothesized that women with a 'gynoid' or 'female' fat distribution of the lower body ('pear' shaped) are at less metabolic risk compared to women who are equally obese, but whose fat distribution is 'android', or 'male' and distributed viscerally ('apple' shaped) (see **Figure 4.4**). Moreover, visceral adipose tissue is composed of enlarged, highly metabolically active, dysfunctional, macrophage-infiltrated adipocytes that secrete a variety of inflammatory cytokines (see **Figure 4.5**).

Ethnic differences in adipose tissue distribution are also relevant. BMI calculations do not take into account waist-hip measurements (visceral adiposity), e.g. some Asian women have a low BMI but a high visceral adiposity (Scarborough et al. 2010), whilst some African women have a high BMI and rates of obesity but their metabolic profile confers protection (Cappuccio 1997).

Women with PCOS are prone to weight gain, poor glycemic control, decreased insulin sensitivity and oligomenorrhea. A reduction in body weight (5–10%) or use of antidiabetic medications, e.g. metformin, have been shown to improve ovulatory function (Tang et al. 2003). This highlights the role for glycemic control and insulin regulation in ovulation. Furthermore, Guerin et al. (2007) showed that high levels of pre-conception blood glucose may be lead to a higher risk of fetal abnormalities, reinforcing the need for strict glycemic control in patients at risk of insulin resistance.

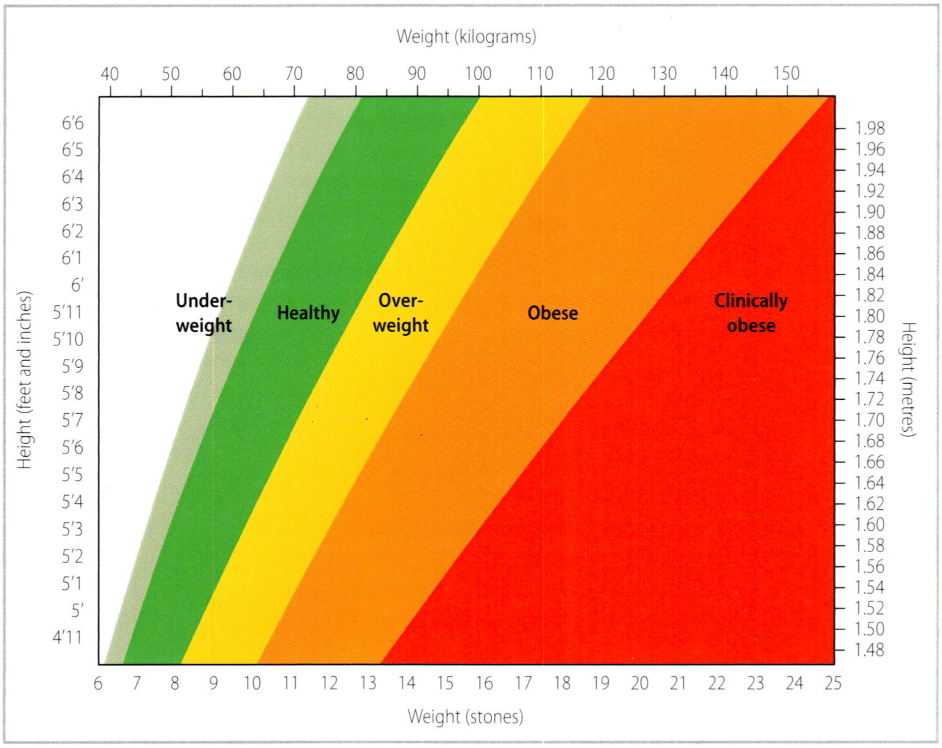

Figure 4.3 A body mass index (BMI) chart. BMI is calculated from weight (kg) and height (m) using the equation BMI = weight/height^2 and expressed as kg/m^2. Using BMI, people can assess their body mass as either underweight, healthy, overweight, obese and clinically obese.

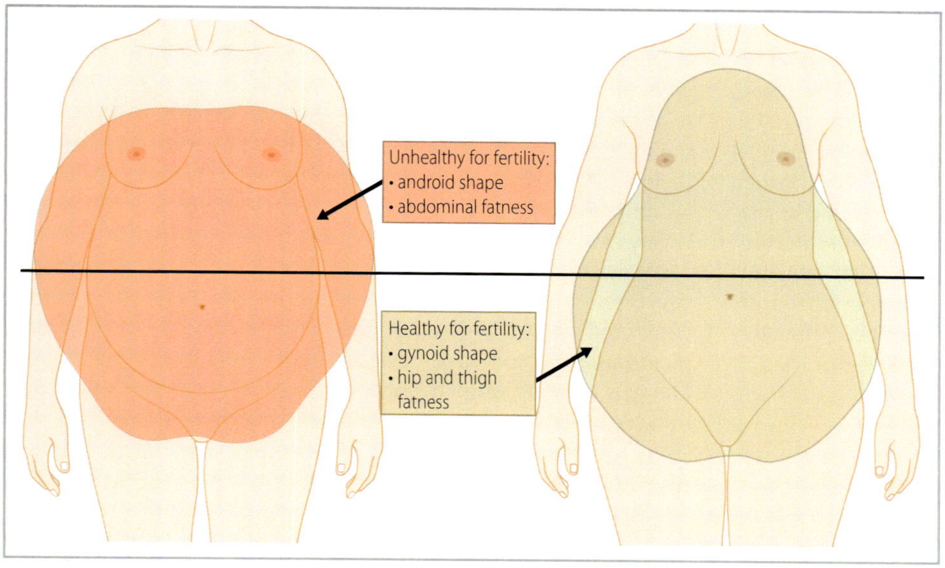

Figure 4.4 Apple versus pear shape. Women can be classified according to fat distribution as either gynoid or 'female' ('pear' shaped/lower body) or an android or 'male' ('apple' shaped/visceral).

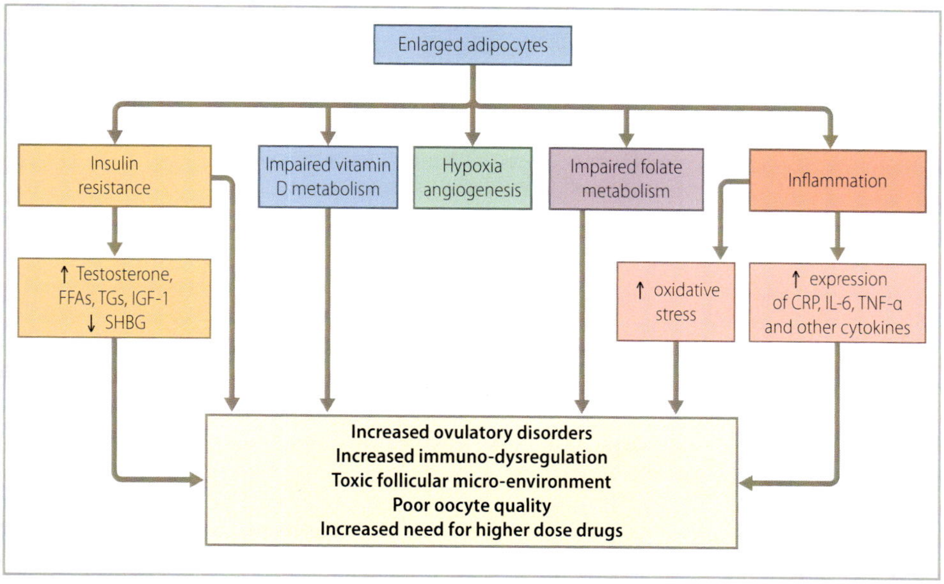

Figure 4.5 Enlarged adipocytes. Visceral adipose tissue is composed of adipocytes that are enlarged, highly metabolically active and possibly dysfunctional. Such adipocytes can lead to insulin resistance, impaired vitamin D and folate metabolism, and inflammation. Regarding fertility, enlarged adipocytes are associated with ovulatory disorders and decreased oocyte quality. CRP, C-reactive proteins; FFAs, free fatty acids; IGF-1, insulin-like growth factor-1; SHBG, sex hormone-binding globulin; TG, triglycerides

Meal timing is also worth considering. Subjects who are dieting and consume most of their daily calories earlier in the day tend to have a greater waist circumference reduction than those who distribute calorie intake throughout the day (Jakubowicz et al. 2013). Obese women are also at risk of specific nutrient deficiencies such as vitamin D and folate, and extra supplementation may be advisable (McMahon et al. 2013, Wortsman et al. 2000).

Underweight

The relationship between under-nutrition and fertility is well recognized. The onset of puberty is closely related to body size, whilst intensive exercise can cause amenorrhea. It has been postulated that menstruation requires ~17% fat/body weight, and that ~22% fat/body weight is necessary for fertility (Frisch 1978).

The amount of body fat influences hormone 'potency', with leaner women making the less potent form of catechol estrogens, and experiencing poor cervical secretions and dryness. Storage of steroid hormones and aromatization of androgens to estrogens in adipocytes is also reduced. If low weight is linked to caloric restriction, there is risk of nutritional deficiencies, e.g. the fat-soluble vitamins A, E, D and K.

Body weight and weight change can highlight psychological and control issues, lack of confidence and body dysmorphic tendencies, all of which accompany the potential stress related to infertility. Therefore, sustained, informed weight management programs and exercise advice can often help to restore fertility, as well as providing a healthy platform for pregnancy. Use of weighing scales that incorporate a body fat monitor may be useful to provide accurate assessment of any changes.

DIET AND ENDOMETRIOSIS

Endometriosis affects up to 50% of infertile women (see Chapter 7). Dietary changes may help to modulate the condition via use of antioxidants and anti-inflammatory compounds, and iron supplementation for dysmenorrhea. Endometriosis may also be exacerbated by exposure to organochlorines, especially dioxins (Sofo et al. 2015) which can induce and maintain inflammation (Sofo et al. 2015).

Dioxins are fat-soluble and found in animal products, meat, fish and dairy. Dairy products also contain levels of IGF-1 and pro-inflammatory arachidonic acid, as well as significant levels of estrogen, all of which may promote endometriosis (Daxenberger et al. 2001). Plant milks can be substituted for dairy, and proteins can be sourced from vegetables rather than meat (e.g. from pulses or Quorn). Fish to consider avoiding include fresh tuna, swordfish, sea bass and bream, since they all may contain high levels of heavy metals and dioxins. However, inclusion of some fish, eggs, minimal dairy like yoghurt and lean red meat once a week is thought to be an important part of a healthy diet. In summary, advising patients to eat a predominately plant-based diet, minimizing red meat, may be beneficial.

Wheat/gluten-free diets

Although many naturopathic therapists advise that wheat or total gluten avoidance can ameliorate the symptoms of endometriosis only a single study of 156 patients, by Marziali and colleagues (2012), has reported that pain was significantly reduced in women with endometriosis who had adhered to a gluten-free diet for 12 months. Whether such a restrictive diet should be followed needs to be explored further.

Supplements

Vitamin D

High levels of vitamin D have been linked to endometriosis, although this association remains speculative (Somigliana et al. 2007). Vitamin D is involved in immune function, cytokine modulation and macrophage activity. Endometrial cells produce an enzyme called 1α-hydroxylase which promotes levels of the active form of vitamin D. Expression of 1α-hydrolxylase is enhanced in endometriosis sufferers. Macrophages, which hydroxylate vitamin D, may further enhance endometriosis-associated inflammation. Measuring vitamin D levels in some patients may be helpful to ensure that undue supplementation does not occur.

Omega three fatty acids

The long chain polyunsaturated ω-3 FAs exhibit potent anti-inflammatory properties that may contribute to pain reduction (Silva et al. 2017). ω-3 FAs block prostaglandin activity in endometrial stromal cells and mediate the release of thromboxanes, interferon, TNFα and cytokines (Marziali et al. 2012). Supplementation may therefore be appropriate.

Resveratrol

Resveratrol is a polyphenol found in the skin of red and black berries and grapes. Resveratrol may benefit women with endometriosis due to its antiestrogenic and anti-inflammatory properties. Resveratrol enhances apoptosis, inhibits vascularization and reduces endometrial cell proliferation (Kolahdouz Mohammadi 2017). It has been proposed that a daily dose of 1000 mg for a 60-kg woman may be beneficial, whilst other trials have used up to 5000 mg/day (Bruner-Tran et al. 2011).

VEGETARIAN AND VEGAN DIETS

Strict vegetarians eat no meat, whilst some eat fish and most eat eggs and dairy products. Vegans eat nothing of animal origin, and may be most at risk of nutrient deficiencies, namely protein, ω-3 FAs, iron, iodine and vitamin B_{12}, so dietary and supplement intervention may be necessary.

Soy protein, beans and lentils, nuts, seeds and protein-rich grains like quinoa provide a mixture of amino acids for protein anabolism. ω-3 FAs are found in dark green leafy vegetables and nuts, in the form of α-linolenic acid (ALA). However, ALA converts poorly to the more metabolically active, anti-inflammatory long chain ω-3 PUFAs eicosapentaenoic acid (EPA) and docosahexaenoic acid (DHA). Since these are important in pregnancy, supplementation of an algae-derived vegan source may be recommended (King & Fewtrell 2008).

Vegetarians need to consume 1.8 times more iron than non-vegetarians, due to lower bioavailability of plant non-heme iron, compared to animal heme iron. However, it should be noted that plant-based carotenoids and vitamin C potentiate absorption (Craig Mangels 2009). In women with endometriosis-related menorrhagia, iron supplementation may be considered.

Iodine is primarily found in fish and dairy foods, so vegans could use an iodised salt to achieve the 250 mg/day recommended in pregnancy. Bio-available vitamin B12 is also exclusively found in foods of animal origin, and supplementation of this is essential to avoid anemia.

DAIRY PRODUCTS

Whether dairy products help or hinder fertility is controversial. Rodent studies suggest that galactose (a dairy carbohydrate) may impair ovulation, and human studies suggest low fat dairy products might be associated with anovulation. By contrast, other studies, e.g. the Nurses Study, report a positive correlation between consumption of full fat dairy products and conception. Full fat dairy consumption is also associated with positive outcomes in relation to IVF treatment (Afeiche et al. 2016). Moreover, full fat dairy products carry a rich source of many fat-soluble nutrients important for fertility, e.g. vitamins A, D, E and K, beta-carotene and oleic acid, as well as protein, calcium and riboflavin. Milk is also one of the principal sources of iodine in the UK.

SOYA PHYTOESTROGENS

Phytoestrogens are found in plants and possess structural and functional similarities to human estrogen. Most phytoestrogens belong to a class of phenols called flavonoids, of which a sub-class, isoflavones share a remarkable similarity to estradiol (see **Figure 4.6**). It has been suggested that phytoestrogens could potentially disrupt natural estrogen production (Jefferson 2010). However, a traditional Asian diet of 1–2 servings of soya (10–50 mg isoflavones/day) does not seem to disrupt ovulation or fertility (Jefferson 2010). Isoflavone levels in foods vary, with some traditional fermented Asian soya foods containing lower levels than 'textured vegetable protein (TVP, a soya vegetarian alternative to meat) but with significantly greater bioavailability (Cassidy et al. 2006). Isoflavone bioavailability also depends on the ability of the gut microbiota to metabolise them.

CAFFEINE

Caffeine is a natural alkaloid found in coffee, tea, cocoa, and some soft drinks and medications. Caffeine is 'probably the most frequently ingested pharmacological substance in the world' (Nawrot et al. 2003). In a Europe-wide study, Bolumar and colleagues (1997) found that women consuming >500 mg of caffeine/day had an increased waiting time to their first pregnancy. They suggested that caffeine might inhibit corpus luteum function through a decrease in serum prolactin,

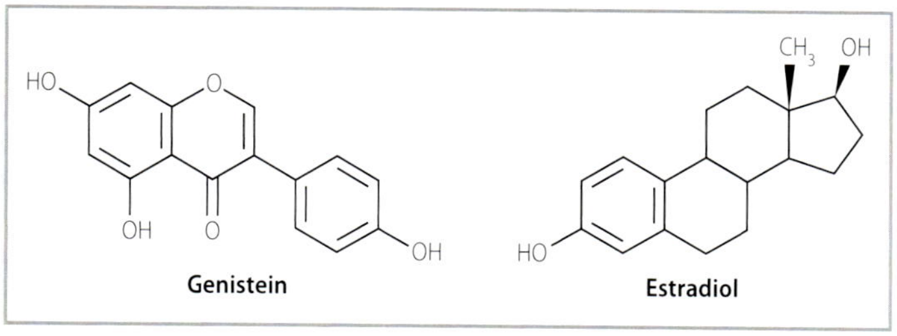

Figure 4.6 The chemical structures of the phytoestrogen genistein and estradiol. Despite phytoestrogens being found in plants, the structures are so similar to human estrogen that is has been suggested that phytoestrogens can mimics human estrodiol but triggering estrogen receptors.

reduced estrogen and subsequent ovarian inhibition.

Recent studies have focused on the effect of caffeine on oocyte transport in the fallopian tubes, with caffeine inhibiting fallopian tube contractility (Dixon et al. 2011). Therefore, women wanting to conceive may benefit from reducing caffeine-containing foods, medications and drinks (Cao et al. 2016; see **Figure 4.7**).

During pregnancy, a maximum caffeine consumption of 200 mg/day is recommended.

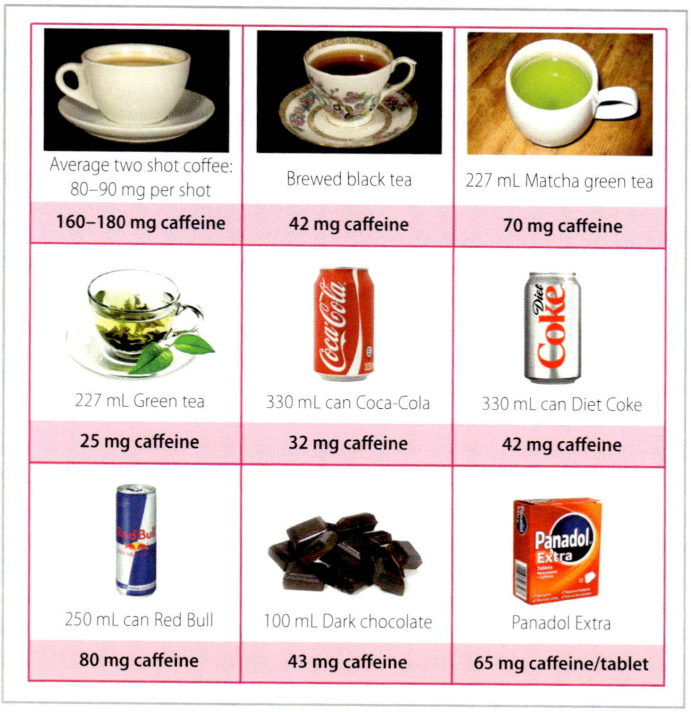
Average two shot coffee: 80–90 mg per shot
160–180 mg caffeine
Brewed black tea
42 mg caffeine
227 mL Matcha green tea
70 mg caffeine
227 mL Green tea
25 mg caffeine
330 mL can Coca-Cola
32 mg caffeine
330 mL can Diet Coke
42 mg caffeine
250 mL can Red Bull
80 mg caffeine
100 mL Dark chocolate
43 mg caffeine
Panadol Extra
65 mg caffeine/tablet

Figure 4.7 Caffeine content of frequently ingested products, such as coffee, tea, coke, chocolate and popular medications.

ALCOHOL

Knowledge of the effects of alcohol ingestion on fertility is inconclusive but it appears to be dose-dependent. Alcohol causes estradiol levels to rise due to competition for hepatic clearance via cytochrome P450 enzymes, which may in turn reduce FSH secretion and suppress folliculogenesis, affecting ovulation. Mikkelsen et al. (2016) found no significant effect of alcohol consumption on fecundability under 14 units a week, but accepted that this study did not distinguish between regular and 'binge' drinking which may be a significant factor if large quantities of alcohol are consumed during the fertile window or post ovulation. Furthermore, alcohol consumption at the time of conception may cause insulin insensitivity and glucose intolerance in offspring (Gårdebjer et al. 2015).

Alcohol consumption before and during IVF treatment is associated with poorer outcomes, particularly if both partners drink (Nicolau et al. 2014). Indeed, women who had at least four drinks per week experienced a lower live birth rate. Thus, woman trying to conceive are advised to drink very moderately (<4 drinks a week) and to abstain altogether upon commencement of an IVF treatment cycle.

SMOKING

Smoking is linked to ovarian follicular depletion, increased time to conception, hormonal dysregulation, DNA mutations, higher oocyte aneuploidy rates and effectively adds 10 years to the biological age of a women's oocytes, having a 'devastating impact on the live birth rate in IVF treatment' (Lintsen et al. 2005). As well as decreasing local protective antioxidant pathways, impairing folliculogenesis and decreasing IVF rates, if continued into pregnancy, smoking can adversely affect the health of the offspring (Camlin et al. 2014).

BISPHENOL A

Bisphenol A (BPA) is an endocrine disruptor that has an affinity with both estrogen, androgen and thyroid receptors. Oocyte quality has been shown to be adversely affected in IVF patients who have high BPA levels (Machtinger et al. 2013). Moreover, a link has been found between urinary BPA levels and IVF implantation failure (Ehrlich et al. 2012). Since BPA is commonly used in the manufacture of plastics and food can linings, women contemplating pregnancy should consider switching to BPA-free alternatives (Rochester 2013).

NOVEL SUPPLEMENTS AND NUTRACEUTICALS

Women are increasingly turning to the internet and alternative therapists for advice on how to improve fertility. As a result, there has been a rise in use of nutraceuticals, even though manufacturer's claims are often unsubstantiated. Below are some novel supplements which may be helpful.

Co-enzyme Q10

Coenzyme Q10 (CoQ10) is a fat-soluble co-enzyme antioxidant involved in energy metabolism. CoQ10 may help maintain mitochondrial integrity and reduce oocyte aneuploidy (Wilding et al. 2003). Rodent studies have shown that CoQ10 supplementation may also delay ovarian reserve depletion and improve oocyte quality (Ben-Meir et al. 2015).

Dehydroepiandrosterone

Dehydroepiandrosterone (DHEA) is a steroid hormone that may improve oocyte quality and ovarian reserve (in both older women and women who have suffered premature ovarian failure) (Fusi et al. 2013). Administration can be for several weeks, with cumulative benefits reported up to 5 months. DHEA combined with CoQ10 has also been reported to improve outcome during IVF treatment (Gat et al. 2016). However, due to potential rises in testosterone, DHEA may not benefit women with PCOS, elevated cholesterol, type II diabetes, cancer and liver or kidney disorders.

Melatonin

Melatonin is used in many countries to counter jet lag and sleep disorders. It is naturally found in follicular fluid where it may act as an antioxidant (Taketani et al. 2007). Ovarian melatonin levels follow the 'light/dark' concentrations in the pineal gland, related to hours of daylight. During IVF cycles, one study has shown that daily oral administration of 3 mg melatonin at night, from day 5 of the previous menstrual cycle to the day of oocyte retrieval, might improve fertilization and pregnancy rates (Tamura et al. 2012).

Both DHEA and melatonin are available over the counter in the USA and the internet. However, both are prescription-only medications in the UK.

L-carnitine and acetyl-L-carnitine

The amino acid carnitine may improve oocyte maturation by upregulating mitochondrial beta-oxidation (Várnagy et al. 2013). Furthermore, carnitine may reduce levels of anti-inflammatory cytokines and ROS to modulate any adverse effects of endometriosis on embryonic development (Mansour et al. 2009). However, carnitine could interfere with thyroxine and cause gastrointestinal disorders, hence long-term use is not recommended.

Myo-inositol

Myo-inositol is a derivative of glucose and may influence insulin receptor sensitivity. Much research relates to its role in relieving PCOS symptoms and restoring ovarian function by improving ovulation and normalizing cycle length and luteal progesterone levels (Gerli et al. 2007). Myo-inositol may also reduce androgenic symptoms of PCOS, e.g. acne and male pattern baldness, and contribute to weight loss through normalizing lipid metabolism and insulin sensitivity.

EXERCISE

Exercise helps to reduce stress and may particularly help women with PCOS, via induced metabolic changes such as improved fasting insulin and insulin-sensitivity, which has positive effects on menstrual cycle regularity and ovulation (Palomba et al. 2008). Exercise may also influence estrogen metabolism and decrease any endometriosis risk, since skeletal muscle contraction induces anti-inflammatory cytokines and reduces oxidative stress (see Chapter 7).

However, women with PCOS who wish to conceive should avoid intense physical activity as this can lead to menstrual irregularities, and increase levels of the stress hormones cortisol and adrenaline, which may inhibit LH production. A low BMI and low fat:high muscle ratio can also disrupt the hypothalamic-pituitary-ovarian axis, resulting in gonadotropin suppression, producing an 'anovulatory, hypoestrogenic state' (Olive 2010).

COMPLEMENTARY AND ALTERNATIVE MEDICINE

Fertility patients may seek complementary and alternative medicine (CAM) either instead of, or to supplement, conventional medical treatment. Female private patients have been shown to be the highest users of CAM, and cite benefits as spending time with someone who was 'really interested' and 'listened carefully to what I was saying' (Coulson & Jenkins 2005). Chinese and Western herbs are two CAMs often used alongside conventional IVF drugs.

Acupuncture

Acupuncturists use specific protocols claimed to enhance IVF success, particularly around the time of oocyte retrieval and embryo transfer (Manheimer et al. 2008). Acupuncture may also improve cycle regulation and pelvic blood flow, and reduce stress. Effects are mediated through neuropeptides, particularly β-endorphins that act on the hypothalamic-pituitary-ovarian hormonal axis. Whilst studies support the use of acupuncture for fertility (Paulus et al. 2002), it has been postulated that a placebo-effect may be partly biasing successful results (Domar 2006).

Herbal medicine

Hormonal disturbances and infertility can be treated using both traditional Western and Chinese herbal medicine. Many herbs contain compounds that mimic hormones with pro- and anti-estrogenic properties, for example agnus castus or chaste berry. Herbs can also be anti-inflammatory, insulin-sensitizing or influence hepatic clearance. However, awareness among conventional medical practitioners remains low (Ried & Stuart 2017).

Patients should be advised that if they start taking a herbal medicine they should inform their clinic as they can interact with fertility drugs. Worryingly, in one study, over a third of ART patients admitted

Table 4.2 Potential interactions between drugs used in fertility treatment and nutrients

Drug	Nutrient	Interaction	Action
Oral contraceptive pill	Magnesium, vitamin B_6, zinc, selenium	Impairment of absorption	Multivitamin
Metformin	Folic acid, B_{12}	Impairment of absorption	Supplement extra folic acid and B_{12}
Thyroxine	Iron	Reduction of thyroxine efficacy	Take thyroxine and iron-containing supplement apart
Prednisalone, dexamethasone	Calcium and vitamin D	Osteoblastic suppression and increased bone resorption Impairment of glycemic control; weight gain Impairment of immune function	Supplementation of calcium and vitamin D Specific dietary advice; low GI Immune supportive diet and lifestyle
Heparin	Calcium and vitamin D	Reduction in bone density	Supplementation of calcium and vitamin D
Proton pump inhibitors	Vitamin B_{12}	Impairment of absorption	Supplementation of vitamin B_{12}
Note: The flavonoid naringenin in grapefruit juice slows hepatic clearance of drugs			

to using herbs in the 3-month period to treatment and yet none had informed their fertility clinic (Shannon et al. 2010).

CONCLUSION

This chapter has highlighted various aspects of diet and lifestyle that can affect female fertility.

Women may wish to make positive changes to both, to enhance the chance of conception and improve pregnancy outcome. They are recommended to seek advice from nutritionists, and also to discuss such matters with fertility clinic staff, to ensure that there are no adverse interactions between diet, supplements and prescribed fertility drugs. Women with specific nutritional needs or those taking specific medications should always discuss these prior to changing diet, as some nutrients may impair absorption or possibly cause adverse reactions (see **Table 4.2**).

Medical professionals and fertility clinics may consider giving patients basic pre-conception nutrition and lifestyle plans so they are better armed to improve their fertility and chances of a successful pregnancy.

REFERENCES

Achebe MM, Gafter-Gvili A. How I treat anemia in pregnancy: iron, cobalamin, and folate. Blood 2017; 129:940–949.

Afeiche MC, Chiu YH, Gaskins AJ, et al. Dairy intake in relation to in vitro fertilization outcomes among women from a fertility clinic. Hum Reprod 2016; 31:563–571.

Anderson JW, Baird P, Davis RH, et al. Health benefits of dietary fiber. Nutr Rev 2009; 67:188–205.

Barker DJ. The fetal and infant origins of adult disease. Br Med J 1990; 301:1111.

Bedaiwy MA, Elnashar SA, Goldberg JM, et al. Effect of follicular fluid oxidative stress parameters on intracytoplasmic sperm injection outcome. Gynecol Endocrinol 2012; 28:51–55.

Bender D. Nutrition and Metabolism, 4th edn. CRC Press London, 2008.

Ben-Meir A, Burstein E, Borrego-Alvarez A, et al. Coenzyme Q10 restores oocyte mitochondrial function and fertility during reproductive aging. Aging Cell 2015; 14:887–895.

Boland MP, Lonergan P, O'Callaghan D. Effect of nutrition on endocrine parameters, ovarian physiology, and oocyte and embryo development. Theriogenology 2001; 55:1323–1240.

Bolumar F, Olsen J, Rebagliato M, Bisanti L. Caffeine intake and delayed conception: a European multicenter study on infertility and subfecundity. European Study Group on Infertility Subfecundity. Am J Epidemiol 1997; 145:324–334.

British Dietetic Association. Food Fact Sheet: Folic Acid. Birmingham: British Dietetic Association, 2010.

Bruner-Tran KL, Osteen KG, Taylor HS, et al. Resveratrol inhibits development of experimental endometriosis in vivo and reduces endometrial stromal cell invasiveness in vitro. Biol Reprod 2011; 84:106–112.

Camlin NJ, McLaughlin EA, Holt JE. Through the smoke: use of in vivo and in vitro cigarette smoking models to elucidate its effect on female fertility. Toxicol Appl Pharmacol 2014; 281:266–275.

Cao H, Ren J, Feng X, Yang G, Liu J. Is caffeine intake a risk factor leading to infertility? A protocol of an epidemiological systematic review of controlled clinical studies. Syst Rev 2016; 5:45.

Cappuccio FP. Ethnicity and cardiovascular risk: variations in people of African ancestry and South Asian origin. J Hum Hypertens 1997; 11:571–576.

Cassidy A, Brown JE, Hawdon A, et al. Factors affecting the bioavailability of soy isoflavones in humans after ingestion of physiologically relevant levels from different soy foods. J Nutr 2006; 136:45–51.

Chavarro JE, Gaskins JA, Afeiche MC. Nutrition and ovulatory function. In: Tremellon K, Pearce K, (Eds). Nutrition, Fertility and Human Reproductive Function. CRP Press Boca Raton FL 2015.

Chavarro JE, Rich-Edwards JW, Rosner BA, Willett WC. A prospective study of dietary carbohydrate quantity and quality in relation to risk of ovulatory infertility. Eur J Clin Nutr 2009; 63:78–86.

Chavarro JE, Rich-Edwards JW, Rosner BA, Willett WC. Iron intake and risk of ovulatory infertility. Obst Gynecol 2006; 108:1145–1152.

Chavarro JE, Rich-Edwards JW, Rosner BA, Willett WC. Protein intake and ovulatory infertility. Am J Obst Gyn 2008; 198:210–e211.

Cobb-Clark DA, Kassenboehmer SC, Schurer S. Healthy habits: The connection between diet, exercise, and locus of control. J Eco Behav Org 2014; 98:1–28.

Coulson C, Jenkins J. Complementary and alternative medicine utilisation in NHS and private clinic settings: a United Kingdom survey of 400 infertility patients. J Exp Clin Ass Reprod 2005; 2:5.

Craig WJ, Mangels AR. Position of the American Dietetic Association: vegetarian diets. J Am Diet Assoc 2009; 109:1266–1282.

Creo AL, Thacher TD, Pettifor JM, Strand MA, Fischer PR. Nutritional rickets around the world: an update. Paediatr Int Child Health 2016; 6:1–15.

Daxenberger A, Ibarreta D, Meyer HH. Possible health impact of animal oestrogens in food. Hum Reprod Update 2001; 7:340–355.

De-Regil LM, Harding KB, Roche ML. Preconceptional nutrition interventions for adolescent girls and adult women: global guidelines and gaps in evidence and policy with emphasis on micronutrients. J Nutr 2016; 146:1461S–70S.

Dinu M, Pagliai G, Casini A, Sofi F. Mediterranean diet and multiple health outcomes: an umbrella review of meta-analyses of observational studies and randomised trials. Eur J Clin Nutr 2018; 72:30–43.

Dixon RE, Hwang SJ, Britton FC, Sanders KM, Ward SM. Inhibitory effect of caffeine on pacemaker activity in the oviduct is mediated by cAMP-regulated conductances. Br J Pharm 2011; 163:745–754.

Domar AD. Acupuncture and infertility: we need to stick to good science. Fertil Steril 2006; 85:1359–1361.

Ehrlich S, Williams PL, Missmer SA. Urinary bisphenol A concentrations and implantation failure among women undergoing in vitro fertilization. Environ Health Perspect 2012; 120:978–983.

Fedorcsák P, Dale PO, Storeng R, et al. Impact of overweight and underweight on assisted reproduction treatment. Hum Reprod 2004; 19:2523–2528.

Food Standards Agency. National Diet and Nutrition Survey (NDNS): results from Years 1 to 4 (combined) of the rolling programme for 2008 and 2009 to 2011 and 2012. London: Public Health England and Food Standards Agency, 2014.

Frisch RE. Nutrition, Fatness and Fertility. In: Moseley WH (Ed). Nutrition and Human Reproduction. Plenum Press, New York 1978:91–121.

Fusi FM, Ferrario M, Bosisio C, Arnoldi M, Zanga L. DHEA supplementation positively affects spontaneous pregnancies in women with diminished ovarian function. Gynecol Endocrinol 2013; 29:940–943.

Gårdebjer EM, Anderson ST, Pantaleon M, Wlodek ME, Moritz KM. Maternal alcohol intake around the time of conception causes glucose intolerance and insulin insensitivity in rat offspring, which is exacerbated by a postnatal high-fat diet. FASEB J 2015; 29:2690–2701.

Gaskins AJ, Mumford SL, Chavarro JE, et al. The impact of dietary folate intake on reproductive function in premenopausal women: a prospective cohort study. PloS One 2012; 7:e46276.

Gat I, Blanco Mejia S, Balakier H, et al. The use of coenzyme Q10 and DHEA during IUI and IVF cycles in patients with decreased ovarian reserve. Gynecol Endocrinol 2016; 21:1–4.

Gerli S, Papaleo E, Ferrari A, Di Renzo GC. Randomized, double blind placebo-controlled trial: effects of myo-inositol on ovarian function and metabolic factors in women with PCOS. Eur Rev Medic Pharm Sciences 2007; 11:347–354.

Gluckman PD, Hanson MA, Cooper C, Thornburg KL. Effect of in utero and early-life conditions on adult health and disease. N Engl J Med 2008; 359:61–73.

Guerin A, Nisenbaum R, Ray JG. Use of maternal GHb concentration to estimate the risk of congenital anomalies in the offspring of women with prepregnancy diabetes. Diabetes Care 2007; 30:1920–1925.

Henderson L, Irving K, Gregory J, et al. The National Diet & Nutrition Survey: adults aged 19 to 64 years. Vitamin and Mineral Intake and Urinary Analytes. London: Food Standards Agency and Department of Health, 2003.

Jakubowicz D, Barnea M, Wainstein J, Froy O. High caloric intake at breakfast vs. dinner differentially influences weight loss of overweight and obese women. Obesity 2013; 21:2504–2512.

Jefferson WN. Adult ovarian function can be affected by high levels of soy. J Nutr 2010; 140:2322S–2325S.
Kolahdouz Mohammadi R, Arablou T. Resveratrol and endometriosis: In vitro and animal studies and underlying mechanisms (review). Biomed Pharmecother 2017; 91: 220-228.
Karuputhula NB, Chattopadhyay R, Chakravarty B, Chaudhury K. Oxidative status in granulosa cells of infertile women undergoing IVF. Syst Biol Repr Med 2013; 59:91–98.
Lerchbaum E, Obermayer-Pietsch B. Mechanisms in endocrinology: Vitamin D and fertility: a systematic review. Eur J Endocrinol 2012; 166:765–778.
Lintsen AM, Pasker-de Jong PC, De Boer EJ, et al. Effects of subfertility cause, smoking and body weight on the success rate of IVF. Hum Reprod 2005; 20:1867–1875.
Lumey LH, Stein AD, Kahn HS, et al. Cohort profile: The Dutch Hunger Winter families study. Int J Epidemeol 2007; 36:1196–1204.
Machtinger R, Combelles CM, Missmer SA, et al. Bisphenol-A and human oocyte maturation in vitro. Hum Reprod 2013; 28:2735–2745.
Mamsen LS, Lutterodt MC, Andersen EW, et al. Cigarette smoking during early pregnancy reduces the number of embryonic germ and somatic cells. Hum Reprod 2010; 25:2755–2761.
Manheimer E, Zhang G, Udoff L. et al. Effects of acupuncture on rates of pregnancy and live birth among women undergoing in vitro fertilisation: systematic review and meta-analysis. Br Med J 2008; 336:545–549.
Mansour G, Abdelrazik H, Sharma RK, et al. L-carnitine supplementation reduces oocyte cytoskeleton damage and embryo apoptosis induced by incubation in peritoneal fluid from patients with endometriosis. Fertil Steril 2009; 91:2079–2086.
Marziali M, Venza M, Lazzaro S, et al. Gluten-free diet: a new strategy for management of painful endometriosis related symptoms? Minerva Chirurgica 2012; 67:499–504.
McMahon DM, Liu J, Zhang H, Torres ME, Best RG. Maternal obesity, folate intake, and neural tube defects in offspring. Birth Defects Res A Clin Mol Teratol 2013; 97:115–122.
Meuvret R. Les crises de subsistence et la démographie de la France d'ancien regime. Population IV 1946:641–650.
Mikkelsen, EM, Riis AH, Wise LA, et al. Alcohol consumption and fecundability: prospective Danish cohort study. BMJ 2016; 354:i4262.
Milman N. Iron prophylaxis in pregnancy – general or individual and in which dose? Ann Hematol 2006; 85:821–828.
Missmer SA, Chavarro JE, Malspeis S, et al. A prospective study of dietary fat consumption and endometriosis risk. Hum Reprod 2010; 25:1528–1535.
Nawrot P, Jordan S, Eastwood J, et al. Effects of caffeine on human health. Food Addit Contam 2003; 20:1–30.
Nicolau P, Miralpeix E, Solà I, Carreras R, Checa MA. Alcohol consumption and in vitro fertilization: a review of the literature. Gynecol Endocrinol 2014; 30:759–763.
Olive DL. Exercise and fertility: an update. Curr Opin Obstet Gynecol 2010; 22:259–263.
Omani Samani R, Maroufizadeh S, Navid B, Amini P. Locus of control, anxiety, and depression in infertile patients. Psychol Health Med 2017; 22:44–50.
Palomba S, Giallauria F, Falbo A, et al. Structured exercise training programme versus hypocaloric hyperproteic diet in obese polycystic ovary syndrome patients with anovulatory infertility: a 24-week pilot study. Hum Reprod 2008; 23:642–650.
Paulus WE, Zhang M, Strehler E, El-Danasouri I, Sterzik K. Role of acupuncture in patients who undergo assisted reproductive therapy. Fertil Steril 2002; 77:721–724.
Rao R, Georgieff MK. Iron in fetal and neonatal nutrition. Semin Fetal Neonatal Med 2007; 12:54–63.
Ried K, Stuart K. Efficacy of Traditional Chinese Herbal Medicine in the management of female infertility: a systematic review. Complementary Ther Med 2017; 19:319–331.
Ried K. Chinese herbal medicine for female infertility: An updated meta-analysis. Complementary Ther Med 2015; 23:116–128.
Rochester JR. Bisphenol A and human health: a review of the literature. Reprod Toxicol 2013; 42:132–155.
Santos JE, Bilby TR, Thatcher WW, Staples CR, Silvestre FT. Long chain fatty acids of diet as factors influencing reproduction in cattle. Reprod Domest Anim 2008; 3:23–30.
Scaramuzzi RJ, Brown HM, Dupont J. Nutritional and metabolic mechanisms in the ovary and their role in mediating the effects of diet on folliculogenesis: a perspective. Reprod Domest Anim 2010; 45:32–41.
Scarborough P, Bhatnagar P, Kaur A, Wickramasinghe K, Rayner M. Ethnic differences in cardiovascular disease. London: British Heart Foundation 2010.
Shannon J, El Saigh I, Tadrous R, Mocanu E, Loughrey J. Usage of herbal medications in patients undergoing IVF treatment in an Irish infertility treatment unit. Ir J Med Sci 2010; 179:63–65.
Silva RV, Oliveira JT, Santos BLR, et al. Long-chain omega-3 fatty acids supplementation accelerates nerve regeneration and prevents neuropathic pain behavior in mice. Front Pharmacol 2017; 17:723.
Sofo V, Götte M, Laganà AS, Salmeri FM, et al. Correlation between dioxin and endometriosis: an epigenetic route to unravel the pathogenesis of the disease. Arch Gynecol Obstet 2015; 292:973–986.
Somigliana E, Panina-Bordignon P, Murone S, et al. Vitamin D reserve is higher in women with endometriosis. Hum Reprod 2007; 22:2273–2278.
Stamets K, Taylor DS, Kunselman A, et al. A randomized trial of the effects of two types of short-term hypocaloric diets on weight loss in women with polycystic ovary syndrome. Fertil Steril 2004; 81:630–637.
Taketani T, Tamura H, Taniguchi K, Maekawa R, Sugino N. Influence of oxidative stress on oocyte quality and protective role of melatonin as an antioxidant. Biol Reprod 2007; 77:218.
Tamura H, Takasaki A, Taketani T, et al. The role of melatonin as an antioxidant in the follicle. J Ovarian Res 2012; 5:5.
Tang T, Lord JM, Norman RJ, Balen AH. Insulin-sensitizing drugs (metformin, troglitazone, rosiglitazone, pioglitazone, D-chiro-inositol) for polycystic ovary syndrome. Cochrane Database Syst Rev 2003:2.
Vague J. Sexual Differentiation, a factor affecting the forms of obesity. Presse Med 1947; 30: 339–340.
Vanderpump MP, Lazarus JH, Smyth PP. British Thyroid Association UK Iodine Survey Group. Iodine status of UK schoolgirls: a cross-sectional survey. Lancet 2011; 377:2007–2012.
Várnagy Á, Bene J, Sulyok E, et al. Acylcarnitine esters profiling of serum and follicular fluid in patients undergoing in vitro fertilization. Reprod Biol Endocrinol 2013; 11:67.
Waterland RA, Michels KB. Epigenetic epidemiology of the developmental origins hypothesis. Ann Rev Nutr 2017; 27:363–388.
WHO Secretariat, Andersson M, de Benoist B, Delange F, Zupan J. Prevention and control of iodine deficiency in pregnant and lactating women and in children less than 2-year-old: conclusions and recommendations of the Technical Consultation. Public Health Nutr 2007; 10:1606–1611.
Wilding M, De Placido G, De Matteo L. Chaotic mosaicism in human preimplantation embryos is correlated with a low mitochondrial membrane potential. Fertil Steril 2003; 79:340–346.
Wortsman J, Matsuoka LY, Chen TC, Lu Z, Holick MF. Decreased bioavailability of vitamin D in obesity. Am J Clin Nutr 2000; 6972:690–693.
Zimmerman MB. Iodine Deficiency. Endocr Rev 2009; 30:376.

Chapter 5 Ovarian reserve and anti-Müllerian hormone

Stamatina Iliodromiti, Scott M Nelson

INTRODUCTION

The ovarian reserve is classically defined as the number of non-growing follicles (NGFs) remaining within the ovary at any specific point in time. Although a wide variety of ovarian reserve biomarkers have been proposed, it is now clear that anti-Müllerian hormone (AMH) demonstrates the most favorable analytical and performance characteristics.

Several large recent systematic reviews of cohort studies and individual patient data meta-analyses have demonstrated a consistent positive association of AMH with oocyte yield, poor and excess response, and live births in in-vitro fertilization (IVF) treatment cycles.

This chapter provides an update on the strengths and weaknesses of AMH as a measure of ovarian reserve. This includes a description of new automated AMH immunoassays and the data underlying the performance characteristics of AMH as a biomarker of ovarian response relative to antral follicle count (AFC). Recent randomized controlled trials (RCTs) will be discussed to show how AMH can be used to tailor ovarian stimulation.

Follicle growth and recruitment

The molecular mechanisms regulating NGF recruitment and selection for continued growth versus atresia are becoming clearer. Key concepts to consider include:

- Recruitment of primordial follicles occurs across a female's reproductive life. This dynamic process, with differential rates of follicular activation at different ages, continuously supplies growing follicles for selection for ovulation (Wallace & Kelsey 2010) and is probably influenced by health status
- Follicles undergo atresia at all stages of development
- The number of activated follicles reflects the total pool of primordial follicles in a variable manner, and this changes in childhood and adult life (Kelsey et al. 2012)
- Ovarian reserve depletion depends on the initial quantity of primordial follicles, and the rate of primordial follicle recruitment

While biomarkers of activated follicles, such as AMH and AFC, reflect the primordial follicle pool (Hansen et al. 2011), they are most useful in indicating the number of follicles that are at late stages of follicular development and therefore capable of responding to exogenous gonadotropins.

Thus, AMH and AFC are of greatest value in reflecting what has been termed the functional, rather than the true, ovarian reserve (Anderson et al. 2012).

ANTI-MÜLLERIAN HORMONE

Factors that can influence anti-Müllerian hormone values

Automated assays

Since the original reports of measuring serum AMH in the 1990s, immunoassays have improved. Although, four manual enzyme-linked immunosorbent assays (ELISA) are still available, their performances are variable. Fully automated assays are significantly more sensitive and provide superior performance, such that manual AMH ELISA assays are nowadays redundant.

Stable automated assays are a critical step in the path to standardization. Agreement of an international human standard developed in accordance with the International Federation of Clinical Chemistry will inevitably now follow to allow external calibration of AMH assays and standardized reporting and clinical interpretation.

Inter-individual variation

As the rate of follicular recruitment declines with female age, so the circulating AMH levels also progressively decline (**Table 5.1**). AMH levels, reach undetectable levels approximately 5 years prior to the cessation of menses. However, for a given age, AMH levels in both normal and infertile populations can vary substantially (Kelsey et al. 2011). This is not surprizing, as primordial follicle counts and follicular activity vary substantially between individuals with vast differences observed in healthy women of the same age (Wallace & Kelsey 2010).

Table 5.1 Anti-Müllerian hormone (AMH) range. The serum AMH level varies among individual women, even when they are healthy and of the same age. This reflects natural variation in follicular activity between individuals

AMH serum level (ng/mL)	Clinical interpretation in women <35 years
> 4.0	High (possible PCOS)
1.5–4.0	Normal
1.0–1.5	Low normal
0.5–1.0	Low
< 0.5	Very low

Ethnicity

Ethnicity affects age-specific AMH levels. For example, African, Chinese, Hispanic and South Asian women have a lower AMH at a given age, compared with Caucasian women. Whether this ethnic disparity reflects accelerated ovarian aging, inherent differences in follicular recruitment and/or differences in AMH secretion per follicle is unclear. It is hoped that analysis of histological ovarian specimens from different ethnic groups, combined with assessment of follicular AMH secretion, may clarify the reason for the differences.

The significance of altered AMH secretion could lead to ethnicity-specific levels whereby different interpretations are needed. However, at present there is little evidence for this, with the AMH to ovarian response relationship similar across multiple different ethnicities.

Obesity

Obesity is not thought to be associated with AMH levels. Initial cross-sectional data in 1,896 non-polycystic ovary syndrome (PCOS) infertile women demonstrated a weak negative correlation between AMH levels and body mass index (BMI). However, the authors did not adjust for age, which would be expected to confound this association (Cui et al. 2014).

This negative association was not replicated in a population-based study of 2,320 pre-menopausal women with high BMI, central adiposity and age-specific AMH percentiles (Dolleman et al. 2013). An analysis of 1,308 adolescent 15-year-old (where fat mass was assessed via X-ray absorptiometry) showed no association of AMH with fat mass or BMI (Fraser et al. 2013). Furthermore, a longitudinal analysis of women undergoing weight loss programs did not demonstrate an alteration in AMH levels.

Increasing body weight does, however, reduce circulating exogenous follicle-stimulating hormone (FSH) levels after gonadotropin injection. Thus, bodyweight needs to be taken into account for when prescribing gonadotropins, but this is independent of any effect on circulating AMH (see **Chapter 8**).

Comorbidities and smoking

Comorbidities are becoming increasingly associated with altered AMH levels. The most established comorbidity is PCOS, which is associated with substantially greater levels of AMH, to the extent that AMH cut-off levels, with optimal sensitivity and specificity, have been suggested for the diagnosis of the syndrome (Iliodromiti et al. 2013).

Other medical disorders have more limited data. Adolescent girls with type 1 diabetes have higher AMH levels than controls (Codner et al. 2011), but in adult life AMH levels are lower, suggesting altered follicular dynamics. Certainly women with type 1 diabetes go through the menopause earlier than healthy controls (Soto et al. 2009). In contrast, in a study of 72 women with recent-onset rheumatoid arthritis, no alteration of AMH levels was observed (Brouwer et al. 2013).

More recently, it has been suggested that AMH production and/or follicular dynamics are altered acutely in response to being unwell. Young girls diagnosed with hematological or other childhood cancers showed lower AMH levels compared with their healthy peers at the time of initial diagnosis (van Dorp et al. 2014). In a cohort of 208 girls with newly diagnosed cancer, AMH was also negatively associated with markers of general health including body temperature and anemia. Similarly, lower AMH levels have been reported in adults with breast cancer, lymphoma and acute onset Crohn's disease than in healthy (though infertile) controls.

Cross-sectional data also suggests that smoking is independently associated with lower age adjusted aggregated levels of AMH.

Therefore, these data indicate the importance of general health in ovarian function, and consequently in interpreting tests of ovarian follicular activity. However, they do not alter the AMH-ovarian response relationship and dosing can be performed accordingly.

In contrast to initial conclusions from cross-sectional studies, AMH levels are also affected by the endocrine environment, which influences follicular activation and development. For example, pregnancy, gonadotropin-releasing hormone (GnRH) analogs and combined hormonal contraceptives (irrespective of whether they are oral, transdermal or vaginal) all reduce AMH concentrations. This reflects suppression of endogenous gonadotropin secretion and altered antral follicular development.

Women would still be expected to respond to exogenous gonadotropins as predicted by their AMH value. Although there is limited data regarding this, it is consistent with the finding that fewer oocytes are obtained from women with a range of malignancies undergoing IVF prior to specific treatment.

Although all of the above factors may contribute to large age-specific variation in AMH, they do not seem to interfere substantially with the consistent robust associations with oocyte yield. Whilst AMH is expressed by granulosa cells from the initiation of follicle growth, expression is almost absent in the final preovulatory stages of development (**Figure 5.1**).

In normal women, it has been estimated that 60% of serum AMH is derived from follicles 5–8 mm in diameter (Jeppesen et al. 2013), with an abrupt decline coincident with selection for dominance. The above factors should, however, be considered as potential confounders when research studies and trials are designed, particularly with respect to studies of future reproductive health outcomes.

Intra-individual variation

In an influential paper, La Marca and colleagues found no evidence for significant fluctuation of AMH across the menstrual cycle, in contrast to the well-established marked variation in both inhibin B and FSH (La Marca et al. 2006). Similar results were found by others although secondary analysis revealed that younger women (who were more likely to have higher AMH) had significantly larger intra-individual variation in AMH levels than older women, with 17 out of 22 women under 38 years showing a variation in AMH concentration >0.5 ng/mL within one cycle (Overbeek et al. 2012).

Evidence of statistically significant differences in mean values across the cycle can be misleading in studies aiming to assess the variation of AMH at the individual level. Analysis of the true

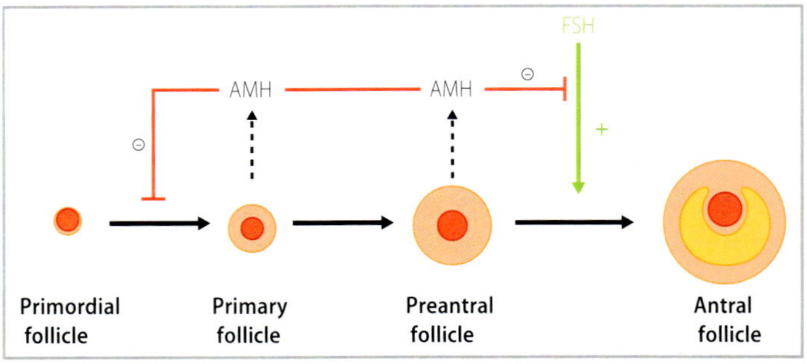

Figure 5.1 Model of anti-Müllerian hormone (AMH) actions in the ovary. AMH is expressed in primary, pre-antral and small antral follicles. Initial recruitment of primordial follicles takes place as a continuous process, whereas cyclic recruitment is driven by a rise in FSH serum levels at the end of a previous menstrual cycle. AMH inhibits (–) the initial recruitment of primary follicles from the resting primordial follicle pool and the stimulatory effect of FSH on the growth of preantral and small antral follicles (+).

intraindividual cycle variation suggests that the intraclass correlation coefficient (ICC) was 0.96. This indicates that the between-subject variation was responsible for the larger proportion of the observed cyclical differences and only 4% of the observed value was true within-subject variation related with the phase of the cycle (Deb et al. 2013).

INTRACLASS CORRELATION COEFFICIENT

The Intraclass Correlation Coefficient (ICC) is a measure of the reliability of measurements or ratings.

The ICC is used to measure a wide variety of numerical data from clusters or groups, including:

- How closely relatives resemble each other with regard to a certain characteristic or traits
- Reproducibility of numerical measurements made by different people measuring the same thing

Studies have confirmed cyclic variation with higher AMH in the late follicular phase, and this is more evident in younger women who have naturally higher mean AMH levels. This cyclical variation in AMH has minimal impact on clinical performance and was not large enough to warrant a shift in clinical practice toward timing AMH measurement.

Circadian variation

To date, only one study has addressed the circadian variation in AMH in a cohort of 19 women (Bungum et al. 2011). AMH was found to be lowest in the early morning hours (between 4 a.m. and 6 a.m.) with a maximum mean difference from its zenith values of 1.9 pmol/L (10.6%). AMH was relatively stable during the daytime, when blood sampling is routinely performed for most women. Thus, this result, though of interest, is not considered to be clinically relevant.

In contrast, the same study demonstrated that FSH levels, where are still used as a marker of ovarian response in some clinics, and other ovarian-derived hormones (E2 and progesterone) exhibited substantial circadian fluctuation even during the daytime (Bungum et al. 2011). Collectively, the data suggest that although AMH can vary across the menstrual cycle, this variability may be of potential value in analyzing follicle growth patterns but is not large enough to warrant restricting AMH measurements to a specific day or phase.

The variability of AMH levels in different menstrual cycles has been evaluated in several studies. When measured over three consecutive cycles, AMH levels had an ICC of 0.89, which was significantly higher than the ICC of FSH, inhibin B or AFC (0.55, 0.76, 0.73 respectively) (Fanchin et al. 2005) indicating lower variability. Age-adjusted ICC for AMH across four consecutive cycles was found to be 0.89 (95% CI, 0.84–0.94), indicating that only 11% of the intercycle variability was attributable to intraindividual fluctuation (van Disseldorp et al. 2010). The ICC of AFC determined at the same time points was significantly lower (0.71, 95% CI 0.63–0.77).

In summary, these analyses suggest that repeat AMH measurements during subsequent cycles are not necessary for accurate patient assessment.

ANTRAL FOLLICLE COUNT AS AN ALTERNATIVE MEASURE OF THE OVARIAN RESERVE

The developmental pathway from primordial follicle to ovulation is associated with approximately a 500-fold increase in follicular diameter (see Figure 1.7). Primordial follicles have a diameter of approximately 30 μm, and cannot be seen using ultrasound. It is only when a fluid-filled antrum develops that detection is possible due to ultrasound reflectivity. Antral follicles need to reach 2–10 mm in diameter before they can be imaged and counted via transvaginal ultrasound (TVS). An AFC can then be undertaken to predict ovarian response. However, some clinics use a more limited range due to the increased variability in number of the larger follicles.

Factors that can influence antral follicle count

Technical issues

The theoretical advantage of an AFC over a biochemical marker is that transvaginal sonography is usually available in a fertility clinic. Hence, an AFC can be readily performed and provides immediate results. However, there are technical issues with using ultrasound that need to be considered. For example, interobserver and intraobserver variability in AFC determination have been robustly analyzed and illustrate a key limitation of this biomarker, as currently performed (Deb et al. 2009).

The commonly used two-dimensional (2D) technique in estimating the AFC has wide limits of agreement varying from +8 to -7 follicles when two consecutive measures are performed by the same operator, or +7 to -5 follicles with two different experienced operators (Deb et al. 2009). This is sufficient to alter clinical management at an individual level and can introduce significant measure bias when pooling data in clinical research.

The reproducibility of the test improves only modestly when three-dimensional (3D) technique and off-line analysis of the stored images is performed (Deb et al. 2009, Jayaprakasan et al. 2008). However, this involves additional analysis, increased workload and loss of the benefit of immediacy.

The limits of agreement between consecutive measurements of AFC become significantly narrower when automatic analysis and counting or post-processing are implemented. However, the drawbacks of longer offline analysis persist and this approach has not been widely adopted. The validity of automated analysis is also questionable, since it only counts approximately one-third of the antral follicles that are counted via manual or the post-processing techniques (Deb et al. 2009).

A consensus statement was expected to resolve the issues of the large variability in AFC measurement by describing in detail the optimal technique with the use of the appropriate ultrasound probe in carefully selected patients (Broekmans et al. 2010). However, this report excluded women with previous ovarian surgery, ovarian endometriosis, a single ovary or irregular cycles, with the latter making up a significant proportion of the patients seen in a fertility clinic. Furthermore, the technical settings of ultrasound, such as depth, gain and focus, were not discussed (Broekmans et al. 2010).

This contrasts with the use of ultrasound-based biomarkers such as nuchal translucency in prenatal diagnosis, which continuously undergo rigorous external quality assessment (EQA) to ensure homogeneity and high accuracy in measurement by certified clinicians. The lack of this standardization for AFC measurement may underlie its limited transportability across different operators, sites and settings. The degree of variation observed, even in the research setting, when the technique is as standardized as possible between centers, illustrates the difficulties that need to be overcome (Arce et al. 2013).

The steady improvement in ultrasound resolution over recent years has led to a re-evaluation of the AFC threshold for diagnosing polycystic ovarian (PCO) morphology, now suggested to increase from ≥12 to ≥25 follicles (Dewailly et al. 2014). The fact that the upper limit for a normal AFC has more than doubled within such a short timeframe is not dissimilar to the issues that faced the AMH assay and its lack of standardization.

The previous AFC threshold of 12 follicles (with currently available high-resolution ultrasound) would classify an expected 'normal' responder as 'high' responder. This could lead to inappropriate selection of AFC stratified ovarian stimulation protocols, and suboptimal stimulation for that patient. Likewise, the cut-off values suggested in studies for predicting poor response have evolved substantially from an AFC of <3 follicles in 1998 to <12 follicles in 2009 (Chang et al. 1998, Melo et al. 2009).

Thus, the current suggested AFC thresholds of expected poor or normal ovarian response (Ferraretti et al. 2011) may not be transferable to future ultrasound machines which will inevitably have higher resolution. This issue is also illustrated by AFC determination by MRI, which gives significantly higher values compared to ultrasound assessment (Leonhardt et al. 2014).

Inevitably, AFC thresholds for clinical practice will always be subject to lagging behind the resolution of the available technology thereby adversely impacting on its potential role as a globally applicable biomarker.

Inter-individual variation

Factors affecting AFC have been understudied relative to AMH, but are likely to be similar given that they both reflect similar stages of follicular activity. In contrast to the large population cohorts for analysis of AMH, assessment of the relationship of AFC with age has previously only been examined in small sample sizes. A recent analysis of infertile women (>10,000) and oocyte donors (5000) has demonstrated that infertile women tend to have a reduced AFC and increased prevalence of low ovarian reserve (**Figure 5.2**; Iliodromiti et al. 2016). An age-related decline in AFC with age was confirmed for all women, accepting that there was also a substantial variation present at each age.

A single cross-sectional study suggested ethnic differences, with the average age-specific AFC in Indian women lower than in Caucasian women. However, the study did not provide 95% confidence intervals for each ethnic specific regression line and was limited by its sample size (n = 229 Caucasians women, n = 236 Indian women) (Iglesias et al. 2014).

Smokers have been reported as having a lower AFC compared with nonsmokers of similar age (Freour et al. 2012). It is unclear whether the cause was a result of accelerated depletion of the primordial follicle pool or modified follicular recruitment among smokers. The former has been suggested in animal models (Tuttle et al. 2009) and may also be relevant in human fetal ovaries (Anderson et al. 2014) and linked with the increased risk of early onset of the menopause among current smokers (Wellons et al. 2013).

It is also now clear that AFC behaves similarly to AMH in response to exogenous hormones. Gonadotropin suppression, caused by use of the contraceptive pill, has been shown to decrease the AFC, particular of follicles measuring >6 mm in diameter (Deb et al. 2012). In line with this, a cross-sectional study showed that women taking the contraceptive pill had a persistently lower AFC compared with women of the same age with natural cycles (Bentzen et al. 2013).

Intra-individual variation

Antral follicle counts exhibit significant variation within and across consecutive cycles (Deb et al. 2013). Assessment of the ICC of AFC showed that it had a modest ICC of 0.71 between two cycles and of 0.69 within one cycle, substantially worse than for AMH; 0.89 and 0.87 respectively (van Disseldorp et al. 2010). The source of this intracycle variability appears to be the variation in the number of the larger follicles (6–10 mm in diameter) (Deb et al. 2013).

Given these concerns, the consensus statement suggested that AFC should be performed from day 2 to day 4 of an pretreatment cycle (Broekmans et al. 2010). However, this recommendation may present a significant limitation and inconvenience to both patient and clinic, and does not apply to women with irregular cycles.

In conclusion, despite being a common test offered by fertility clinics, an AFC has limited clinical use. This is because AFC is most accurate when applied to well-selected patients only, has limited flexibility in relation to the phase of the cycle and exhibits substantial operator- and instrument-dependent performance.

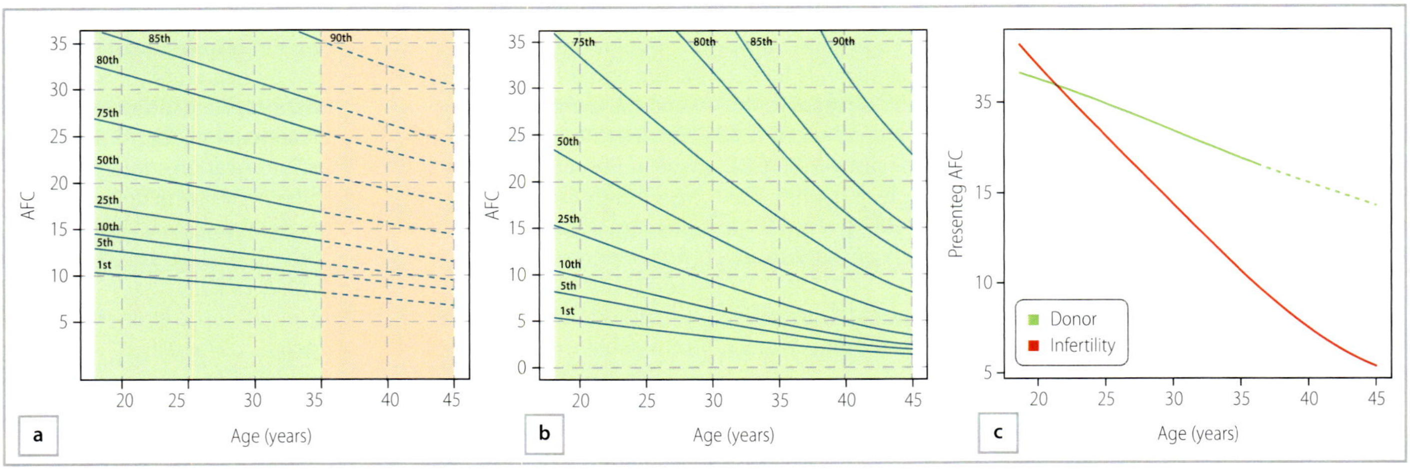

Figure 5.2 Comparison of age specific decline in antral follicle counts (AFCs) from oocyte donors and infertile patients. (a) Age specific ranges of AFC in potential oocyte donors. Black lines represent percentiles as labeled. The gray shaded areas in A for donors over the age of 35 years have resulted from extrapolation of the spline prediction model. (b) Age specific ranges of AFC in women seeking fertility treatment. (c) Spline prediction decline of AFC with aging in potential donors (blue line) and infertility patients (red line). (Data from Iliodromiti et al. 2016).

COMPARISON OF AMH AND AFC PERFORMANCE IN PREDICTING OVARIAN RESPONSE

The AMH and AFC have often been considered as interchangeable biomarkers for the prediction of ovarian response prior to starting any ovarian stimulation. Acceptance of this is highlighted by their recent inclusion as alternative independent markers, combined with age, in the European Society of Human Reproduction and Embryology (ESHRE) consensus statement on the definition of expected poor response (Ferraretti et al. 2011).

At the other end of the ovarian response spectrum, despite excessive ovarian response not having an equivalent consensus statement definition, stratified stimulation algorithms with indicative starting gonadotropin doses have been developed, based on specific cut-offs of either single biomarker, in order to avoid production of high follicle numbers and oocyte yields >15–20 oocytes (La Marca et al. 2013, La Marca et al. 2012, Nelson 2013).

Given that many fertility clinics may have limited access to both biomarkers or exhibit preference for one or the other, there has been limited consideration of their potential overlap and their relative strengths.

Observational cohort data assessing predictive performance of AMH and AFC

Over 40 cohort studies and an individual patient data (IPD) meta-analyses have examined the performance of AMH in the prediction of poor ovarian response (La Marca & Sunkara, 2014). Widely ranging threshold values for apparent optimal trade-off between sensitivity and specificity have been proposed. The range of threshold values for AMH (from 0.1 ng/mL to 2.97 ng/mL) primarily arises from the considerable heterogeneity introduced by the use of three different manual AMH assays, the inconsistencies in the definition of poor response and variable baseline characteristics, and fertility potentials of the participants across the studies.

Despite these limitations, the majority of the pooled studies reported that AMH has sensitivity >70% and specificity >70% in predicting poor response in women undergoing fertility treatment (La Marca and Sunkara 2014). Similarly, 22 cohort studies and one IPD meta-analyses have assessed the performance of AFC (La Marca & Sunkara 2014). The performance characteristics of AFC varied substantially among the studies, with threshold values ranging from 3 to 12 follicles.

Single center studies evaluating both biomarkers for the prediction of poor response have also not revealed significant differences in their performance. Different studies either claim superiority of AFC over AMH, or AMH over AFC. A systematic review assessing the performance of each biomarker echoed the above findings, summarizing that both biomarkers have equivalent receiver-operating curves (ROC) in the prediction of poor response (Broer et al. 2009). This finding was replicated in a recent IPD analysis which demonstrated that the area under the curve (AUC) of the age adjusted ROC curve for AMH in predicting poor response was 0.77 (95% CI: 0.70–0.83), practically identical to that of AFC (AUC 0.79, 95% CI: 0.73–0.85) (Broer et al. 2013).

For excessive response, the same issues have been observed. There have been over 16 cohort studies and one IPD meta-analyses for AMH with a diverse range of threshold values and associated performance characteristics reported. For AFC, there have been seven cohort studies and one IPD meta-analysis, but again no consensus on an overall threshold and anticipated performance. Cumulative analyses suggest comparable accuracy of AMH and AFC in predicting excessive ovarian response (La Marca & Sunkara 2014).

Collectively, the above data provide apparent confirmation that both markers are equally effective at predicting poor and excessive ovarian response.

Issues of study design are relevant, particularly if AMH is measured at a central diagnostic laboratory, while AFC is derived locally: this will inherently favor AMH. However, compared to ultrasound imaging, the relative ease of standardization of hormone assay, with established quality control systems such as the UK National External Quality Assessment Service (NEQAS), is an inherent potential advantage of AMH in determining clinically relevant cut-off values for widespread use.

Randomized controlled trials assessing predictive performance of AMH and AFC

Initial doubts about the equivalence of AFC and AMH in response prediction started appearing when the pharmaceutically-sponsored international multicenter Xpect trial failed to show an independent association between AFC and the number of retrieved oocytes (Andersen et al. 2011). In contrast, AMH was the only robust predictor of ovarian response in univariate and multivariate models. When poor or excessive response was assessed as dichotomous outcomes, AMH has remained a significant predictive variable, unlike AFC.

Notably, the specific purpose of this trial was to identify factors capable of predicting ovarian response in patients undergoing their first treatment cycle with a daily dose of 200IU recombinant FSH (rFSH) in a GnRH antagonist protocol, further strengthening the conclusion that AMH was the superior biomarker.

A subsequent pharmaceutically-sponsored international multicenter RCT of two gonadotropin preparations (MEGASET trial) added significant weight to the above findings. This study demonstrated a significant association between AMH and oocyte yield, number of blastocysts and cumulative live birth. However, surprisingly it did not detect a significant univariate association between AFC and any of these outcomes (Arce et al. 2013). Consequently, only AMH was associated with oocyte yield in multivariate models.

Although the findings of the trial were initially criticized as potentially being attributable to marked operator variability across centers, secondary analysis demonstrated that there were only weak associations between AFC and oocyte yield within individual centers (Arce et al. 2013).

Retrospective analysis of another multicenter RCT (MERIT trial) comparing two different gonadotropins in a long GnRH agonist protocol has also demonstrated that AMH had consistently greater association with ovarian response compared with AFC across different sites (Nelson et al. 2015). This site-specific analysis of the correlation of AFC and AMH with oocyte yield overcomes objections that the superior performance of AMH over AFC in these two multicenter trials may have been attributed to marked sonographer-dependent variability across the study sites and integrated data evaluation rather than by the actual performance at each study center (**Figure 5.3**) (Nelson et al. 2015).

Multivariate analysis confirmed that knowledge of AFC did not enhance the predictive power of AMH in these two trials (MEGASET and MERIT). Apparent conflicting findings resulted from the retrospective analysis of the 'Engage' trial, a double-blind RCT assessing the ongoing clinical pregnancy rate after a bolus dose of corifollitropin alfa versus daily rFSH injections, which supported the inclusion of

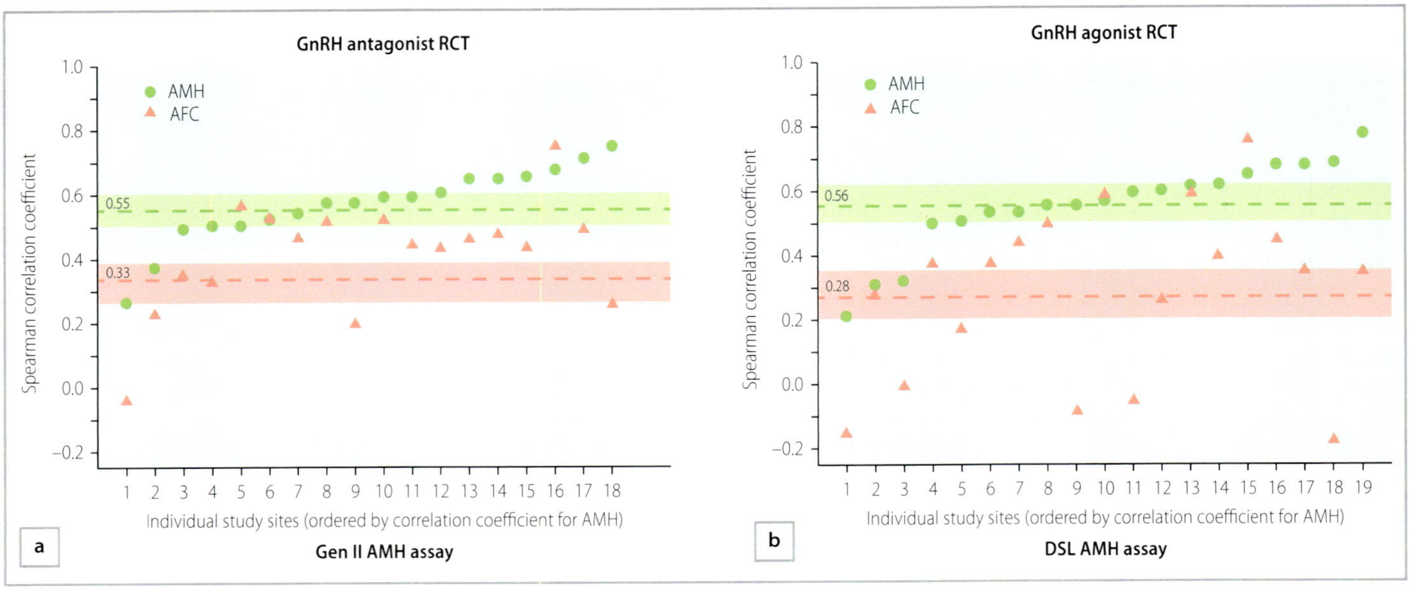

Figure 5.3 Correlations between basal values of anti-Müllerian hormone (AMH) and antral follicle count (AFC), respectively, and number of oocytes retrieved in patients treated (a) in a gonadotropin-releasing hormone (GnRH) antagonist trial and (b) a long GnRH agonist trial at individual IVF clinics. The dotted lines show the overall mean ±95% confidence intervals correlation coefficients of AMH and AFC for the whole cohorts. AMH was a stronger predictor of oocyte yield (i.e. a difference in correlation coefficient of >0.10) in 13 of 19 study clinics in the long GnRH agonist trial, and in 12 of 18 study clinics in the GnRH antagonist trial. Data from Nelson et al. 2015.

Table 5.2 Performance characteristics of prognostic models for ovarian response resulted from analyses of randomised controlled trial (RCT) data. AUC: area under the curve of receiving operator curve

Trials	Low ovarian response		High ovarian response	
	Predictor variables	**Performance characteristics**	**Predictor variables**	**Performance characteristics**
Xpect	AMH AMH & smoking	AUC: 0.84 AUC: 0.85	AMH AMH & AFC	AUC: 0.77 AUC: 0.80
MEGASET	AMH AFC	AUC: 0.78/0.90† AUC: 0.67/0.74†	AMH AFC	AUC: 0.77/0.81† AUC: 0.64/0.65†
Engage*	Age Age & AFC	AUC: 0.63 AUC: 0.75	Age Age & AFC	AUC: 0.64 AUC: 0.75
Pursue	Age Age & AMH Age & AMH & AFC	AUC: 0.61 AUC: 0.87 AUC: 0.88	Age Age & AMH Age & AMH & AFC	AUC: 0.61 AUC: 0.86 AUC: 0.88
Oocyte yield				
MERIT	AMH AFC AMH &AFC	R2: 0.29 R2: 0.07 R2: 0.30		
MEGASET	AMH AFC AMH &AFC	R2: 0.23 R2: 0.07 R2: 0.23		
* AMH was not measured. † Performance in each treatment arm				

AFC in prognostic models for high and low response (Broekmans et al. 2014); however, AMH was not measured.

Retrospective analysis of the 'pursue' trial, similar to 'engage' trial in design, has shown that models incorporating only age and AMH have optimal characteristics in predicting high and low responders, whereas inclusion of AFC only minimally improved model performance (Oehninger et al. 2015). **Table 5.2** summarizes the performance characteristics of the univariate or composite models, which include AMH or AFC as predictor variables from the above trials.

In a phase II trial of a novel rFSH (follitropin delta), a range of biomarkers were considered for prediction of ovarian response (NCT01426386). Of those examined (age, AMH, AFC, FSH, inhibin B), AMH predicted best the ovarian response with no or negligible explanation to the variation in oocytes retrieved by the addition of the other markers (Arce et al. 2016). Utilizing this information, a novel dosing algorithm that incorporated AMH and bodyweight to individualize follitropin dose was associated with a reduction in iatrogenic complications, while maintain pregnancy and live birth rates as compared to conventional ovarian stimulation (NCT01956110).

These consistent data from several large scale RCTs assessing biomarker performance in the prediction of ovarian response indicate the inherent limitations of AFC to predict ovarian response in a multicenter context. AMH, when centrally analyzed, is the more accurate biomarker under those conditions.

TAILORING TREATMENT BASED ON OVARIAN BIOMARKERS

Individually tailoring treatment based on ovarian biomarkers aims to offer the best treatment for a patient's age and unique characteristics, thus optimising oocyte yield (**Figure 5.4a**), maximizing success, eliminating iatrogenic risks, such as OHSS, and minimizing the risk of cycle cancellation (**Figure 5.4b**).

Although personalization of IVF treatment may lead to an improvement in patient compliance and better clinical practice, clinicians have largely struggled to achieve this. The difficulty derives from the vast number of drugs and choices available for ovarian stimulation, such as the GnRH analogs, the gonadotropin preparations and other adjuvant therapies, and from the lack of a clear evidence-based therapeutic approach for different subgroups of patients.

To date, a variety of protocols of approaches have been proposed based on pretreatment AMH levels and/or AFCs, but these have broadly classified patients based on absolute thresholds of the AMH or AFC or have been small single center studies with no external validation (La Marca et al. 2012, Nelson et al. 2009, Yates et al. 2011).

Despite these limitations, there is now widespread agreement that, for those identified with a high functional ovarian reserve, GnRH antagonist controlled strategies are preferable. This reflects their altered follicular recruitment patterns, lower risk of OHSS and ability to trigger final maturation with a GnRH agonist rather than hCG if required.

There is, however, still considerable debate on the optimal protocol for those patients with a low ovarian reserve or the value of GnRH agonist versus GnRH antagonist controlled cycles for those at low risk of developing an excessive ovarian response.

The rationale for the creation of a unique algorithm that encompassed AMH and bodyweight for individualization of the follitropin delta dose in the ESTHER-1 study (Arce et al. 2016) recognized that:

- The starting dose of gonadotropin is critical
- There is a strong association of baseline AMH with ovarian response
- Bodyweight modifies the exposure to exogenous gonadotropins

This landmark trial confirmed the benefit of obtaining an AMH level before treatment begins. This enables anticipation of the likely ovarian response and individualization of the FSH dose to modify oocyte yield while maintaining efficacy. This sets the new benchmark for ovarian stimulation, with additional phenotyping of patients potentially improving identification of those who will benefit from alterations in this simple algorithm.

CONCLUSION

Significant changes have occurred in the measurement techniques for both AMH and AFC over the last decade. Reference values for both biomarkers have changed substantially, and further change is anticipated.

Both reflect a very similar ovarian follicle population, which, if perfectly measured, would be expected to have similar value. This underpins the classical viewpoint that these biomarkers exhibit equivalent performance characteristics for the prediction of ovarian response.

However, it appears likely that this equivalence has been overstated and inflated by study design. Emerging data from large scale multicenter RCTs indicate a substantially better performance of AMH. International standardization of AMH, combined with a robust automated assay, is likely to enhance its status as the biomarker of ovarian response of choice. However, ultrasound will continue to have an important role due to advantages of immediate structural assessment.

Clinicians will inevitably continue to assess and debate the value of individual ovarian reserve biomarkers, but there is clear evidence that AMH can facilitate individualization of treatment and improve outcomes.

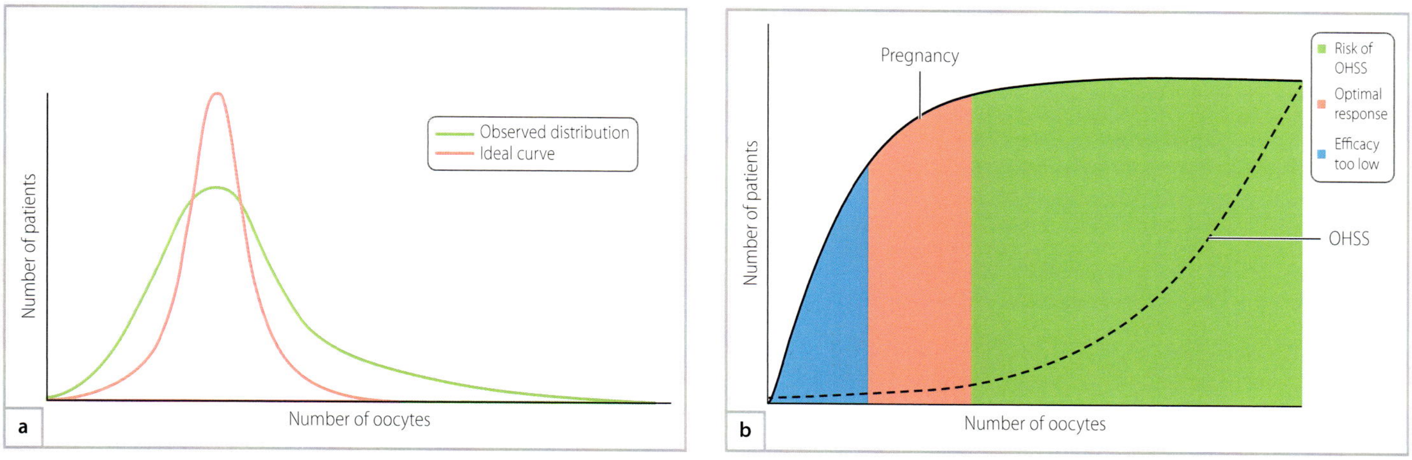

Figure 5.4 Optimization of ovarian response to reduce iatrogenic complications. (a) Treatment is tailored to optimize the number of viable oocytes a patient can produce, but the observed distribution never meets the ideal curve. (b) Care needs to be taken to maximize the chance of success, whilst minimizing iatrogenic risks, such as OHSS or cycle cancellation.

REFERENCES

Andersen AN, Witjes H, Gordon K, Mannaerts B. Predictive factors of ovarian response and clinical outcome after IVF/ICSI following a rFSH/GnRH antagonist protocol with or without oral contraceptive pre-treatment. Hum Reprod 2011; 26:3413–3423.

Anderson RA, McIlwain L, Coutts S, et al. Activation of the aryl hydrocarbon receptor by a component of cigarette smoke reduces germ cell proliferation in the human fetal ovary. Mol Hum Reprod 2014; 20:42–48.

Anderson RA, Nelson SM, Wallace WH. Measuring anti-Mullerian hormone for the assessment of ovarian reserve: when and for whom is it indicated? Maturitas 2012; 71:28–33.

Arce JC, Klein BM, Erichsen L. Using AMH for determining a stratified gonadotropin dosing regimen for IVF/ICSI and optimizing outcomes. In: Seifer DB and Tal R (eds) Anti-Müllerian Hormone: Biology, role in ovarian function and clinical significance. Nova Science Publishers Hauppauge, NY 2016:83–102.

Arce JC, la Marca A, Klein BM, Nyboe Andersen A, Fleming R. Reply of the authors. Fertil Steril 2013; 100:e10.

Arce JC, La Marca A, Mirner Klein B, Nyboe Andersen A, Fleming R. Antimullerian hormone in gonadotropin releasing-hormone antagonist cycles: prediction of ovarian response and cumulative treatment outcome in good-prognosis patients. Fertil Steril 2013; 99:1644–1653.

Bentzen JG, Forman JL, Johannsen TH, et al. Ovarian antral follicle subclasses and anti-müllerian hormone during normal reproductive aging. J Clin Endocrinol Metab 2013; 98:1602–1611.

Broekmans FJ, de Ziegler D, Howles CM, et al. The antral follicle count: practical recommendations for better standardization. Fertil Steril 2010; 94:1044–1051.

Broekmans FJ, Verweij PJ, Eijkemans MJ, Mannaerts BM, Witjes H. Prognostic models for high and low ovarian responses in controlled ovarian stimulation using a GnRH antagonist protocol. Hum Reprod 2014; 29:1688–1697.

Broer SL, Mol BWJ, Hendriks D, Broekmans FJM. The role of antimüllerian hormone in prediction of outcome after IVF: comparison with the antral follicle count. Fertil Steril 2009; 91:705–714.

Broer SL, van Disseldorp J, Broeze KA, et al. Added value of ovarian reserve testing on patient characteristics in the prediction of ovarian response and ongoing pregnancy: An individual patient data approach. Hum Reprod Update 2013; 19:26–36.

Brouwer J, Laven JS, Hazes JM, Schipper I, Dolhain RJ. Levels of serum anti-Müllerian hormone, a marker for ovarian reserve, in women with rheumatoid arthritis. Arthritis Care Res (Hoboken) 2013; 65:1534–1538.

Bungum L, Jacobsson AK, Rosen F, et al. Circadian variation in concentration of anti-Mullerian hormone in regularly menstruating females: relation to age, gonadotrophin and sex steroid levels. Hum Reprod 2011; 26:678–684.

Chang MY, Chiang CH, Hsieh TT, Soong YK, Hsu KH. Use of the antral follicle count to predict the outcome of assisted reproductive technologies. Fertil Steril 1998; 69:505–510.

Codner E, Iniguez G, Hernandez IM, et al. Elevated anti-Mullerian hormone (AMH) and inhibin B levels in prepubertal girls with type 1 diabetes mellitus. Clin Endocrinol (Oxf) 2011; 74:73–78.

Cui Y, Shi Y, Cui L, et al. Age-specific serum antimüllerian hormone levels in women with and without polycystic ovary syndrome. Fertil Steril 2014; 102:230–236.

Deb S, Campbell BK, Clewes JS, et al. Intracycle variation in number of antral follicles stratified by size and in endocrine markers of ovarian reserve in women with normal ovulatory menstrual cycles. Ultrasound Obstet Gynecol 2013; 41:216–222.

Deb S, Campbell BK, Pincott-Allen C, et al. Quantifying effect of combined oral contraceptive pill on functional ovarian reserve as measured by serum anti-Mullerian hormone and small antral follicle count using three-dimensional ultrasound. Ultrasound Obstet Gynecol 2012; 39:574–580.

Deb S, Jayaprakasan K, Campbell BK, et al. Intraobserver and interobserver reliability of automated antral follicle counts made using three-dimensional ultrasound and SonoAVC. Ultrasound Obstet Gynecol 2009; 33:477–483.

Dewailly D, Lujan ME, Carmina E, et al. Definition and significance of polycystic ovarian morphology: a task force report from the Androgen Excess and Polycystic Ovary Syndrome Society. Hum Reprod Update 2014; 20:334–352.

Dolleman M, Verschuren WM, Eijkemans MJ, et al. Reproductive and lifestyle determinants of anti-Mullerian hormone in a large population-based study. J Clin Endocrinol Metab 2013; 98:2106–2115.

Fanchin R, Taieb J, Lozano DH, et al. High reproducibility of serum anti-Mullerian hormone measurements suggests a multi-staged follicular secretion and strengthens its role in the assessment of ovarian follicular status. Hum Reprod 2005; 20:923–927.

Ferraretti AP, La Marca A, Fauser BC, et al. ESHRE consensus on the definition of 'poor response' to ovarian stimulation for in vitro fertilization: the Bologna criteria. Hum Reprod 2011; 26:1616–1624.

Fraser A, McNally W, Sattar N, et al. Prenatal exposures and anti-Mullerian hormone in female adolescents: the Avon Longitudinal Study of Parents and Children. Am J Epidemiol 2013; 178:1414–1423.

Freour T, Masson D, Dessolle L, et al. Ovarian reserve and in vitro fertilization cycles outcome according to women smoking status and stimulation regimen. Arch Gynecol Obstet 2012; 285:1177–1182.

Hansen KR, Hodnett GM, Knowlton N, Craig LB. Correlation of ovarian reserve tests with histologically determined primordial follicle number. Fertil Steril 2011; 95:170–175.

Iglesias C, Banker M, Mahajan N, et al. Ethnicity as a determinant of ovarian reserve: differences in ovarian aging between Spanish and Indian women. Fertil Steril 2014; 102:244–249.

Iliodromiti S, Kelsey TW, Anderson RA, Nelson SM. Can anti-Mullerian hormone predict the diagnosis of polycystic ovary syndrome? A systematic review and meta-analysis of extracted data. J Clin Endocrinol Metab 2013; 98:3332–3340.

Iliodromiti S, Sanchez CI, Messow CM, Cruz M, Garcia-Velasco JA. Excessive age- related decline in functional ovarian reserve in infertile women: prospective cohort of 15,500 women. J Clin Endocrinol Metab 2016; 101:3548–3554.

Jayaprakasan K, Campbell BK, Clewes JS, Johnson IR, Raine-Fenning NJ. Three-dimensional ultrasound improves the interobserver reliability of antral follicle counts and facilitates increased clinical work flow. Ultrasound Obstet Gynecol 2008; 31:439–444.

Jeppesen JV, Anderson RA, Kelsey TW, et al. Which follicles make the most anti-Mullerian hormone in humans? Evidence for an abrupt decline in AMH production at the time of follicle selection. Mol Hum Reprod 2013; 19:519–527.

Kelsey TW, Anderson RA, Wright P, Nelson SM, Wallace WH. Data-driven assessment of the human ovarian reserve. Mol Hum Reprod 2012; 18:79–87.

Kelsey TW, Wright P, Nelson SM, Anderson RA, Wallace WHB. A Validated model of serum anti-mullerian hormone from conception to menopause. PLoS One 2011; 6:e22024.

La Marca A, Grisendi V, Giulini S, et al. Individualization of the FSH starting dose in IVF/ICSI cycles using the antral follicle count. J Ovarian Res 2013; 6:11.

La Marca A, Papaleo E, Grisendi V, et al. Development of a nomogram based on markers of ovarian reserve for the individualisation of the follicle-stimulating hormone starting dose in in vitro fertilisation cycles. BJOG 2012; 119:1171–1179.

La Marca A, Stabile G, Artenisio AC, Volpe A. Serum anti-Mullerian hormone throughout the human menstrual cycle. Hum Reprod 2006; 21:3103–3107.

La Marca A, Sunkara SK. Individualization of controlled ovarian stimulation in IVF using ovarian reserve markers: from theory to practice. Hum Reprod Update 2014; 20:124–140.

Leonhardt H, Gull B, Stener-Victorin E, Hellstrom M. Ovarian volume and antral follicle count assessed by MRI and transvaginal ultrasonography: a methodological study. Acta radiologica (Stockholm, Sweden: 1987) 2014; 55:248–256.

Melo MA, Garrido N, Alvarez C, et al. Antral follicle count (AFC) can be used in the prediction of ovarian response but cannot predict the oocyte/embryo quality or the in vitro fertilization outcome in an egg donation program. Fertil Steril 2009; 91:148–156.

Nelson SM. Biomarkers of ovarian response: current and future applications. Fertil Steril 2013; 99: 963–969.

Nelson SM, Klein BM, Arce JC. Comparison of antimüllerian hormone levels and antral follicle count as predictor of ovarian response to controlled ovarian stimulation in good-prognosis patients at individual fertility clinics in two multicenter trials. Fertil Steril 2015; 103:923–930.

Nelson SM, Yates RW, Lyall H, et al. Anti-Mullerian hormone-based approach to controlled ovarian stimulation for assisted conception. Hum Reprod 2009; 24:867–875.

Oehninger S, Nelson SM, Verweij P, Stegmann BJ. Predictive factors for ovarian response in a corifollitropin alfa/GnRH antagonist protocol for controlled ovarian stimulation in IVF/ICSI cycles. Reprod Biol Endocrinol 2015; 13:117.

Overbeek A, Broekmans FJ, Hehenkamp WJ, et al. Intra-cycle fluctuations of anti-Mullerian hormone in normal women with a regular cycle: a re-analysis. Reprod Biomed Online 2012; 24:664–669.

Soto N, Iniguez G, Lopez P, et al. Anti-Mullerian hormone and inhibin B levels as markers of premature ovarian aging and transition to menopause in type 1 diabetes mellitus. Hum Reprod 2009; 24:2838–2844.

Tuttle AM, Stampfli M, Foster WG. Cigarette smoke causes follicle loss in mice ovaries at concentrations representative of human exposure. Hum Reprod 2009; 24:1452–1459.

van Disseldorp J, Lambalk CB, Kwee J, et al. Comparison of inter- and intra-cycle variability of anti-Mullerian hormone and antral follicle counts. Hum Reprod 2010; 25:221–227.

van Dorp W, van den Heuvel-Eibrink MM, de Vries AC, et al. Decreased serum anti-Mullerian hormone levels in girls with newly diagnosed cancer. Hum Reprod 2014; 29:337–342.

Wallace WH, Kelsey TW. Human ovarian reserve from conception to the menopause. PLoS One 2010; 5:e8772.

Wellons MF, Bates GW, Schreiner PJ, et al. Antral follicle count predicts natural menopause in a population-based sample: the Coronary Artery Risk Development in Young Adults Women's Study. Menopause 2013; 20:825–830.

Yates AP, Rustamov O, Roberts SA, et al. Anti-Müllerian hormone-tailored stimulation protocols improve outcomes whilst reducing adverse effects and costs of IVF. Human Reprod 2011; 26:2353–2362.

Chapter 6 Polycystic ovary syndrome

Roy Homburg

INTRODUCTION

Polycystic ovary syndrome (PCOS) is a prevalent condition of women in their reproductive years and 5–10% are afflicted by two or more symptoms. Importantly, PCOS is linked to 75% of all anovulatory disorders causing infertility. In 1935, the condition was described by Stein and Leventhal in seven obese anovulatory women (see Azziz & Adashi 2016). Since then, PCOS has become a syndrome which has attracted the attention of researchers in a wide range of medical specialties. Despite this, the exact etiology still escapes us, but we have progressed considerably regarding the treatment of the reproductive consequences of the syndrome. This chapter provides an overview of PCOS and the management of anovulatory infertility associated with the syndrome.

DEFINITION

The 2003 Rotterdam Consensus Meeting of the European Society of Human Reproduction and Embryology (ESHRE) and the American Society for Reproductive Medicine (ASRM) proposed the following definition of PCOS, which has been widely adopted ever since (Fauser et al. 2004). Any two of the three are sufficient to confirm the diagnosis:

1 Oligo- or anovulation
2. Hyperandrogenism (biochemical or clinical)
3. Polycystic ovaries on ultrasound examination

Syndromes with similar presenting features, e.g. congenital adrenal hyperplasia, androgen-secreting tumors or Cushing's syndrome, should be excluded.

The 'ultrasound definition' of a polycystic ovary is the presence of twelve or more follicles in either ovary measuring 2–9 mm in diameter and/or increased ovarian volume (>10 mL). This definition has become a bone of contention as improved resolution of new ultrasound scanners has enabled clearer imaging of smaller follicles. This may mean the number of twelve follicles may have to be upgraded in the future.

Although not essential for an initial diagnosis, a serum concentration of anti-Müllerian hormone (AMH) >40 pmol/L will usually confirm PCOS, and can aid in the planning of ovarian stimulation accordingly (see Table 5.1).

ETIOLOGY AND PATHOPHYSIOLOGY

Although PCOS is a hereditable syndrome in the majority of cases, the search for associated genes has not yet borne fruit. Present thinking leans more toward an epigenetic phenomenon involving a hyperexposure of the female fetus in-utero to testosterone. This influences the expression of genes, particularly those concerned with ovarian steroid production, insulin action and gonadotropin-releasing hormone (GnRH) pulsatility.

This developmental theory of the origin of PCOS has been mainly conceived by the seminal work of Abbott and colleagues (2005) who injected pregnant monkeys with testosterone at two stages during their pregnancy. When the offspring were followed up beyond puberty and compared with controls, many of the monkeys developed polycystic ovaries, insulin resistance and showed high concentrations of luteinizing hormone (LH) in their serum (for review, see Abbott et al. 2016).

Further credence for the ability of high levels of maternal testosterone during pregnancy to influence adult life are evidenced by the fact that girls so exposed during intrauterine life exhibit more male behavior (Hines et al. 2002, Homburg et al. 2017), an increased prevalence of autism spectrum disorders (Kosidou et al. 2015) and high AMH serum levels in adolescence (Hart et al. 2010).

Whatever the etiology, PCOS is a very heterogeneous syndrome as regards both clinical presentation and laboratory manifestations. The basic dysfunction seems to lie within the ovary and an over-production of androgens. However, the clinical expression and severity of the symptoms are dependent on extraovarian factors such as obesity, insulin resistance and LH concentrations.

The pathophysiology of the syndrome can be seen as a self-perpetuating 'androgen circle' (Homburg 2009). Almost every enzymatic action within the polycystic ovary which encourages androgen production is accelerated. The androgen excess is probably responsible for the fact that 6–8 times more preantral and small antral follicles are present in the polycystic ovary compared with the normal ovary. Although the follicles arrest in development at a diameter size of 2–9 mm and have a slow rate of atresia, they remain sensitive to exogenous injections of gonadotropins containing follicle-stimulating hormone (FSH). The large number of small follicles and the fact that each follicle produces more AMH than its same-sized counterpart in the normal ovary, are responsible for the raised serum AMH concentrations seen in women who suffer with PCOS. As the number of small follicles increases, so does the AMH level and the severity of the symptoms (Garg & Tal 2016).

Hyperinsulinemia, due to insulin resistance, occurs in 80% of women with PCOS and central obesity, but also in 30–40% of lean women with PCOS. This is thought to be due to a postreceptor defect affecting glucose transport and is unique to women with PCOS. Insulin resistance is significantly exacerbated by obesity and the compensatory hyperinsulinemia exacerbates androgen production.

High serum concentrations of LH are detected in 40–50% of women with PCOS, more commonly in lean rather than obese women. Although FSH serum concentrations are often within the lower portion of the normal range, an intrinsic inhibition of FSH action may be present.

MANAGEMENT

The management of PCOS depends on the presenting symptoms. The first-line treatment for overweight women must be to lose weight, regardless of whether the symptoms are hirsutism, acne, oligo-/amenorrhea or anovulatory infertility.

Weight loss

Diet and exercise ('lifestyle changes') can be effective in reducing the increased truncal-abdominal fat in women with PCOS, since this exacerbates insulin resistance and hyperandrogenism, and, consequently, the severity of the ovulatory irregularity (see Chapter 4). The loss of just 5% of body weight is capable of restoring menstrual regularity, ovulation and inducing a spontaneous pregnancy. An explanation of these facts should be given at the first consultation with the female patient, to induce motivation; a referral to a clinic dedicated to lifestyle changes is also recommended.

Antiestrogens

Clomifene citrate

Clomifene citrate (CC) is capable of inducing a release of FSH from the anterior pituitary gland, which is often enough to reset the cycle of events leading to ovulation. CC blocks hypothalamic estrogen receptors, signaling a lack of circulating estrogen to the hypothalamus and setting the negative feedback mechanism into motion (**Figure 6.1**).

CC is given orally in a dose of 50–150 mg/day for 5 days from day 2, 3, 4 or 5 of spontaneous or induced bleeding (i.e. the period), starting with the lowest dose and raising the dose by increments of 50 mg/day per cycle until an ovulatory cycle is achieved.

There is no apparent advantage of using a daily dose of >150 mg (Homburg 2003). A course of 4–6 ovulatory cycles is usually sufficient to know whether pregnancy will be achieved using CC, as approximately 75% of the pregnancies achieved with CC occur within the first three cycles of treatment (Homburg 2003).

Although CC has been shown to restore ovulation in approximately 80% of patients, it will result in pregnancy in only about 35–40%, and about 20% will not respond at all and are considered to be CC-resistant (Homburg 2009). CC is less likely to induce ovulation in patients who are obese, insulin-resistant, hyperandrogenic or if they have a high LH level at the beginning of their cycles.

The risk of multiple gestation with CC is 8–10% (Homburg 2003). The risk may be reduced considerably by ultrasound monitoring and withholding human chorionic gonadotropin (hCG), intrauterine insemination (IUI) or intercourse if more than two follicles >14 mm in diameter are detected (Homburg 2003).

The discrepancy between ovulation and pregnancy rates in patients treated with CC may be partly explained by the peripheral antiestrogenic effects of CC, particularly at the level of the endometrium (see Chapter 11). These antiestrogenic effects are apparently idiosyncratic as they are unrelated to the dose or duration of treatment. A poor endometrial thickness of <7 mm at ovulation (as assessed by ultrasonography) rarely yields a successful pregnancy (Molina et al. 2018). If this low endometrial thickness is observed in the first cycle of treatment with CC, a step-up to other forms of ovulation induction is recommended.

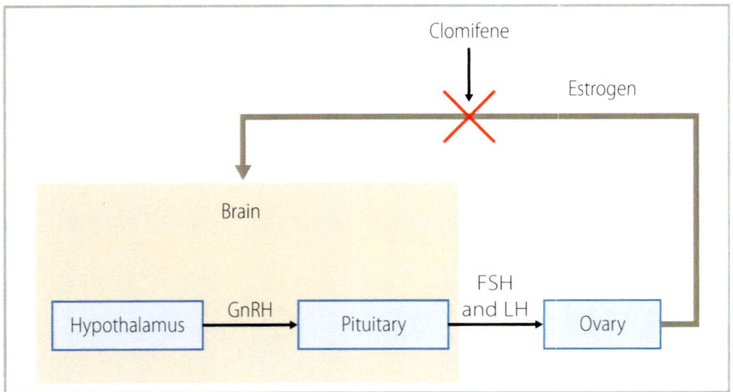

Figure 6.1 How clomiphene citrate (CC) works. CC blocks estrogen receptors in the brain which tricks the hypothalamus into thinking that there is a lack of circulating estrogen. As a result the hypothalamus secretes more GnRH. This causes the pituitary to secrete more FSH and LH. In turn, this causes the ovaries to produce more follicles.

Monitoring of at least the first CC cycle by ultrasound evaluation of follicular growth and endometrial thickness on day 12–14 of the cycle is justified by a cumulative conception rate of 48% compared with 35% for those who have unmonitored cycles ref needed. The routine addition of a mid-cycle exogenous injection of hCG may be useful for scheduling the timing of insemination (intercourse or IUI), particularly if given when an ultrasonically demonstrated leading follicle attains a diameter of 19–24 mm. The addition of dexamethazone as an adjunct to CC therapy is only really justified for those who have congenital adrenal hyperplasia as a cause for their anovulation (Homburg 2003).

If CC leads to an increase in serum LH levels, this may compromise pregnancy rates, since LH levels are often already high in women with PCOS. We have demonstrated that pretreatment with micronized progesterone is capable of modulating LH pulsatility, reducing LH concentrations and inducing a more favorable environment for ovulation induction with CC (Homburg et al. 1988). This treatment improved response to CC and yielded consequent pregnancies.

Aromatase inhibitors

Letrozole is an aromatase inhibitor, a nonsteroidal compound that suppresses estrogen biosynthesis by blocking the action of aromatase, which converts androstenedione to estrogens. Mainly employed for the treatment of postmenopausal women with advanced breast cancer, it can be given orally in a dose of 2.5 mg–5 mg/day and is almost free of side-effects. The efficient estrogen lowering properties of letrozole are utilized to temporarily release the hypothalamus from the negative feedback effect of estrogen allowing an increased release of FSH from the pituitary.

Although the final effect is common to both letrozole and CC, their mechanism of action is very different and this would seem to confer several advantages to letrozole for the induction of ovulation (Mitwally & Casper 2003). Unlike CC, letrozole has no direct effect on estrogen receptors and so has no deleterious effects on endometrium. The main reason for the gap between ovulation and pregnancy rates using CC can theoretically be avoided when letrozole is used. A further hypothetical advantage of aromatase inhibitors is that estrogen production is advanced by the FSH release, contrasting to the use of CC, whereby the hypothalamus is able to respond to estrogen with a negative feedback mechanism. This modulates an excessive secretion of FSH and the result is more likely to be a monofollicular ovulation. Together with a much shorter half-life (about 2 days) than CC, the prevalence of multiple pregnancies is therefore expected to be less than that witnessed with the use of CC for ovulation induction.

The theoretical advantages of letrozole have proved to be practical in a large randomized controlled trial (RCT) conducted by Legro and colleagues (2014) showing the superiority of letrozole over CC. This RCT comprised 750 women with anovulatory PCOS who were randomized to receive either CC or letrozole. A 44% increase in pregnancy rate was achieved by letrozole over CC (27.5% versus 19.5%). The twinning rate was not significantly higher in those women who received CC (7.4% versus 3.2%) with no significant difference in the rate of congenital abnormalities.

However, the use of letrozole for induction of ovulation is still 'off-label' due to questions of possible teratogenicity. This concern was raised by one, unpublished, congress presentation of an increased incidence of locomotor and cardiac anomalies in infants whose pregnancy was induced with letrozole, compared with a control group of spontaneously conceiving women with an absolutely normal pregnancy. Despite the scientific mistake in selection of the comparators, the incidence of all malformations was not different between the two groups (Biljan et al. 2005).

Subsequent studies have quashed these unsubstantiated doubts by reporting a lesser incidence of both minor and major congenital anomalies (Tulandi et al. 2006, Legro et al. 2014). The first study compared a large group of women ($n = 911$) who conceived using letrozole compared with those who used CC (Tulandi et al. 2006). Further reassuring information was provided in a very large series of women who received letrozole for ovulation induction with no preponderance of congenital abnormalities (Legro et al. 2014). In the light of this data, it remains a mystery why letrozole is still contraindicated for ovulation induction in almost every country in the world.

Insulin sensitizers

Insulin resistance is frequently associated with PCOS, occurring in 60% of women with PCOS and central obesity, but also in 30–40% of lean women with PCOS (Sam 2015). The insulin resistance in women with PCOS is due to a post-receptor defect affecting glucose transport; this is unique to women with PCOS and differs from the insulin resistance associated with diabetes type II. Hyperinsulinemia is invoked as a compensatory mechanism, counteracting the reduction in insulin sensitivity. This is of prime importance in the pathophysiology of PCOS as hyperinsulinemia is an important factor in the pathogenesis of hyperandrogenism. The more severe the insulin resistance, the more severe the ovulatory disturbance and the symptoms of hyperandrogenism.

Metformin is an oral biguanide (an organic compound with the formula $HN(C(NH)NH_2)_2$ that dissolves in water to give a highly basic solution, slowly hydrolysing to ammonia and urea), well established for the treatment of hyperglycemia. It reduces insulin resistance and secretion and, more importantly, has a direct action on ovarian theca cells to decrease androgen production. The sum total of its actions is a decrease in insulin levels and a lowering of circulating total and free androgen levels with a resulting improvement of the clinical sequelae of hyperandrogenism.

Taken orally in a dose of 1500–2500 mg, metformin causes gastrointestinal side-effects in about 15–20% of patients. Metformin has been shown to have a direct action on ovarian cells in vitro, decreasing androgen production and the difficulties of accurately measuring insulin sensitivity in all PCOS patients. This has encouraged 'blanket' treatment with metformin to all PCOS patients in many centers. The wisdom of this strategy has not been ratified!

The initial enthusiasm for the use of metformin, particularly for ovulation induction, has been curtailed by the publication of a number of RCTs. There are now a large number of studies published on the effect of metformin in a dose of 1500–2550 mg/day in women with PCOS (Morley et al. 2017). The majority of these studies demonstrated an improvement in insulin concentration, insulin sensitivity, and serum androgen concentration accompanied by decreased LH and increased SHBG concentrations and restoration of regular ovulation.

Fleming and colleagues (2002), in a randomized placebo-controlled trial, demonstrated a significantly increased frequency of ovulation with metformin (850 mg, twice a day) compared to placebo in a group of 92 oligomenorrheic women with PCOS.

However, in a large North American RCT, CC was found to be superior to metformin, as there was a significant difference in the number of clinical pregnancies and live full-term singleton births (22.6% versus 7.2%) when using CC (Legro et al. 2007). A meta-analysis examining the use of metformin for ovulation induction in women with PCOS concluded that it could not be recommended for this indication (Tang et al. 2009). An ESHRE-ASRM consensus meeting therefore concluded that insulin sensitizers should not be used as first-choice agents for induction of ovulation in women with PCOS, while their administration does not appear to decrease the incidence of early pregnancy losses.

Metformin may be useful for women with CC-resistance and this combination is worth trying before proceeding to the much more expensive low-dose gonadotropin therapy.

Gonadotropin therapy

Low-dose gonadotropin therapy is designed to induce ovulation and conception while minimizing the complications due to multifollicular development, ovarian hyperstimulation syndrome (OHSS) and multiple pregnancies. The prevalence of both multiple pregnancy and OHSS during ovulation induction is almost entirely dependent on the number of follicles that develop as a result of ovarian stimulation.

The best course of action to prevent complications of gonadotropin therapy for anovulation is to encourage the growth of one dominant follicle only. This can be largely achieved by using a chronic low dose protocol (in preference to the conventional protocol that was previously popular). Any dose of FSH overstepping the threshold of the polycystic ovary will produce multifollicular development and impending danger of multiple pregnancy and OHSS. The regimen of chronic low-dose gonadotropin therapy is dependent on the threshold theory, which demands the attainment and maintenance of follicular development with exogenous FSH without exceeding the threshold requirement of the ovary.

The principle of the classic chronic low dose regimen (**Figure 6.2**), is to employ a low starting dose for a minimum of 14 days with no dose change, and then use small incremental dose rises (usually 25–37.5 IU) when necessary, at intervals of not less than 7 days, until follicular development is initiated. The dose that initiates follicular development is continued until the criteria for giving hCG are attained. The purpose of this form of therapy is to achieve the development of a single dominant follicle rather than the development of many large follicles, and so avoid the risk of OHSS and multiple pregnancies.

Using a starting dose of 50–75 IU/day of FSH or human menopausal gonadotropins (hMG) without a change of dose for the first 7–14 days and only small incremental dose rises of 25–37.5 IU for a minimum of 7 days where necessary, pregnancy rates of >20% per cycle may be expected, while OHSS is almost completely eliminated and multiple pregnancy rates are <6% (Homburg & Howles 1999).

A compilation of reported results from the literature using a chronic low dose protocol identical to that described above is presented in **Table 6.1**. It should be noted that there is a remarkably consistent rate of uniovulatory cycles of around 70% in each series. The pregnancy rates are acceptable judging from past experiences with conventional therapy and taking into account that many of the patients comprising these series received only one cycle of therapy. Benefits of the chronic low dose protocol are the extraordinarily low prevalence of OHSS, which was almost completely eliminated, and the low multiple pregnancy rate of 5.7%. The majority of patients (90%) on a low dose protocol develop a single large follicle, and meet hCG administration criteria mid-cycle without any change in the initial dose.

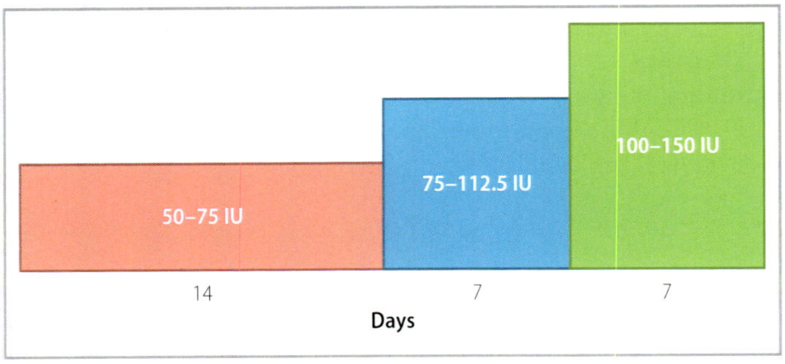

Figure 6.2 The 'classic' chronic low-dose protocol for gonadotropin induction of ovulation for women with anovulatory PCOS.

The step-up protocol illustrated here has produced better results than a step-down version. The low-dose, step-up, gonadotropin therapy is virtually the only correct way to utilize gonadotropins for anovulatory patients with PCOS. Small starting doses in the first cycle, preferably for a 14-day initial period without a dose change, and then a small incremental dose rise if required, produce the best results.

Laparoscopic ovarian drilling

The original treatment for PCOS, proposed by Stein and Levanthal in 1935, was bilateral wedge resection of the ovaries. This met with remarkable success regarding resumption of ovulation, but was abandoned because of the high probability of inducing pelvic adhesions.

The advent of a medical means to induce ovulation also arose. Thanks to modern technology, the same effect of decreasing the amount of active ovarian tissue is achieved. Laparoscopic ovarian drilling (LOD), by diathermy or laser, now presents a further treatment option for women with anovulatory infertility associated with PCOS (see Figure 2.5). LOD has proved effective in restoring ovulation and inducing pregnancy, particularly in women of normal weight and with high serum concentrations of LH. The main advantages of laparoscopic ovarian drilling (LOD) are:

- Very high prevalence of monofollicular ovulation and therefore a significant reduction in multiple pregnancy rates compared with gonadotropin therapy
- Often successful 'one-off' procedure which may avoid the use of expensive medical therapy
- The exclusion of ovarian hyperstimulation syndrome (OHSS)

Some units employ LOD when CC-resistance is apparent; most others following failure of gonadotropin therapy. The multiple pregnancy rate is also low after LOD (Farquhar et al. 2012).

The LOD has most popularly employed a bipolar coagulating current, but unipolar diathermy is less traumatic to the ovary. Laser puncture of the ovary produces similar results. Using electrocautery, 40W for 4 seconds for each puncture is a good rule of thumb. Between four and ten punctures to a depth of 2–4 mm on each ovary should be made. Less than four punctures per ovary can result in poorer pregnancy rates but more than ten may cause ovarian damage that will do more harm than good. Ten punctures of the ovary should only be used on very large ovaries. Over-heating of the ovaries can be prevented by flushing the ovary with normal saline or an antiadhesion preparation.

A Cochrane data base analysis of four RCTs comparing LOD with gonadotropin therapy, showed similar cumulative ongoing pregnancy rates 6–12 months after LOD, and after 3–6 cycles of gonadotropin therapy (Farquar et al. 2012). However, gonadotropin therapy was preferable (with a significant odds ratio of 1.48) when comparing ongoing cumulative pregnancy rates after 6 months following ovarian cautery versus 6 cycles of gonadotropin therapy.

If ovulation is not forthcoming within 2–3 months following LOD, then ovulation induction can often be more successfully employed than preceding the operation with CC (or FSH if CC fails to induce ovulation). However, in a large number of cases spontaneous ovulation has been induced even for several years following LOD in a similar fashion to ovarian wedge resection (the 'predecessor' of LOD).

A study of long-term follow-up after LOD showed that 54/110 women (49%) conceived spontaneously within a year and a further 42 women (38%) within 1–9 years following the operation (Amer et al. 2002). For those who respond to LOD but relapse into anovulation, a repeat procedure has been shown to be effective, although this has not been widely adopted.

The immediate and long-term effects of a surgical procedure are few but exist nevertheless. We have encountered some reticence to undergo this procedure from patients who, on the whole, seem to prefer a medical induction of ovulation rather than an operative procedure. Women with anovulatory PCOS who are of normal weight and have high LH concentrations seem to have the most favorable prognosis.

Table 6.1 A summary of study results based on the efficacy of low-dose gonadotropin therapy to induce ovulation

Condition	Result (1040 patients; 2472 cycles)
Pregnancies	411 (40%)
Fecundity/ovulation cycle	23%
Uniovulation	71%
Ovarian hyperstimulation syndrome (OHSS)	0.14%
Multiple pregnancies	5.1%

In vitro fertilization

The anovulation associated with PCOS is not an indication per se for patients to consider treatment via in vitro fertilization (IVF). When anovulation is the sole cause of infertility, the vast majority of women with PCOS will ovulate and conceive following ovulation induction therapy. Those who fail to do so very often have an additional factor, whether it be male, mechanical or endometriosis (which may have gone undetected). While results of IVF for women with PCOS are generally satisfactory compared with those with normal ovaries, ovarian stimulation protocols must be adapted to avoid the major pitfall of OHSS in these women.

Women with polycystic ovaries will almost inevitably yield more oocytes than those with normal ovaries. However, the fertilization rate of the oocytes from polycystic ovaries is lower. The resultant yield of embryos available for transfer is thus often similar and there is little difference in the outcome of IVF for women with normal or polycystic ovaries, whether calculated per started cycle, oocyte retrieval or embryo transfer.

Compared with ovulation induction for PCOS, the multiple pregnancy rate can be better controlled in IVF by regulating the number of embryos transferred.

A milder stimulation protocol should be employed for women with polycystic ovaries undergoing IVF. For the first cycle at least, it is recommended that the starting dose of gonadotropins should be lower than that usually employed for women with normal ovaries in order to avoid possible over-stimulation. We have found that, for the first cycle, a starting dose of 150 IU of gonadotropins is often adequate and even less may be used. To be forewarned of potential 'hyperstimulators', we have found AMH a very useful indicator (although an antral follicle count may also serve the purpose). Whether the gonadotropins used are urinary or recombinant FSH, hMG or a combination, does not seem to unduly influence the outcome and usually depends on local circumstances.

The main bone of contention has been the choice between GnRH agonist or antagonist for these women. For many years, the long GnRH agonist protocol was the standard choice. However, advantages of using the GnRH antagonist have more recently become apparent:

- It is a shorter cycle and therefore more 'patient friendly.'
- It requires less gonadotropin stimulation than with the agonist and this reduces the risks of overstimulation, cancellation of the cycle or OHSS.
- It offers the alternative of substituting the hCG triggering of ovulation and maturation of oocytes with one injection of a GnRH agonist. This almost prevents OHSS and avoids cycle cancellation.

It should be noted that the LH peak released by the agonist trigger has a relatively shorter duration of action than hCG. This means that in order to overcome the luteal phase deficiency a mandatory heavy supplementation of the luteal phase with added progesterone and estrogen and even small doses of hCG is needed. Alternatively, a policy of freezing all embryos with replacement in a future natural cycle should be employed to avoid lower pregnancy rates.

The use of metformin in IVF cycles for women with PCOS has shown some benefit when given as an adjunct treatment. Although not changing IVF parameters, an increase in pregnancy rate has been claimed in women of normal weight but the most important result was a decrease in OHSS rates. Adjunct-treatment with metformin appears to dampen the response to gonadotropin stimulation.

SUMMARY

The optimistic conclusion of this review is that, for women faced with infertility associated with PCOS, there is a good prognosis. The plethora of ovulation induction methods suited to anovulatory PCOS described here, and performed in sensible order, can produce excellent pregnancy results.

REFERENCES

Abbott DH, Barnett DK, Bruns CM, Dumesic DA. Androgen excess fetal programming of female reproduction: a developmental aetiology for polycystic ovary syndrome? Hum Reprod Update 2005; 11:357–374.

Abbott DH, Levine JE, Dumesic DA. Translational insight into polycystic ovary syndrome (pcos) from female monkeys with pcos-like traits. Curr Pharm Des 2016; 22:5625–5633.

Azziz R, Adashi EY. Stein and Leventhal: 80 years on. Am J Obstet Gynecol 2016; 214:247.e1–247.e11.

Amer SA, Gopalan V, Li TC, et al. Long term follow-up of patients with polycystic ovarian syndrome after laparoscopic ovarian drilling: clinical outcome. Hum Reprod 2002; 17:2035–2042.

Biljan MM, Hemmings R, Brassard N. The outcome of 150 babies following the treatment with letrozole or letrozole and gonadotropins. Fertil Steril 2005; 84:S95.

Farquhar C, Brown J, Marjoribanks J. Laparoscopic drilling by diathermy or laser for ovulation induction in anovulatory polycystic ovary syndrome. Cochrane Database Syst Rev 2012:CD001122.

Fauser B, Tarlatzis B, Chang J, Azziz R, et al. The Rotterdam ESHRE/ASRM-sponsored PCOS consensus workshop group. Revised 2003 consensus on diagnostic criteria and long-term health risks related to polycystic ovary syndrome (PCOS). Hum Reprod 2004; 19:41–47.

Fleming R, Hopkinson ZE, Wallace AM, Greer IA, Sattar N. Ovarian function and metabolic factors in women with oligomenorrhea treated with metformin in a randomized double blind placebo-controlled trial. J Clin Endocrinol Metab 2002; 87:569–574.

Garg D, Tal R. The role of AMH in the pathophysiology of polycystic ovarian syndrome. Reprod Biomed Online 2016; 33:15–28.

Hart R, Sloboda DM, Doherty DA, et al. Circulating maternal testosterone concentrations at 18 weeks of gestation predict circulating levels of anti-müllerian hormone in adolescence: a prospective cohort study. Fertil Steril 2010; 94:1544–1547.

Hines M, Golombok S, Rust J, Johnston KJ, Golding J. Testosterone during pregnancy and gender role behavior of preschool children: a longitudinal, population study. Child Dev 2002; 73:1678–1687.

Homburg R. Androgen circle of polycystic ovary syndrome. Hum Reprod 2009; 24:1548–1555.

Homburg R. The management of infertility associated with polycystic ovary syndrome. Reprod Biol Endocrinol 2003. 14; 1:109.

Homburg R, Howles CM. Low dose FSH therapy for anovulatory infertility associated with polycystic ovary syndrome: rationale, reflections and refinements. Hum Reprod Update 1999; 5:493.

Homburg R, Gudi A, Shah A, M Layton A. A novel method to demonstrate that pregnant women with polycystic ovary syndrome hyper-expose their fetus to androgens as a possible stepping stone for the developmental theory of PCOS. A pilot study. Reprod Biol Endocrinol 2017; 15:61.

Homburg R,Weissglas L,Goldman J. Improved treatment for anovulation in polycystic ovarian disease utilizing the effect of progesterone on the inappropriate gonadotrophin release and clomophine response. Human Reprod 1998; 3:285–288.

Kosidou K, Dalman C, Widman L, et al. Maternal polycystic ovary syndrome and the risk of autism spectrum disorders in the offspring: a population-based nationwide study in Sweden. Mol Psychiatry 2015; 10:183:1–8.

Legro RS, Barnhart HX, Schlaff WD, et al. Clomiphene, metformin, or both for infertility in the polycystic ovary syndrome. N Engl J Med 2007; 356:551–566.

Legro RS, Zhang H. Eunice Kennedy Shriver NICHD Reproductive Medicine Network. Letrozole or clomiphene for infertility in the polycystic ovary syndrome. N Engl J Med 2014; 371:119–129.

Mitwally MF, Casper RF. Aromatase inhibitors for the treatment of inferftility. Expert Opin Investig Drugs 2003; 12:353–371.

Molina A, Sánchez J, Sánchez W, Vielma V. Platelet-rich plasma as an adjuvant in the endometrial preparation of patients with refractory endometrium. JBRA Assist Reprod 2018; 22:42–48.

Morley LC, Tang T, Yasmin E, Norman RJ, Balen AH. Insulin-sensitising drugs (metformin, rosiglitazone, pioglitazone, D-chiro-inositol) for women with polycystic ovary syndrome, oligo amenorrhoea and subfertility. Cochrane Database Syst Rev 2017; 11:CD003053.

Tang T, Lord JM, Norman RJ, Yasmin E, Balen AH. Insulin-sensitising drugs (metformin, rosiglitazone, pioglitazone, D-chiro-inositol) for women with polycystic ovary syndrome, oligo amenorrhoea and subfertility. Cochrane Database of Syst Rev 2009; 3:CD003053.

Tulandi T, Martin J, Al-Fadhli R. et al. Congenital malformations among 911 newborns conceived after infertility treatment with letrozole or clomiphene citrate. Fertil Steril 2006; 85:1761–1765.

Chapter 7 Endometriosis

Simone Ferrero, Annalisa Racca, Umberto Leone Roberti Maggiore

INTRODUCTION

Endometriosis is a benign, estrogen-dependent, chronic gynecological disorder, defined as the presence of endometrial glands and stroma outside the uterus (**Figure 7.1**). It can be categorized in three different forms: superficial endometriosis, deep infiltrating endometriosis (lesions penetrating ≥5 mm under the peritoneal surface) and ovarian endometriosis.

Endometriotic lesions may have various locations. They are commonly observed on the pelvic peritoneum, on the ovaries, in the rectovaginal septum, on the uterosacral ligaments and in the vesico-uterine fold; whilst they are more rarely observed in the bowel, diaphragm, umbilicus, pericardium, pleura, and even in the brain (**Figure 7.2**). Endometriosis is usually associated with pain symptoms and infertility.

EPIDEMIOLOGY

Since endometriosis is a disease that is dependent on reproductive hormones, it is chiefly found in women of a reproductive age. However, it has also been described in adolescent and post-menopausal women, although this is a rarity. The diagnosis of endometriosis is based on surgical visualization and histological confirmation of the disease. These criteria have hampered epidemiological investigations aiming to estimate the true prevalence of endometriosis, since it is not ethical to expose a random sample of women to laparoscopy.

Limited data are available on the prevalence of the disease in women without a specific pathology. Italian researchers have shown that the prevalence of symptomatic endometriosis among pre-menopausal women is estimated to be 3–4% (Ferrero et al. 2010). However, a United Kingdom study based on the national general practice research database reported a lower prevalence of diagnosed endometriosis of 1.5% (Ballard et al. 2008).

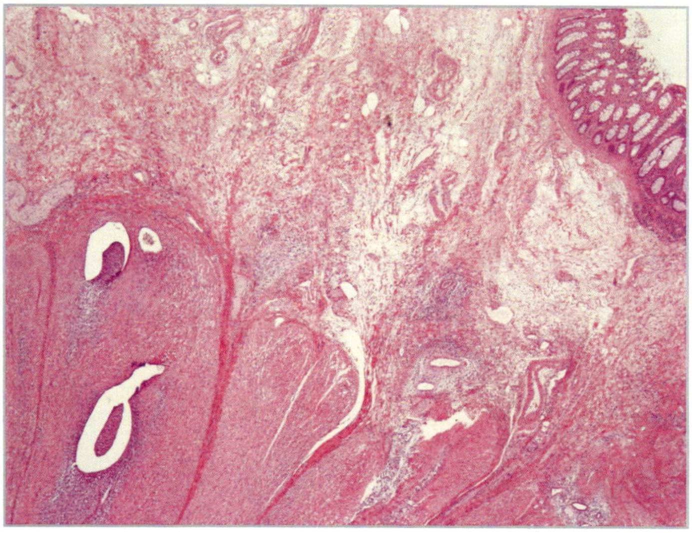

Figure 7.1 Histology of a deep endometriotic nodule. The hematoxylin and eosin stain shows multiple foci of endometriosis located in the muscularis mucosa of the rectum with a mild disarray of the muscular fibers and perilesional fibrosis.

In the United States, extensive data has been collected via a prospective cohort study of US nurses that began in 1989, called the Nurses' Health Study (Missmer et al. 2004). This study collect data over a 10 year-period, from which a total of 90,065 female nurses contributed 726,205 'person-years' to the analysis. The reported incidence of endometriosis, regardless of infertility status, was 298 per 100,000 person-years. Among women with a history of infertility, the incidence of diagnosis of laparoscopically confirmed endometriosis was recorded as 1380 per 100,000 person-years (Missmer et al. 2004).

In general, it is estimated that endometriosis is found in up to:

- 20% of asymptomatic women
- 30% of women with infertility
- 50% of those with pain symptoms

In part, these large variations can be explained by differences in the indications for laparoscopy and laparotomy, or merely by the differing degrees of attention paid by surgeons to the accurate identification of endometriotic lesions.

SYMPTOMS

Endometriosis is typically associated with pain symptoms and infertility, although women with endometriosis can be asymptomatic. Pain symptoms include:

- Dysmenorrhea
- Dyspareunia
- Non-cyclic lower abdominal pain
- Lower back pain
- Dyschezia

The severity of symptoms correlates poorly with the extent of the disease. However, some studies have shown a correlation between pain symptoms and the anatomic location of the endometriotic lesions.

Severe dysmenorrhea is associated with pouch of Douglas adhesions and nodules, whilst dyspareunia is correlated with endometriotic lesions of the uterosacral ligaments. Lower urinary tract symptoms are more frequent when endometriosis involves the bladder. Deep endometriotic lesions infiltrating the bowel wall can cause severe intestinal symptoms (such as subocclusive symptoms, which causes blockages, and heavy transit disturbances) or less severe disturbances mimicking the irritable bowel syndrome. Pleuritic chest pain, pleural effusion, pneumothorax, or cyclic hemoptysis may be due to pulmonary involvement. Endometriotic nodules in the retroperitoneal space may cause sciatica.

DIAGNOSIS

Physical findings may sometimes be suggestive for endometriosis. Thickened, nodular uterosacral ligaments or rectovaginal nodules may be palpable. Adnexal enlargement or tenderness may reflect ovarian involvement. Retroverted fixation of the uterus may be noted with obliteration of the posterior pouch of Douglas. Examination with a

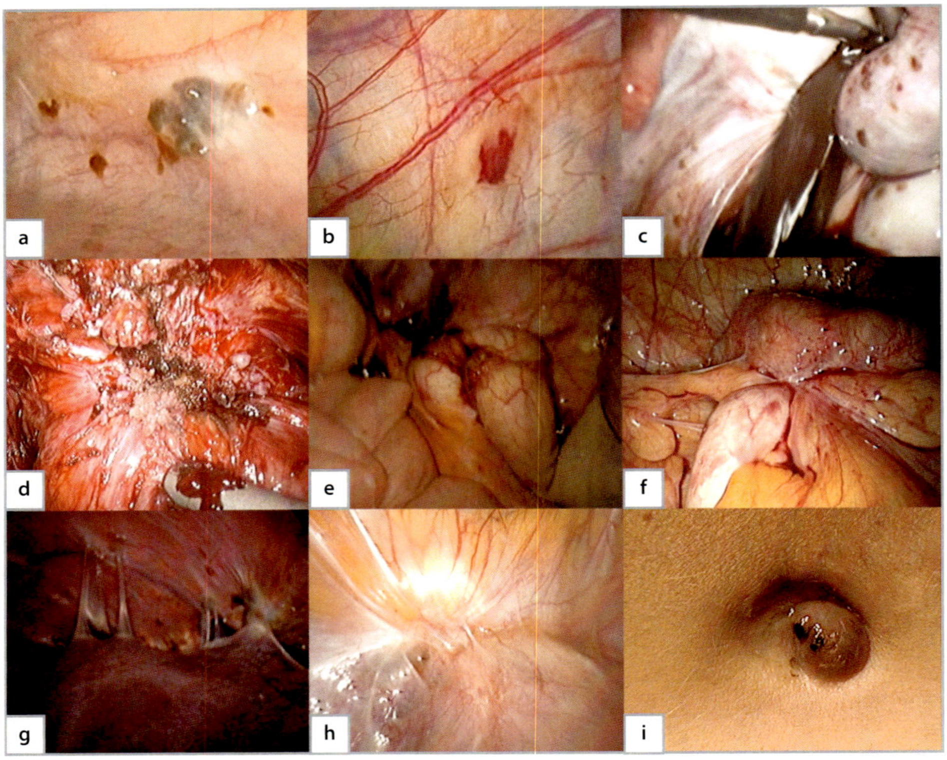

Figure 7.2 Endometriotic lesions. (a) Peritoneal brown-black endometriotic deposit. (b) Peritoneal flame-like endometriotic lesion. (c) Ovarian endometriotic cyst. (d) Deep rectal endometriotic nodule. (e) Appendiceal endometriotic nodule. (f) Deep ileal endometriotic nodule. (g) Hepatic superficial endometriotic lesions. (h) Deep bladder endometriotic nodule. (i) Umbilical endometriotic nodule.

speculum may reveal either a normal vaginal mucosa or a protruded endometriotic nodule in the posterior vaginal fornix.

Several blood markers (e.g. CA125, CA19-9, and serum protein PP14) have been used to screen for endometriosis. However, these tests lack the sensitivity and specificity required for clinical application.

Imaging techniques have been widely used to diagnose endometriosis. Transvaginal ultrasonography (TVS) is the first-line investigation for the assessment of the pelvic cavity and can assist in accurately diagnosing deep and ovarian endometriosis. At TVS, ovarian endometrioma appear as a mass with circular homogeneous, hypoechogenic 'tissue' without papillary proliferations; there is typically a clear demarcation from the ovarian parenchyma (**Figure 7.3**).

Transvaginal ultrasonography also allows identification of endometriotic nodules of the uterosacral ligaments, rectovaginal septum, rectosigmoid colon, bladder and vagina (**Figure 7.3**). However, the accuracy of TVS in the diagnosis of endometriosis is dependent on the experience of the ultrasonographer.

Magnetic resonance imaging may be used as an alternative imaging technique to obtain an overview of all potential locations of pelvic endometriosis. However, the gold standard for the diagnosis of endometriosis is the visualization of the lesions by laparoscopy and the histologic confirmation of the excised nodules (Dunselman et al. 2014).

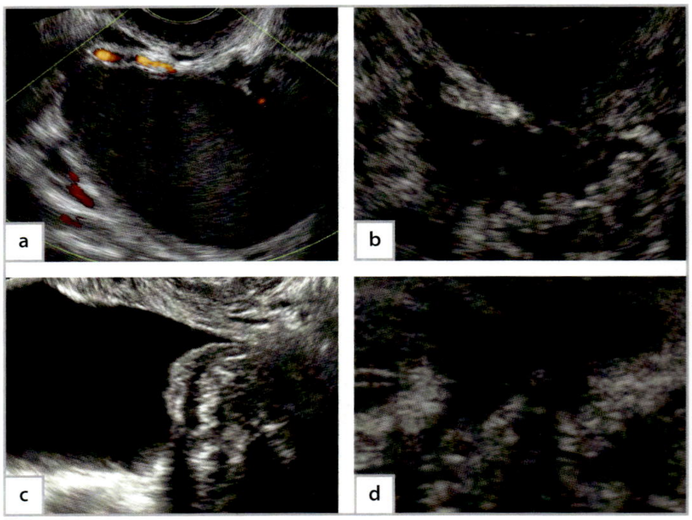

Figure 7.3 Ultrasonographic diagnosis of endometriosis. (a) Ovarian endometriotic cyst. The cyst has homogeneous, hypoechoic content without papillary proliferations; it can be clearly demarcated from the ovarian parenchyma. (b) Rectal endometriotic nodule. It appears as a nodular, solid, hypoechoic lesion penetrating the rectal muscularis propria and causing a thickening of the intestinal wall; some hyperechoic foci are present within the nodule. (c) Bladder endometriotic nodule. The hypoechoic nodule infiltrates the bladder detrusor and protrude into the bladder lumen. (d) Umbilical endometriotic nodule. It appears as a hypo-echoic mass with irregular margins and no blood vessels at Doppler examination.

SEVERITY CLASSIFICATION

The severity of endometriosis is usually classified using a system designed by the former American Fertility Society, now the American Society for Reproductive Medicine (ASRM, 1997) (**Figure 7.4**). Four anatomic areas (peritoneum, fallopian tubes, ovaries and pouch of Douglas) are examined for the presence of endometriosis and adhesions; a weighted point system is then used to determine the stage. Although obliteration of the pouch of Douglas automatically results in a severe score, this classification is deficient in its description for women with pain symptoms.

Lesions are scored according to the depth of infiltration of endometriosis under the peritoneal surface. Endometriotic lesions penetrating ≥5 mm are defined as deeply infiltrating endometriosis; with deeper implants having a higher score than superficial implants, according to the ASRM classification.

STAGE I (Minimal)

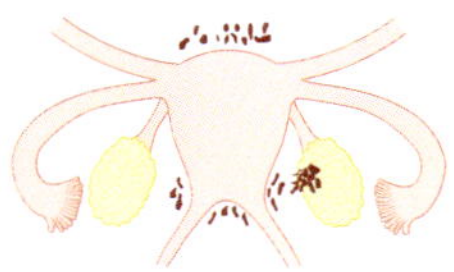

Peritoneum		
Superficial endo	1–3 cm	2
Right ovary		
Superficial endo	<1 cm	1
Filmy adhesions	1/3	1
Total points		4

STAGE II (Mild)

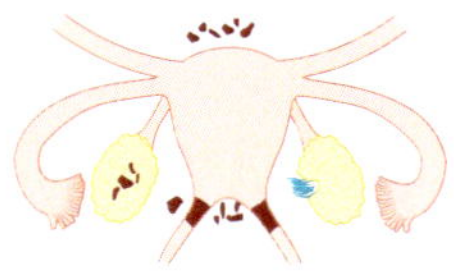

Peritoneum		
Deep endo	>3 cm	6
Right ovary		
Superficial endo	<1 cm	1
Filmy adhesions	<1/3	1
Left ovary		
Superficial endo	<1 cm	1
Total points		9

STAGE III (Moderate)

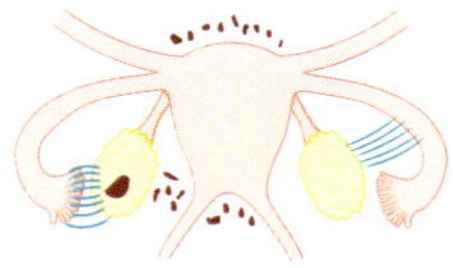

Peritoneum		
Deep endo	>3 cm	6
Cul de sac		
Partial obliteration		4
Left ovary		
Deep endo	1–3 cm	16
Total points		26

STAGE III (Moderate)

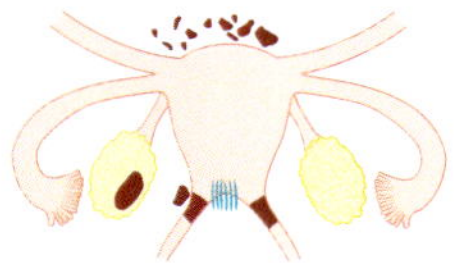

Peritoneum		
Superficial endo	>3 cm	4
Right tube		
Filmy adhesions	<1/3	1
Right ovary		
Filmy adhesions	<1/3	1
Left tube		
Dense adhesions	<1/3	16*
Left ovary		
Deep endo	1–3 cm	4
Dense adhesions	<1/3	4
Total points		30

STAGE IV (Severe)

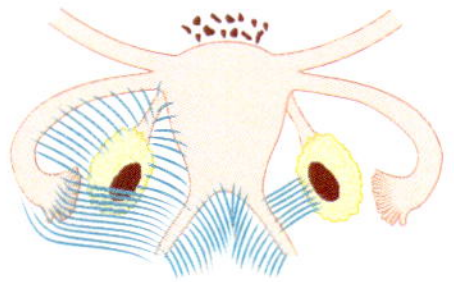

Peritoneum		
Deep endo	>3 cm	6
Culdesac		
Complete obliteration		40
Right ovary		
Deep endo	1–3 cm	16
Dense adhesions	<1/3	4
Left tube		
Dense adhesions	>2/3	16
Left ovary		
Deep endo	1–3 cm	16
Dense adhesions	>2/3	16
Total points		114

STAGE IV (Severe)

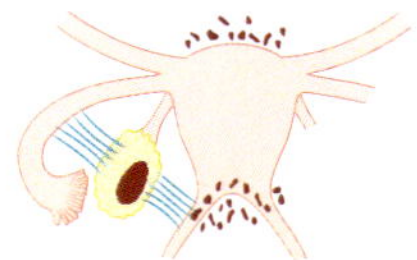

Peritoneum		
Superficial endo	>3 cm	4
Right ovary		
Deep endo	<1 cm	32**
Dense adhesions	<1/3	8**
Left tube		
Dense adhesions	<1/3	8*
Total points		52

* Point assignment change to 16   ** Point assignment doubled

Figure 7.4 The different classification of endometriosis, Stages I to IV (adapted from the original American Society for Reproductive Medicine 1996).

A limitation of the ASRM classification system is the inability to effectively predicting clinical outcomes of treatment, especially pregnancy rates in infertile patients. In this regard, in 2010, a clinical tool that aimed to predict pregnancy rates in patients with surgically documented endometriosis who attempt non-in vitro fertilization (non-IVF) conception was developed: the endometriosis fertility index (EFI) (Adamson & Pasta 2010).

The EFI scoring system includes evaluation of:

- Historical factors at the time of surgery (age, duration of infertility and pregnancy history)
- Adnexal function at conclusion of surgery (functional score of fallopian tubes, fimbriae and ovaries bilaterally)
- The extensiveness of endometriosis (rAFS endometriotic lesion score and total rAFS score)

The EFI is considered a simple, robust, and validated clinical tool that predicts pregnancy rates after endometriosis surgical staging and it has been currently externally validated in three European studies (Belgium, France and Italy).

ETIOLOGY

The precise etiology of endometriosis remains unknown, and over the last century, three theories have been proposed to explain the establishment of this condition. No single theory can account for the location of the ectopic endometrium in all patients with endometriosis, but rather, each may play some role. The three theories are as follows.

The retrograde menstruation theory

This is the most widely accepted theory on the pathogenesis of endometriosis. In the mid-1920s, John Sampson, a gynecologist working in New York, USA, is credited with coming up with the term 'endometriosis'. Sampson noticed the low frequency of endometriosis in amenorrheic or hysterectomized women and observed the retrograde reflux of menstrual fluid. Based on this, he proposed that the disorder originated from retrograde menstruation of viable endometrial tissue through the fallopian tubes into the peritoneal cavity where it implanted on the peritoneal surface or pelvic organs.

The coelomic metaplasia theory

This theory states that endometriosis results from spontaneous metaplastic change in mesothelial cells derived from the coelomic epithelium (located in the peritoneum and the pleura). During gonadal development, coelomic epithelium develops into peritoneum, pleura and the surface of the ovary. As such, the coelomic metaplasia theory may help to explain the distant sites of endometriosis within the body.

The vascular–lymphatic theory

It has also been suggested that endometriosis may result from lymphatic and hematogenous dissemination of endometrial cells which somehow find their way into ther vascular-lymphatic system. This theory also helps to explain how endometrioisis can occur at distant sites such as the lymph nodes and lungs.

RISK FACTORS

Epidemiological studies show that women with early menarche, and short and heavy menstrual cycles are at a higher risk, whereas parity seems to be inversely associated with the risk of endometriosis. A systematic review of the literature suggests that patients with endometriosis consume fewer vegetables and omega-3 polyunsaturated fatty acids and more red meat and saturated fats (Parazzini et al. 2013). Contradictory results have been reported on the association between alcohol consumption and endometriosis risk. Furthermore, there is no evidence for an association between the risk of endometriosis and caffeine consumption or tobacco smoking.

Leisure physical activity in early adolescence, teenage years and adulthood may, to some extent, decrease the risk of endometriosis. Overweight women have a lower risk of suffering endometriosis, while women with endometriosis tend to be thinner and have a lower body mass index (BMI) (Vigano et al. 2012). This may be explained by the higher rates of irregular menstrual cycles and anovulatory cycles in women with higher BMI.

It is unclear whether there is an association between oral contraceptive use and endometriosis. A systematic review and meta-analysis found that the risk of endometriosis seems to be reduced during oral contraceptive use. However, the authors concluded that the apparent protective effect of oral contraceptive against endometriosis may be the result of postponement of surgical evaluation due to temporary improvement of pain symptoms (Vercellini et al. 2011).

The causes of endometriosis are likely to involve multiple environmental and genetic factors. Environmental contaminants may be involved in the pathogenesis of the disease. Animal studies have shown that environmental toxicants (e.g. dioxin and dioxin-like compounds) are potent modulators of the immune and endocrine function critical to the development of endometriosis (Rier & Foster 2003). Furthermore, chemicals present in the environment and in food may contribute to the development of endometriosis. There is also a hypothesis that disruption of development during fetal and infant periods may increase the risk of endometriosis in adulthood (Upson et al. 2015).

Several studies on heritability have shown familial accumulation, high concordance in monozygotic twins, and an increased risk (3–15 fold) in first-degree relatives of patients with endometriosis compared with women in the general population. In 2015, an analysis of self-reported data from a nationwide population-based twin registry in Sweden (including a total of 28,370 women of whom 1,228 had a history of endometriosis) revealed a contribution of 47% by additive genetic factors and the remaining 53% attributed to unique environmental effects. This supports the hypothesis that genes have a concrete influence on phenotypic manifestations of endometriosis (Saha et al. 2015).

ENDOMETRIOSIS AND INFERTILITY

Although the association between endometriosis and infertility is well established, the mechanisms by which endometriosis causes infertility are complex and not well understood. Anatomic distortion of the pelvic viscera caused by endometriosis is probably involved in the pathogenesis of infertility. Adhesions of the ovaries and the fallopian tubes may affect tubal motility and impair the access of the ovulated oocyte to the fallopian tube. Similarly, large endometriomas may change the anatomical position of the ovary, thus influencing oocyte pickup.

However, in women with minimal or mild endometriosis, the reasons for infertility are unclear because the anatomical changes described above are not present. Therefore, other molecular factors may contribute to the pathogenesis of infertility in women with endometriosis. The peritoneal fluid (PF) of women with endometriosis is known to contain elevated concentrations of macrophages and these cells may contribute to infertility. PF macrophages may have a phagocytotic activity against sperm and this can increase the level of nitric oxide (NO) in PF. Higher PF NO levels may have a negative effect on sperm function and sperm-oocyte interaction, be toxic for the embryo, and impair the chance of implantation (Germeyer & Giudice 2004).

In addition, superficial endometriotic lesions may release inflammatory cytokines and growth factors into the PF that may also be detrimental to the oocyte, impairing the chance of fertilization in the distal part of the fallopian tube.

Despite the normal histology of the endometrium of women with endometriosis, several molecular differences have been noted in the eutopic endometriums from women with and without endometriosis (**Table 7.1**). These differences may adversely affect the attachment, intrusion and invasive phases of implantation.

It has also been shown that endometriosis may impair the ciliary activity of the fallopian tubes (Papathanasiou et al. 2008). Furthemore, endometriomas may affect folliculogenesis and oocyte quality. In fact, the content of endometriotic cysts is a source of toxic molecules (e.g. reactive oxygen species, iron, proteolytic enzymes and inflammatory cytokines) that are detrimental to the surrounding ovarian heathy tissue (Sanchez et al. 2014).

Finally, endometriosis-related deep dyspareunia may interfere with normal sexual function, thus decreasing the frequency of intercourse and the probability of conceiving.

Table 7.1 Molecular changes in the eutopic endometrium of women with endometriosis that may cause infertility

Molecular change in eutopic endometrium of women with endometriosis	Potential biological consequences
Decreased expression of HOX-A10 and HOX-A11 during the secretory phase	Lower implantation rate
Decreased expression of $\alpha_V\beta_3$ integrin	Lower implantation rate
High levels of Claudin-4 in the implantation window	Lower implantation rate
High FoxP3+ T regulatory cells expression in peri-implantation phase	Lower implantation rate
Aberrant expression of glutathione peroxidase and catalase, elevated levels of manganese and copper superoxide dismutase → increased free radicals in the endometrium	Toxic environment for the developing embryo
Progesterone receptor isoform A-dominant state	Alterations of implantation and the establishment and maintenance of pregnancy
Progesterone receptor isoform B variation in the mid-secretory phase	Lower implantation rate
Decreased expression of Mucin-1, Mucin-4 and Mucin-16 in the mid-secretory phase	Lower implantation rate

TREATMENT OF ENDOMETRIOSIS-ASSOCIATED PAIN

Pain is the cardinal symptom of endometriosis and represents the main indication for treatment. The management of endometriosis is challenging because of the need for a chronic therapy, the partial relief of pain symptoms that are often treated with easily-available therapies, and the recurrence of pain symptoms after the suspension of any hormonal treatment.

Hormonal treatment

Since endometriosis is dependent on sex steroids, hormonal medications aim to suppress ovarian function and the stimulatory effects of sex steroids. These therapies are not cytoreductive, but rather cytostatic. Therefore, when ovulation and menstruation are restored, symptoms typically recur while the quiescent ectopic and eutopic endometrium resumes metabolic activity.

First-line therapies for the treatment of endometriosis-associated pain are combined hormonal contraceptives and progestogens (**Table 7.2**). Hormonal therapies should be tailored to the patient to balance the efficacy of improving pain symptoms with the treatment-related adverse events. This approach facilitates the compliance of patients to treatment.

For this reason some effective compounds that have notable side effects [e.g. danazol and gonadotropin-releasing hormone (GnRH) agonists] should be considered only if first-line therapies do not work (Ferrero et al. 2015) (**Figure 7.5**).

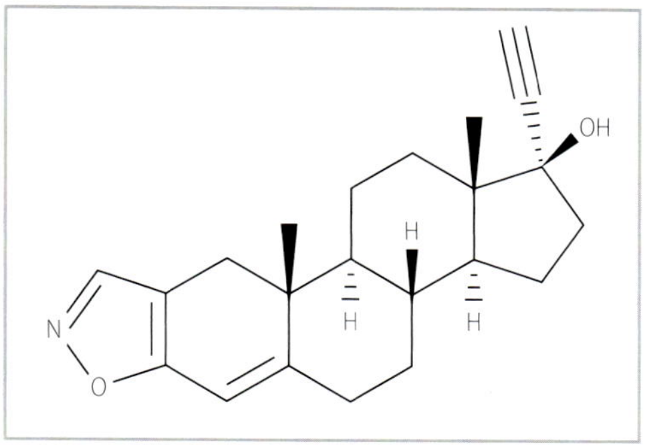

Figure 7.5 Danazol is a synthetic steroid that is used in the treatment of endometriosis and is the derivative of ethisterone with the chemical name 17α-ethynyl-17β-hydroxy-4-androsten-[2,3-d] isoxazole. It was the first drug approved by the US Food and Drug Administration to specifically treat endometriosis in 1971. Its use is limited due to its masculinizing side effects. An alternative to danazol is gonadotropin-releasing hormone (GnRH) agonists. Brand names for danazol include Danazol, Danatrol, Danocrine, Danol, Danoval and Cyclomen.

Surgical treatment

Surgical treatment for endometriosis should only be considered if:

- Hormonal therapies fail
- Patients refuse other therapies
- Patients have contraindications to hormonal therapies

Surgery has been shown to be highly effective in alleviating endometriosis-associated pain (**Table 7.2**), although it may not be cost-effective and risks intraoperative complications. On the basis of current evidence no difference has been shown between open and laparoscopic techniques; however, laparoscopy should be considered the gold standard because of the unquestionable advantages of its minimal invasiveness.

Different techniques (e.g. excision or ablation) have been proposed to treat endometriotic lesions. However, no one technique has been demonstrated to be superior over the other. Surgery may be associated with severe intraoperative complications such as visceral and neural lesions bringing to long-standing consequences. For this reason, patients with deep infiltrating endometriosis should only undergo surgery when strictly necessary and should be referred to tertiary centers to minimize the risk of incomplete treatment of endometriosis and repeated surgical procedures (Duffy et al. 2014, Ferrero et al. 2015).

TREATMENT OF ENDOMETRIOSIS-ASSOCIATED INFERTILITY

Different treatment options [including hormonal therapies, surgery and assisted reproductive techniques (ART)] have been proposed for improving fertility (and increasing the spontaneous pregnancy rate) in patients with endometriosis.

Table 7.2 Main advantages, disadvantages and grade of recommendation for the use of medical and surgical treatments for endometriosis-associated pain

Class of drugs	Cytostatic effect	Cost-effective	Contraceptive	Well-tolerated	Available in different formulations	Long-term use	Grade of recommendation
NSAIDs	-	+	-	+	+	+	D
Progestogens	+	+	+	+	+	+	A
Combined hormonal contraceptives	+	+	+	+	+	+	A
GnRH agonists	+	-	+	-	+	-	B
Danazol	+	+	+	-	-	+	A
Aromatase inhibitors	+	-	+	-	-	-	B
Surgery	N/A	-	-	-*	N/A	N/A	A/B

Abbreviations: GnRH, gonadotropin-releasing hormone; N/A, not applicable; NSAIDs, non-steroidal anti-inflammatory drugs
*Risk of intraoperative complication

Hormonal treatment

Hughes and collegues (2007) performed a systematic review to evaluate the efficacy of ovulation suppression agents (e.g. danazol, progestogens, GnRH analogs and oral contraceptives) in the treatment of endometriosis-associated subfertility to improve pregnancy outcome. Twenty-five randomized controlled trials (RCTs) comparing an ovulation suppression agent with placebo or no treatment, or a suppressive agent with danazol or a GnRH analog with oral contraception, were detected. This systematic review demonstrated that there is no evidence to support the use of hormonal therapies to suppress the ovarian function with the aim of improving fertility in minimal to mild endometriosis. It should be noted that no data was available on the use of these therapies in patients with severe endometriosis and only two of the studies reported on live births (Hughes et al. 2007).

Surgical treatment

Surgical treatment of minimal-mild endometriosis has been demonstrated to be more effective than diagnostic laparoscopy in improving ongoing pregnancy rates. Laparoscopic surgery is associated with higher live birth or ongoing pregnancy rate (odds ratio [OR] 1.94, 95% [CI] 1.20 to 3.16) and increased clinical pregnancy rate (OR 1.89, 95% CI 1.25 to 2.86) compared with diagnostic laparoscopy (Duffy et al. 2014). One prospective controlled cohort study suggested that CO_2 laser vaporization of endometriosis may have superior benefits in terms of postoperative cumulative pregnancy rate compared with monopolar electrocoagulation, diagnostic laparoscopy, and diagnostic laparoscopy followed by 3 months treatment with danazol (Chang et al. 1997).

No controlled study has compared the reproductive outcome of women with moderate-severe endometriosis after surgery or after expectant management. However, two prospective cohort studies reported crude spontaneous pregnancy rates of 57–69% in women with moderate endometriosis and of 52–68% in women with severe endometriosis after laparoscopic surgery (Nezhat et al. 1989, Vercellini et al. 2006). Furthermore, another prospective cohort study demonstrated a significantly lower crude pregnancy rate of 25% in women with moderate endometriosis and no pregnancies in women with severe endometriosis after expectant management (Olive et al. 1985).

Assisted reproductive techniques

A recent systematic review and meta-analysis assessed the impact of endometriosis on ART outcomes and whether the surgical treatment of endometriosis before ART may influence these outcomes (**Table 7.3**). Thirty-six studies were included for data synthesis for a total of 29,454 women of whom 16.5% (4,852) had endometriosis. Patients undergoing IVF/ICSI with endometriosis versus those without the disease had similar live birth rates per woman (OR 0.94, 95% confidence interval [CI] 0.84–1.06) and similar miscarriage rates per woman (OR 1.26, 95% CI 0.92–1.70). However, patients with endometriosis had a lower clinical pregnancy rate per woman (OR 0.78, 95% CI 0.65–0.94) and a lower mean number of oocytes retrieved per cycle (mean difference -1.98, 95% CI -2.87 to -1.09).

A subgroup analysis, in accordance to the ASRM stages, showed that in women with less severe endometriosis (ASRM stages I–II), all of the outcomes were comparable to women with no endometriosis; this included live birth rate (OR 0.96, 95% CI 0.82–1.12), clinical pregnancy rate (OR 0.84, 95% CI 0.69–1.03), and mean number of oocytes retrieved per cycle (mean difference -0.58, 95% CI -1.16 to 0.01).

Conversely, women with more severe endometriosis (ASRM III–IV) had a lower mean number of oocytes retrieved per cycle (mean difference -1.76, 95% CI -2.73 to 0.79), less cinical pregnancies (OR 0.60, 95% CI 0.44–0.81) and less live births (OR 0.77, 95% CI 0.64–0.92), when compared to women without endometriosis.

Only one study investigated the effect of surgery before ART, suggesting some evidence of benefit for treating less severe endometriosis (ASRM I–II). However, the availability of only one study is insufficient to draw definitive conclusions on the potential benefits of surgery for endometriosis in patients who may undergo ART (Hamdan et al. 2015).

The surgical treatment of ovarian endometrioma to improve fertility is a controversial topic. Patients with unilateral endometriomas have been shown to have similar ovulation rates in the healthy and in the affected ovary (Leone Roberti Maggiore et al. 2015). In addition, patients with unilateral endometriotic ovarian cysts and without a history of infertility demonstrated a high rate (43%) of spontaneous conception (Leone Roberti Maggiore et al. 2015). Indications for surgery may be represented by patients complaining of pain symptoms, preferably with an intact ovarian reserve, unilateral cysts, not trying to conceive or in the case of suspicion for malignancy. Before considering any surgery, it is important that physicians inform women with endometriomas about the risk of the possible loss of the ovary and also the possiblity of reduced ovarian function after surgery.

The decision to perform surgery should be considered carefully in patients who have had previous ovarian surgery.

ART should be considered for inpatients who are:

- Asymptomatically infertile
- Older (>35 years of age)
- With reduced ovarian reserve
- With bilateral endometriomas
- With history of prior ovarian surgery

Hamdan and colleagues (2015) performed a systematic review and meta-analysis (on thirty-three studies) aiming to evaluate the impact of endometriomas on IVF/ICSI outcomes. They assessed the impact of surgery for endometriomas and determined the effect of different

Table 7.3 Effects of different types of endometriosis on outcomes following assisted conception treatment

Variables	Mild-moderate endometriosis	Moderate severe endometriosis	Endometrioma	Previous surgical treatment for endometrioma
Higher cycle cancellation rate	N/A	N/A	+	N/A
Decreased number of oocytes retrieved	–	+	+	–
Lower clinical pregnancy rate	–	+	–	–
Lower live birth rate	–	+	–	–
Abbreviation: N/A, not applicable				

surgical techniques (**Table 7.3**). Compared to women without endometriomas, women with endometriomas had similar live birth rates (OR 0.98; 95% CI 0.71 to 1.36, 5 studies, 928 women), similar clinical pregnancy rates [OR 1.17; 95% CI 0.87 to 1.58), 5 studies, 928 women], lower mean numbers of oocytes retrieved (standardized mean difference -0.23; 95% CI -0.37 to -0.10, 5 studies, 941 cycles) and a higher cycle cancellation rate (OR 2.83; 95% CI 1.32 to 6.06, 3 studies, 491 women).

Patients who underwent previous surgical treatment for their endometrioma before IVF/ICSI in comparison with those without surgical treatment, had similar live birth rates (OR 0.90; 95% CI 0.63 to 1.28, 5 studies, 655 women), similar clinical pregnancy rate (OR 0.97; 95% CI 0.78 to 1.20, 11 studies, 1512 women) and similar number of oocytes retrieved (standardized mean difference -0.17; 95% CI -0.38 to 0.05, 9 studies, 810 cycles) (Hamdan et al. 2015).

Hamdan and colleagues (2015) concluded that surgical treatment of endometriomas did not alter the outcome of IVF/ICSI treatment compared with those who did not receive surgical intervention. Furthermore, they considered that a reduced ovarian reserve may be attributed to the presence of endometriomas per se, such that individualization of care for women with endometrioma is optimal prior to IVF/ICSI treatment, to ensure such ART is worthwhile.

SUPPORT GROUPS

Support groups can offer much needed information, support and friendship for anyone affected by endometriosis (see Chapter 13).

One example is the Endometriosis Association (www.endometriosisassn.org). This is an independent self-help organization for women with endometriosis. It is also a useful reference group for heathcare professionals. The Endometriosis Association was founded in the USA in 1980 by Mary Lou Ballweg and Carolyn Keith, and is now a worldwide, independent organization. The success of this support group has led to a network of chapters, groups, sponsors, and women with endometriosis in 66 countries. Furthermore, they provide literature of endometriosis in 28 different languages.

Joining a local support group is encouraged as it can give those whose lives are affected by endometriosis the chance to meet and talk with others who share and understand their situation.

REFERENCES

Adamson GD, Pasta DJ. Endometriosis fertility index: the new, validated endometriosis staging system. Fertil Steril 2010; 94:1609–1615.

American Society for Reproductive Medicine (ASRM). Revised American Society for Reproductive Medicine classification of endometriosis: 1996. Fertil Steril 1997; 67:817–821.

Ballard KD, Seaman HE, de Vries CS, Wright JT. Can symptomatology help in the diagnosis of endometriosis? Findings from a national case-control study – Part 1. BJOG 2008; 115:1382–1391.

Chang FH, Chou HH, Soong YK, et al. Efficacy of isotopic $13CO_2$ laser laparoscopic evaporation in the treatment of infertile patients with minimal and mild endometriosis: a life table cumulative pregnancy rates study. J Am Assoc Gynecol Laparosc 1997; 4:219–223.

Duffy JM, Arambage K, Correa FJ, et al. Laparoscopic surgery for endometriosis. Cochrane Database Syst Rev 2014; 4:CD011031.

Dunselman GA, Vermeulen N, Becker C, et al. ESHRE guideline: management of women with endometriosis. Hum Reprod 2014; 29:400–412.

Ferrero S, Alessandri F, Racca A, Leone Roberti Maggiore U. Treatment of pain associated with deep endometriosis: alternatives and evidence. Fertil Steril 2015; 104:771–792.

Ferrero S, Arena E, Morando A, Remorgida V. Prevalence of newly diagnosed endometriosis in women attending the general practitioner. Int J Gynaecol Obstet 2010; 110:203–207.

Germeyer A, Giudice LC. How does endometriosis cause infertility? In: Tulandi T and Redwine DB (eds) Endometriosis advances and controversies. Marcel Dekker, New York, 2004:151–165.

Hamdan M, Omar SZ, Dunselman G, Cheong Y. Influence of endometriosis on assisted reproductive technology outcomes: a systematic review and meta-analysis. Obstet Gynecol 2015; 125:79–88.

Hamdan M, Dunselman G, Li TC, Cheong Y. The impact of endometrioma on IVF/ICSI outcomes: a systematic review and meta-analysis. Hum Reprod Update 2015; 21:809–825.

Hughes E, Brown J, Collins JJ, et al. Ovulation suppression for endometriosis. Cochrane Database Syst Rev 2007:CD000155.

Leone Roberti Maggiore U, Scala C, Venturini PL, et al. Endometriotic ovarian cysts do not negatively affect the rate of spontaneous ovulation. Hum Reprod 2015; 30:299–307.

Missmer SA, Hankinson SE, Spiegelman D, et al. Incidence of laparoscopically confirmed endometriosis by demographic, anthropometric, and lifestyle factors. Am J Epidemiol 2004; 160:784–796.

Nezhat C, Crowgey S, Nezhat F. Videolaseroscopy for the treatment of endometriosis associated with infertility. Fertil Steril 1989; 51:237–240.

Olive DL, Stohs GF, Metzger DA, Franklin RR. Expectant management and hydrotubations in the treatment of endometriosis-associated infertility. Fertil Steril 1985; 44:35–41.

Papathanasiou A, Djahanbakhch O, Saridogan E, Lyons RA. The effect of interleukin-6 on ciliary beat frequency in the human fallopian tube. Fertil Steril 2008; 90:391–394.

Parazzini F, Vigano P, Candiani M, Fedele L. Diet and endometriosis risk: a literature review. Reprod Biomed Online 2013; 26:323–336.

Rier S, Foster WG. Environmental dioxins and endometriosis. Semin Reprod Med 2003; 21:145–154.

Saha R, Pettersson HJ, Svedberg P, et al. Heritability of endometriosis. Fertil Steril 2015; 104:947–952.

Sanchez AM, Vigano P, Somigliana E, et al. The distinguishing cellular and molecular features of the endometriotic ovarian cyst: from pathophysiology to the potential endometrioma-mediated damage to the ovary. Hum Reprod Update 2014; 20:217–230.

Upson K, Sathyanarayana S, Scholes D, Holt VL. Early-life factors and endometriosis risk. Fertil Steril 2015; 104:964–971.

Vercellini P, Eskenazi B, Consonni D, et al. Oral contraceptives and risk of endometriosis: a systematic review and meta-analysis. Hum Reprod Update 2011; 17:159–170.

Vercellini P, Fedele L, Aimi G, et al. Reproductive performance, pain recurrence and disease relapse after conservative surgical treatment for endometriosis: the predictive value of the current classification system. Hum Reprod 2006; 21:2679–2685.

Viganò P, Somigliana E, Panina P, et al. Principles of phenomics in endometriosis. Hum Reprod Update 2012; 18:248–259.

Chapter 8 Drug-induced ovulation

Kieren Wilson, William Ledger

INTRODUCTION

The first successful in-vitro fertilization (IVF) pregnancy, leading to the birth of Louise Brown in 1978, involved tracking the growth of a natural dominant follicle during an unstimulated menstrual cycle. This was followed by a laparoscopic oocyte collection, once the surge in luteinizing hormone (LH) was detected. However, success rates using this 'natural cycle' approach remained very low and it was only after introduction of the use of medications to stimulate follicular growth in the ovaries, and thereby make more than one mature follicle, that pregnancy rates began to rise.

Ovarian stimulatory medications fall into two categories, oral and injectable, and have two purposes. In classical ovulation induction, medication is used to treat a woman who is infertile due to anovulation. This is commonly due to polycystic ovary syndrome (PCOS), for which ovulation induction followed by timed sexual intercourse is often all that is needed to achieve a pregnancy. However, ovarian stimulatory medications are now used much more often to induce superovulation in women who ovulate normally, but who are being prepared for a fertility treatment such as IVF, or possibly intrauterine insemination (IUI) for unexplained or mild male factor infertility.

Pregnancy rates after IVF treatment are improved if several oocytes can be collected, inseminated, fertilized and cultured. Injectable gonadotropins containing follicle-stimulating hormone (FSH) are now used to induce growth of a cohort of ovarian follicles. Providing fertilization is successful, this allows for the production of a cohort of embryos, from which the most viable embryos can be selected for either transfer or cryopreservation.

OVULATION INDUCTION

The aim of classical ovulation induction is to induce the development of one or, at most, two mature follicles. This results in the release of one or two mature oocytes that are capable of being fertilized and producing a single, or occasional, twin pregnancy. The medications commonly used in ovulation induction are oral selective estrogen receptor modulators (e.g. letrozole), inhibitors of estrogen synthesis [e.g. clomifene citrate (CC) and tamoxifen] and injectable gonadotropins (e.g. FSH).

Many women with PCOS will ovulate and conceive after treatment with 25–150 mg daily of CC in the early part of their menstrual cycle. If a woman is naturally amenorrheic or severely oligomenorrheic, menses can be induced with oral progestogens, e.g. Provera (a tablet containing medroxyprogesterone acetate, which is a synthetic form of the naturally occurring female sex hormone, progesterone).

The mechanism of action of CC is to increase pituitary FSH secretion by reducing negative estrogen feedback. Thus, CC does not directly stimulate ovulation but rather amplifies the sequence of events that are physiological of a normal cycle.

Although CC will restore ovulation in approximately 75–90% of patients, it will result in pregnancy in only about 35–40% (Lambalk et al. 2005). 75% of conceptions occur during the first three CC cycles and if a pregnancy is not achieved within six CC cycles alternative therapy should be considered. Side effects include ovarian cyst formation and mood depression, vasomotor flushes, abdominal distension, bloating, breast discomfort, nausea and vomiting.

The use of CC can also lead to a twin pregnancy in about 9% of cases (Diamond et al. 2015). The risk of multiple pregnancy should be explained to patients ahead of treatment. Cycle tracking, using blood tests and ultrasound scanning during the follicular phase of the CC cycle, can identify those women with more than one mature follicle. Judicious cancellation can then reduce, but not entirely prevent, the likelihood of twin or higher order gestations.

More recently, letrozole, an aromatase inhibitor, has been used in preference to CC. Success rates appear comparable, and letrozole may be preferred as it is eliminated more quickly from the body and does not deplete estrogen receptors, thereby having no adverse effect on endometrium (Fouda & Sayed 2011).

Ovulation induction with injectable gonadotropins uses low doses of FSH, with frequent monitoring to avoid over-stimulation and the risk of multiple pregnancy. Success rates amongst patients with PCOS-associated anovulation are high, provided that there is bilateral tubal patency and reasonable sperm quality. Following gonadotropin stimulation, 'triggering' with a single injection of human chorionic gonadotropin (hCG) is necessary to ensure final oocyte maturation and ovulation. hCG is usually administered when a leading follicle of 17–20 mm in mean diameter is measured via transvaginal ultrasound (TVS).

SUPEROVULATION AND IVF

Superovulation strategies use injectable gonadotropins, given over 10–15 days from the start of menses, to induce multifollicular growth. Injectable FSH was originally derived from human pituitary gonadotropin, then from the urine of postmenopausal women, as human menopausal gonadotropin (hMG) (Eshkol & Lunenfeldm 1967). In the 1990s, FSH became commercially available as a recombinant glycoprotein, using a bio-reactor which holds a culture of cells transfected with the gene for human FSH [recombinant FSH (rFSH)] (Loumaye et al. 1995).

Superovulation leads to increasing levels of circulating estradiol, such that they reach supraphysiological concentrations. This would naturally induce an LH surge, leading to premature ovulation and loss of the oocytes before they could be collected. Hence, since the late 1980s, gonadotropin releasing hormone (GnRH) agonists, and later antagonists, have been used to prevent the LH surge and allow growth of a cohort of follicles up to the time of oocyte collection (**Figure 8.1**).

Long protocols

The GnRH agonists are usually used in the 'long' protocol stimulation regime, which involves starting the agonist in the mid-luteal phase of the preceding menstrual cycle. This allows the initial 'flare' of agonist-induced FSH and LH to subside, before FSH injections are started after the woman's menstrual period. The long protocol was used successfully for many years, but came with an increased risk of ovarian hyperstimulation syndrome (OHSS) (see below) and side effects of menopausal symptoms and ovarian cyst formation.

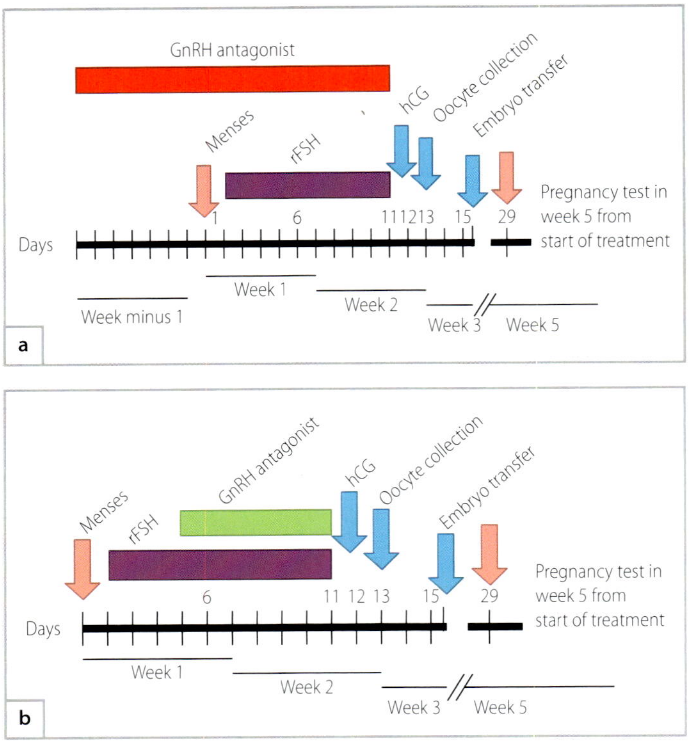

Figure 8.1 Superovulation protocols with timelines to show when superovulatory drugs need to be administered at the various stages. (a) GnRH agonist (long protocol). Patients begin administration of GnRH agonist 1 week before menses is due, and this continues for a duration of 11 days once menses begins. Administration of rFSH antagonist is simultaneously introduced on day 2 to day 11. Administration of hCG takes place between day 11 and day 12, with the oocyte collection taking place 36 hours post-hCG. Depending on fertilization and embryo development, embryo transfer may take place from day 16 (8-cell embryo) to day 18 (blastocyst). Confirmation of pregnancy takes place at the beginning of week 5 of the treatment. (b) GnRH antagonist protocol. Patients begin administration of recombinant follicle-stimulating hormone (rFSH) on day 2 following menses, for a duration of 11 days. Administration of GnRH antagonist is simultaneously introduced on day 5 to day 11. Administration of human chorionic gonadotropin (hCG) takes place between day 11 and day 12, with the oocyte collection taking place 36 hours post-hCG. Depending on fertilization and embryo development, embryo transfer may take place from day 16 (8-cell embryo) to day 18 (blastocyst). Confirmation of pregnancy takes place at the beginning of week 5 of the treatment.

Short protocols

The GnRH antagonists can be started several days after initiation of FSH treatment, since suppression of the LH release from the anterior pituitary gland is immediate. There are significant advantages to the antagonist protocol, recently described in a Cochrane meta-analysis (Al-Inany et al. 2016). This showed a statistically significant reduction in severe OHSS with antagonists versus agonist cycles and statistically significantly fewer interventions to prevent OHSS (e.g. coasting, cycle cancellation), thus making the antagonist cycle more attractive. From a patient perspective, the antagonist cycle is shorter with less time and expense, side effects and injections, improving compliance. The 2016 Cochrane review comparing GnRH agonists with antagonists found no significant differences in pregnancy and live birth rates between the two protocols (Al-Inany et al. 2016).

Cycle monitoring

The ovarian response to FSH is monitored using measurements of serum estradiol and TVS to assess follicle growth. Once preset criteria are met (conventionally three follicles of maximum mean diameter >17 mm), an hCG 'trigger' injection is given. This mimics the natural LH surge, since the alpha subunit of hCG and LH are identical and equally recognized by the ovary.

The trigger induces final oocyte maturation, allowing oocytes to progress from Meiosis I to Meioisis II, with arrest at the metaphase II stage, as observed by extrusion of the first polar body (see Figure 9.3). Transvaginal oocyte collection is then carried out approximately 36 hours after the hCG trigger is given. It is important to avoid an excessive delay in the oocyte collection time, as this might lead to ovulation with loss of the oocytes.

The yield of oocytes after superovulation is variable, depending on dose of medications and the woman's ovarian reserve at the time of stimulation. Recent analyses suggest that a target of 10–15 oocytes is optimum for chance of pregnancy, both from fresh embryo transfer and cumulatively after fresh and frozen transfers (Drakopoulos et al. 2016). However, others argue the cumulative pregnancy rate after milder stimulation seems to also be comparable to that of conventional protocols (Alper & Fauser 2017).

If more than 15 oocytes are collected, this carries an increased risk of OHSS without further increment in pregnancy rate, so the clinician is sensible to be cautious in prescription of gonadotropins, particularly in the first stimulation cycle or if the woman has a high serum AMH (see Chapter 5).

Following collection, each cumulus-oocyte-complex is available for the oocyte to be fertilized, either by IVF or intracytoplasmic sperm injection (ICSI). If fertilization is successful, then embryo transfer can take place 2–5 days later, with a pregnancy test 10–14 days later.

Success rates following IVF treatment depend largely on patient factors (e.g. female age, ovarian reserve, lifestyle factors), and on laboratory quality (e.g. a clean room environment giving higher chances of developing good quality embryos) (Morbeck 2015). Much depends on the experience of the center, with large and long established centers usually achieving the highest success rates, beyond the differences explained by patient mix (Lintsen et al. 2010).

The success rate from good quality centers in Australia and New Zealand, for a 36-year-old woman, is approximately 35%, given as the chance of having a healthy child after fresh transfer of a single blastocyst (**Figure 8.2**). The cumulative success rate (calculated as the success rate following both the fresh and subsequent frozen embryo transfers) increases to over 65% from one treatment cycle.

OVARIAN HYPERSTIMULATION SYNDROME

OHSS is an iatrogenic systemic disease resulting from an excessive ovarian response to gonadotropin stimulation. The disease is mediated by increased vascular permeability, arteriole vasodilation and ovarian enlargement. Vascular endothelial growth factor (VEGF), originally known as vascular permeability factor, is a signal protein produced by cells that stimulates vasculogenesis and angiogenesis. VEGF is believed to be the principal mediator of the increase in capillary permeability seen in OHSS.

The main clinical features are ascites and pleural and pericardial effusions accompanied by intravascular dehydration (**Figure 8.3**). The consequences of severe OHSS are thromboembolism (1–10%), renal dysfunction (oliguria 30%) and acute respiratory distress syndrome.

Thrombotic events usually occur in the first cycle of treatment (85%), at early stage of OHSS in 43% and late stage in 57% of cases (Mor & Schenker 2014). Venous thrombotic events have been recorded in unusual sites, including the jugular, and subclavian veins.

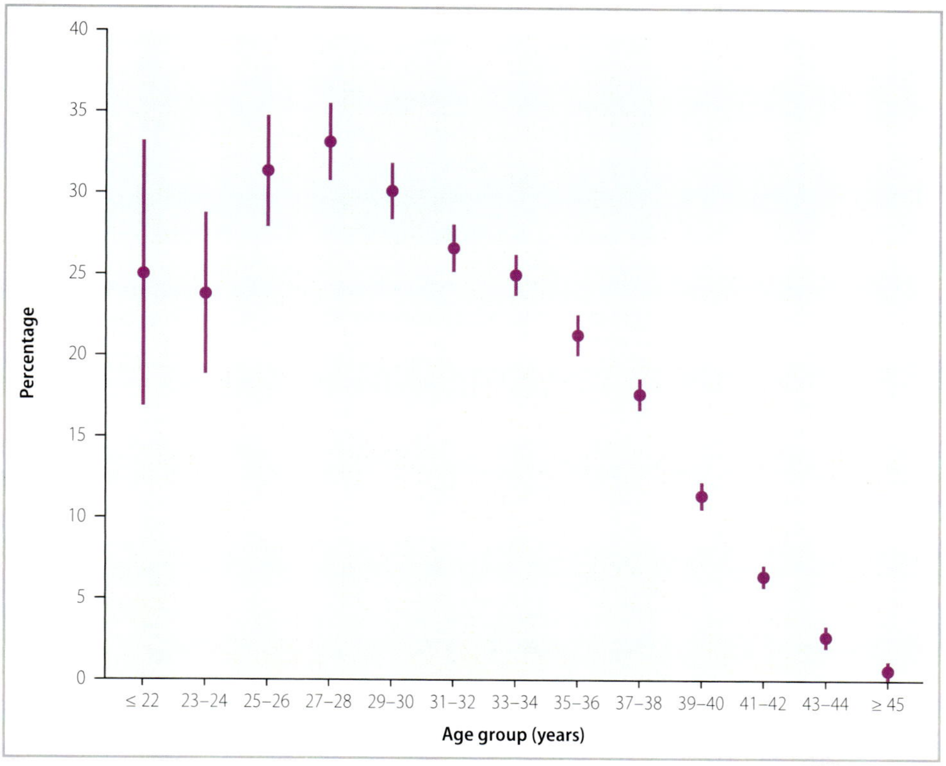

Figure 8.2 Live delivery rate (with 95% confidence interval) per initiated autologous fresh IVF cycle (excluding freeze-all) by women's age at start of a treatment cycle, Australia and New Zealand, 2014. With permission from Harris et al., University of New South Wales, 2016.

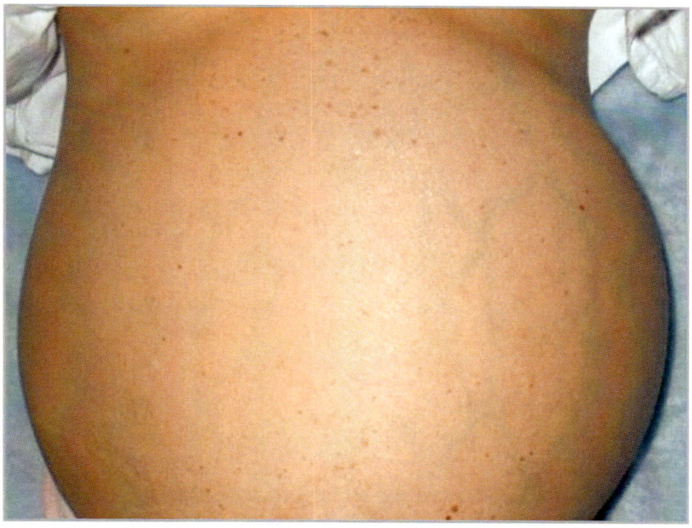

Figure 8.3 Abdominal ascites seen in patients with severe ovarian hyperstimulation syndrome (OHSS).

Prevention of OHSS begins with the identification of patients who are at high risk, and then using risk reducing medication protocols in individual cases. Use of an antagonist protocol with a GnRH agonist trigger, rather than an hCG trigger, almost entirely removes risk of severe OHSS. However, due to inadequacy of the luteal phase, most centers opt to freeze all embryos rather than perform a fresh embryo transfer. These frozen embryos can then be thawed and transferred in a later cycle. Alternative luteal phase strategies involve use of low dose hCG supplementation but this caries a risk of reigniting the OHSS process, albeit with lower frequency.

Women who are at high risk of developing OHSS include those with polycystic ovaries with increased antral follicle count and AMH, younger women and those who have previously experienced OHSS.

The management of the condition depends on the grade of the OHSS. Mild and moderate cases can be managed as outpatients with attention being paid to fluid balance, thromboprophylaxis and analgesia. Women with severe OHSS require intensive care monitoring and active maintenance of intravascular volume, anticoagulation and consideration of drainage of ascetic fluid to reduce intra-abdominal pressure and improve renal perfusion.

For women who are not pregnant, the syndrome will usually resolve after 7–10 days. However, the rising hCG associated with early pregnancy can cause 'late OHSS' with recurrence of the severe form of the disease with occasionally life-threatening consequence (Nouri et al. 2014).

LUTEAL SUPPORT AFTER SUPEROVULATION

Superovulated cycles, whether controlled with GnRH agonists or antagonists, require pharmacological support, as physiological secretion of progesterone from the corpus luteum is frequently impaired. The most commonly used luteal support is vaginal progesterone (either as a pessary or gel), started after oocyte retrieval and continued until the patient is pregnant. Some clinicians continue luteal support to 8–10 weeks of gestation, whereas others, with equivalent success rates, stop provision of luteal support as soon as hCG is detectable in serum, since this is indicative of adequate support for the corpora lutea.

Side effects of vaginal progesterone include vaginal irritation, discharge and dyspareunia (pain during sexual intercourse). Alternatives include injection of intramuscular progesterone (although this is a painful injection) and injection of hCG (to be used only where there is not a significant risk of OHSS).

REFERENCES

Al-Inany HG, Youssef MA, Ayeleke RO, et al. Gonadotrophin-releasing hormone antagonists for assisted reproductive technology. Cochrane Database Syst Rev 2016; 4:CD001750.

Alper MM, Fauser BC. Ovarian stimulation protocols for IVF: is more better than less? Reprod Biomed Online 2017; 34:345–353.

Diamond MP, Legro RS, Coutifaris C, et al. For the NICHD Reproductive Medicine Network (2015) Letrozole, Gonadotropin, or Clomiphene for Unexplained Infertility. N Engl J Med 2015; 373:1230–1240.

Drakopoulos P, Blockeel C, Stoop D, et al. Conventional ovarian stimulation and single embryo transfer for IVF/ICSI. How many oocytes do we need to maximize cumulative live birth rates after utilization of all fresh and frozen embryos? Hum Reprod 2016; 31:370–376.

Eshkol A, Lunenfeld B. Purification and separation of follicle stimulating hormone (FSH) and luteinizing hormone (LH) from human menopausal gonadotrophin (HMG) Part III. Acta Endocrinol 1967; 54:919.

Fouda UM, Sayed AM. Extended letrozole regimen versus clomiphene citrate for superovulation in patients with unexplained infertility undergoing intrauterine insemination: A randomized controlled trial. Reprod Biol Endocrinol 2011; 9:84.

Lambalk, CB, Huirne JAF, Macklon NS, Fauser BCJM, Homburg R. Ovulation induction with clomiphene or gonadotropins. International Congress Series 2005; 1279:16–23.

Lintsen AM, Braat DD, Habbema JD, Kremer JA, Eijkemans MJ. Can differences in IVF success rates between centres be explained by patient characteristics and sample size? Hum Reprod 2010; 25:110–117.

Loumaye E, Campbell R, Salat-Baroux J. Human follicle-stimulating hormone produced by recombinant DNA technology: a review for clinicians. Hum Reprod 1995; 1:188–199.

Mor YS, Schenker JG. Ovarian hyperstimulation syndrome and thrombotic events. Am J Reprod Immunol 2004; 72:541–548.

Morbeck DE. Air quality in the assisted reproduction laboratory: a mini-review. J Assist Reprod Genet 2015; 32:1019–1024.

Nouri K, Tempfer CB, Lenart C, et al. Predictive factors for recovery time in patients suffering from severe OHSS. Reprod Biol Endocrinol 2014; 12:59.

Chapter 9 The human oocyte: characteristics, collection and fertilization

Bryan Woodward

INTRODUCTION

The oocyte is the essential foundation for life. Whilst natural fertilization requires a sperm, it is the oocyte that provides the autonomous support for embryo development during the first few days of life. An oocyte can theoretically support life without a sperm, if induced by assisted reproduction technologies (ART) such as parthenogenetic activation, or via cloning and somatic cell nuclear transfer. As such, an oocyte exhibits pluripotency, since it can develop into all cell types of the adult organism (see Chapter 17 for a detailed discussion on potency).

A mature oocyte can be produced in either a natural menstrual cycle (as discussed in Chapter 1) or more commonly via a superovulation 'stimulated' cycle, whereby several oocytes are produced (as discussed in Chapter 8). If oocytes are surgically collected from the ovaries, they can either be used fresh for fertilization, via in-vitro fertilization (IVF) or intracytoplasmic sperm injection (ICSI), or be cryopreserved for future use (see Chapter 20). Oocytes can be utilized by the patients themselves, to create their own offspring, or they can be donated to help others to have a family (see Chapter 10). Whatever pathway to parenthood is taken, the quality of oocytes is fundamental.

Unlike sperm, the oocyte is produced in limited quantity but with more biological investment (see Chapter 1). As the larger of the two gametes, the oocyte not only provides the female chromosomal complement, but also provides endogenous nutrients to support fertilization and early developmental. All of the organelles and constituents of the developing embryo arise from the oocyte, with paternal chromatin being the only contribution from the sperm.

This chapter will begin by discussing the biological structure of the human oocyte, and then look at ways by which embryologists assess oocyte quality. The in vitro processing of the oocytes in the IVF laboratory, from the point of oocyte retrieval to the point of insemination, will then be covered.

BIOLOGICAL STRUCTURE OF THE OOCYTE

As a haploid female gamete, the oocyte has several unique features and organelles, including a zona pellucida (ZP), an oolemma, an ooplasm and cortical granules. Generic organelles such as the centrosome, mitochondria and endoplasmic reticulum are present, but these are specialized within the oocyte to support its exclusive role.

The oolemma

The oolemma is the phospholipid bilayer plasma membrane that surrounds the oocyte and protects the interior of the cell (the ooplasm) from the outside milieu. The oolemma has several functions including: localizing the ultrastructure within the ooplasm; acting as a selective barrier and transporter of substances to and from the cell; maintaining a membrane potential to optimize cell volume; and controlling communication with other cells (e.g. with follicular cells during oogenesis, and with sperm during fertilization).

The ooplasm

The ooplasm is a gel-like cytoplasm contained by the oolemma. In simple terms, it is made up of a mixture of water, nutrients, enzymes, dissolved gases and waste products from metabolism. This matrix contains all of the oocyte's organelles, including the endoplasmic reticulum (smooth and rough), the Golgi, ribosomes, lysosomes, peroxisomes, and mitochondria, all held within a cytoskeleton. The ooplasm also contains the maternal genome, either in a condensed or decondensed state, depending on the stage of the meiotic cell cycle. When observed microscopically, the ooplasm of a viable mature human oocyte tends to appear consistently granular. If the ooplasm is agranular, vacuolated (**Figure 9.1c**) or has an unusually dark area (**Figure 9.6b**); this is usually indicative of poor quality.

The zona pellucida

The name 'zona pellucida' comes from Latin, and translates as 'transparent zone'. During oogenesis, the ZP forms as an extracellular porous spherical translucent matrix around the oocyte (see **Figure 9.1**). Both the oocyte and the granulosa cells are known to be involved in forming the ZP, since ZP proteins have been detected in both the oocyte and granulosa cells at the primordial follicle stage (Gook et al. 2008).

As the oocyte grows within the follicle, specialized granulosa cell-oocyte intercellular connections develop. These links are called gap junctions. Within gap junctions are proteins, known as connexins, which help to supply the oocyte with smaller biochemicals (e.g. glycosaminoglycans, steroid hormones, nutrients, antioxidants, and other factors) that are essential for both nuclear and cytoplasmic development during folliculogenesis. Signals from the oocyte, known as 'diffusible oocyte secretory factors', are also passed to the granulosa cells (Freitas et al. 2017). As the ZP forms, the granulosa cell-oocyte connections continue as transzonal projections (TZPs) (**Figure 9.2**).

Granulosa cells surrounding the ZP develop into functionally-distinct cumulus cells and maintain communication with the ooplasm. This connection is severed just before ovulation. At this stage, a fully formed ZP surrounds the oolemma, separated by an area of fluid called the perivitelline space (PVS). A viable oocyte usually has a regular PVS which is equidistant between the oolemma and the ZP. Polar bodies are extruded into the PVS during meiosis I and II, causing this area of the PVS to be slightly larger (**Figure 9.3**).

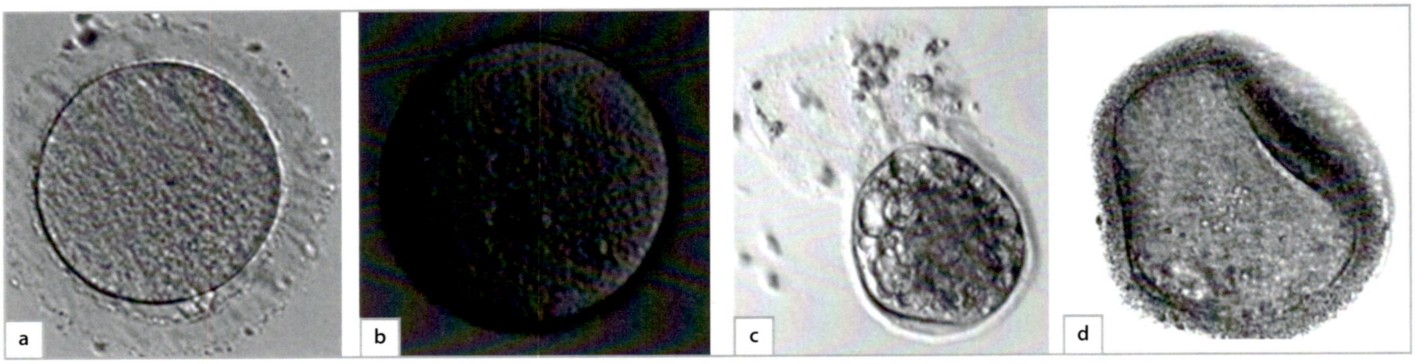

Figure 9.1 Oocytes with zonae pellucida (ZP) of different thickness. (a) An oocyte with a translucent and regular ZP. (b) An oocyte with an ultra-thin zona, only visible under high magnification. (c) A highly vacuolated oocyte with an irregular ZP; (d) An oocyte with an uneven ZP. Courtesy of the Department of Reproductive Medicine, St Mary's Hospital, Manchester, UK.

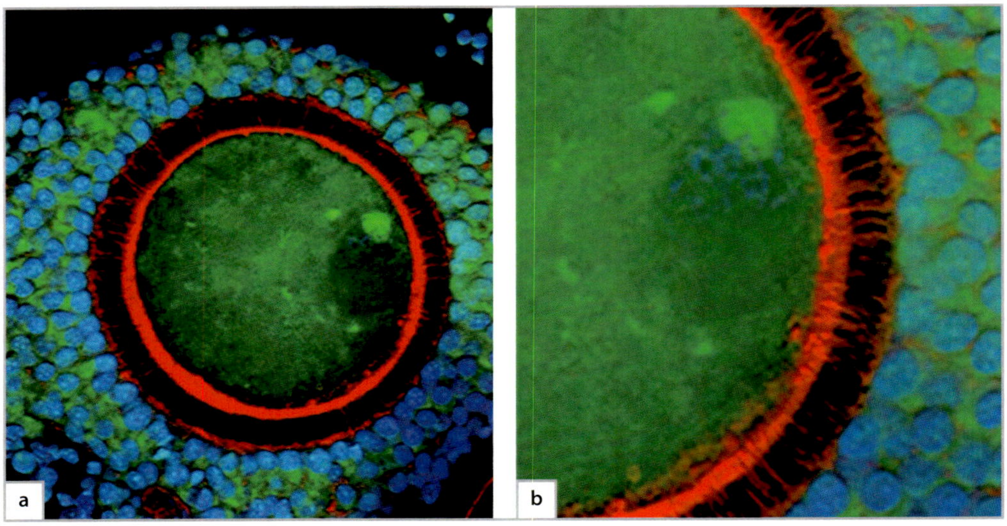

Figure 9.2 During oogenesis, transzonal projections (TZPs) form between the granulosa cells and the oocyte. The TZPs traverse through the zona and attach to the oolemma. Following oocyte maturation, the TZPs become less dense. Images show the TZPs (orange) from an immature oocyte, surrounded by dense cumulus cells (blue). (a) depicts the whole immature oocyte isolated from a Graafian follicle; (b) depicts the same image at higher magnification, where the numerous foci at the oocyte cell surface are clearly visible, representing terminal connections with corona TZPs. Courtesy of Professor David Albertini, New York, USA.

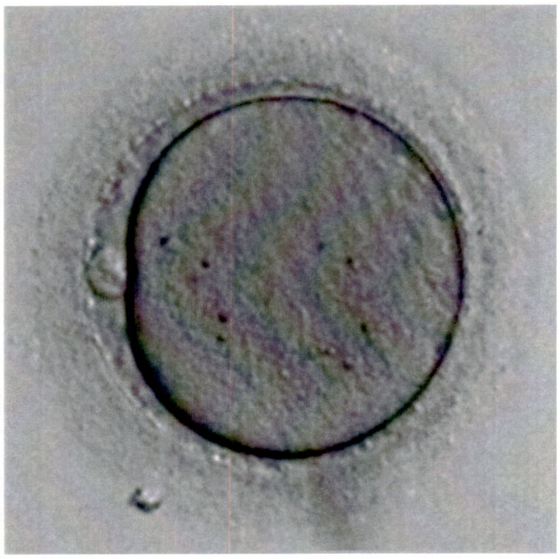

Figure 9.3 A good quality oocyte with a regular zona pellucida and perivitelline space, consistent granularity of the ooplasm, and a single unfragmented polar body (positioned at 9 o'clock).

In the human, the ZP is composed of four glycoproteins: ZP1, ZP2, ZP3 and ZP4. As well as providing a physical barrier to protect the oocyte, these glycoproteins also have a role in sperm-binding: ZP1, ZP3 and ZP4 are involved in inducing the acrosome reaction; whilst ZP2 binds the acrosome-reacted sperm (Petit et al. 2014). Sperm-binding is species-specific, so that only human sperm are capable of fertilizing a human oocyte. Once a single sperm has entered the oocyte, a block is induced to alter the ZP structure and prevent further sperm penetration (known as polyspermy). If the oocyte has a defective ZP, then polyspermy may take place, leading to abnormal fertilization by multiple sperm.

The cortical granules

The block to polyspermy involves small secretory membrane-bound vesicles called cortical granules (CGs). A mature oocyte, at the metaphase II (MII) stage of meiosis, has thousands of CGs located close to the oolemma. CGs are equidistantly spaced under the whole oolemma, apart from an area directly over the MII spindle, where no CGs are found (**Figure 9.4**). This CG-free area is thought to be linked to the presence of chromatin on the spindle.

When a sperm enters an oocyte, CGs undergo exocytosis, whereby they release their contents into the PVS. This calcium-dependent secretory process is called the cortical reaction and causes a structural change in the ZP, to block further sperm from fusing with the oolemma (Liu 2011).

The centrosome

The maternal centrosome is an organelle that helps to organize the spindle dynamics during meiosis. Meiosis I and II result in asymmetric cell divisions, with the formation of the first and second polar body

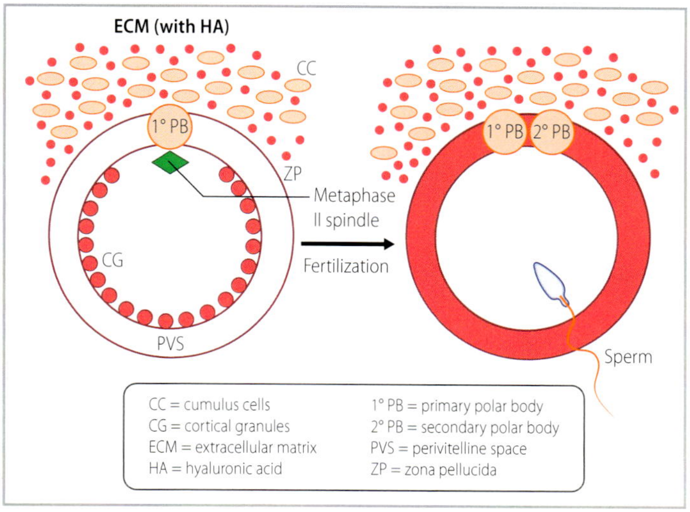

Figure 9.4 Cortical granule location within the mature metaphase II oocyte, and after the cortical reaction which takes place after sperm penetration.

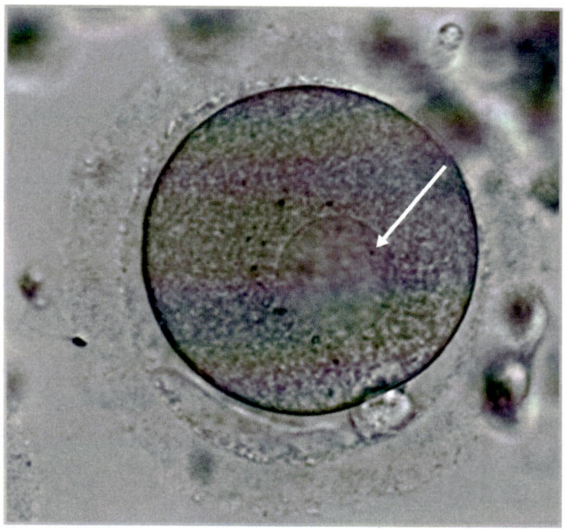

Figure 9.5 An oocyte with a smooth endoplasmic reticulum (SER) disc (arrow shows the SER disc).

with respective divisions. The centrosome aids in the asymmetric positioning of the meiotic spindle for these processes to take place.

A competent centrosome ensures accurate chromosomal separation. The slightest centrosome dysfunction may lead to inaccurate microtubule organization and chromosome alignment such that chromosomes may separate unequally during the anaphase stage of the cell cycle. This is called nondisjunction and is the primary cause of oocyte aneuploidy. Nondisjunction can happen either during meiosis I or meiosis II, although errors in meiosis I appear to be the main reason for oocyte aneuploidy (Eichenlaub-Ritter 2012).

It has been estimated that up to 30% of fertilized oocytes are aneuploid, compared to only 1–2% of sperm (MacLennan et al. 2015). As a result, aneuploid embryos arise primarily due to the inheritance of maternally-derived aneuploidies. Interestingly, whilst aneuploidy has been reported in other species (Hornak et al. 2012), human oocytes have the highest frequency of aneuploid in any species so far studied. Furthermore, this rate significantly rises with advanced maternal age.

Mitochondria

Mitochondria are the powerhouses of the oocyte: they produce energy via adenosine triphosphate (ATP) synthesis to drive all activities. During oogenesis, mitochondria undergo morphogenetic changes, changing from round-shaped to oval-shaped (see Chapter 17). These changes correspond to the increased metabolic demands that are placed on the oocyte, and prepare for the transformation into a zygote following fertilization.

Smooth endoplasmic reticulum (SER) and SER discs

The smooth endoplasmic reticulum (SER) is the oocyte's main calcium store. As such, the SER impacts on oocyte quality as it helps control calcium release. Calcium ions play crucial roles throughout oogenesis, fertilization and embryo development, as they modulate the actin cytoskeleton, and act as a second messenger for cellular events, particularly at the time of fertilization, when calcium oscillations take place.

Within the ultrastructure of the oocyte, the SER is a continuous membranous network throughout the ooplasm. However, at the final stages of oocyte maturation, the SER reorganizes itself in preparation for fertilization. Clusters of SER form in the oocyte cortex, opposite the meiotic spindle (Mann et al. 2010).

Occasionally, the SER aggregates to form an SER disc which is visible within an MII oocyte using standard light microscopy, appearing as a large vacuole (**Figure 9.5**). SER discs can be observed in denuded oocytes, either before ICSI or after conventional IVF insemination. They are distinct from pronuclei (PN), since they do not contain nucleoli.

SER discs can adversely affect calcium release and cell metabolism. In 2011, two professional bodies recommended that oocytes containing SER discs should not be inseminated (the Alpha Scientists in Reproductive Medicine and the ESHRE Embryology Special Interest Group, 2011). However, since then, others have demonstrated that healthy offspring can result from fertilisation of oocytes that contained SER discs, with perinatal complications occurring at a frequency of 9.4% (16/171) (Shaw-Jackson et al. 2014). Thus, provided patients are advised of the risks, oocytes with SER discs can be used for ART.

ASSESSING OOCYTE QUALITY

Oocyte quality plays a pivotal role in determining ART outcomes. Initial grading can be performed on the cumulus-oocyte complex (COC), which includes the oocyte, obscured by its multiple surrounding layers of cumulus cells. At ovulation, the COC aids movement of the oocyte into the oviduct, where the cumulus cells control sperm access to the oocyte, and it is COCs that are retrieved at the oocyte collection procedure.

The COC grading is based on overall size and the level of cumulus cell expansion away from the ZP. Immature COCs tend to have tightly packed, unexpanded cumulus cells that are usually darker than other COCs, and the oocytes are often at the germinal vesicle stage. Mature COCs usually contain cumulus cells that have expanded away from the ZP and appear as a translucent 'cloud' of cells at oocyte collection. Post-mature COCs tend to have hardly any cumulus cells, as the majority have expanded and dispersed away from the oocyte; these oocytes are less competent due to ZP hardening (due to partial CG exocytosis), mitochondrial dysfunction, and loss of chromosomal integrity (Lord & Aitken 2013).

However, COC grading remains imprecise. Discrepancies have been reported between COC appearance and the nuclear maturity of the corresponding oocyte, such that 26% of COCs graded as 'immature' actually contained MII oocytes, whilst 11% of COCs graded as 'mature' contained immature oocytes (Ebner et al. 2008). A proper examination of the oocyte can only take place once the cumulus cells are removed, either before ICSI or at the time of checking for fertilization after conventional IVF.

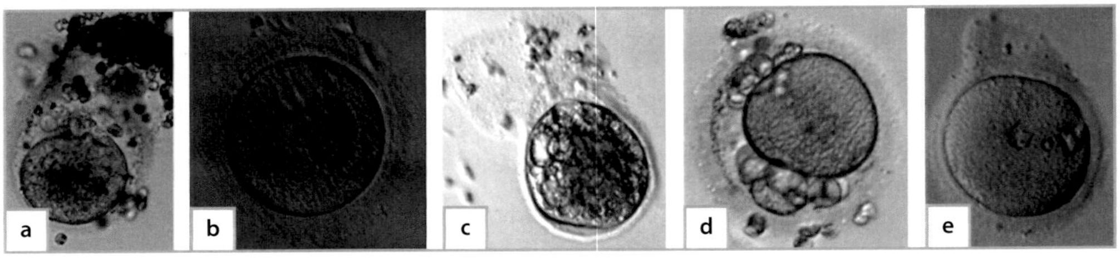

Figure 9.6 Oocytes with various dysmorphism. (a) unusually large PVS; (b) a central area of darkened ooplasm; (c) a vacuolated ooplasm; (d) abnormal fragmented polar body; (e) abnormal zona pellucida. (Courtesy of Embryology Department, St Marys Hospital, Manchester, UK).

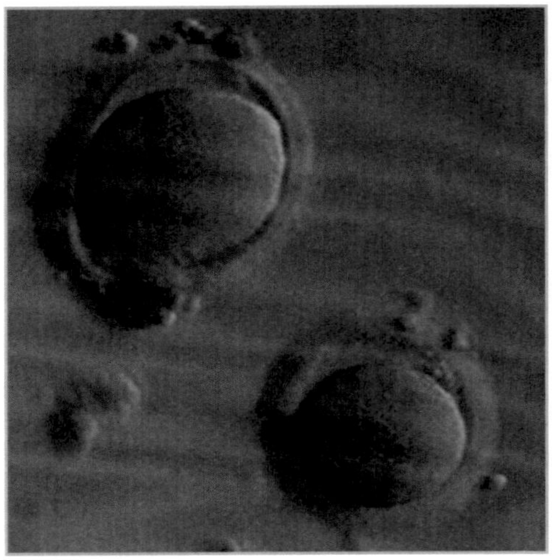

Figure 9.7 The oocyte on the left-hand side is known as a 'giant oocyte', which is approximately twice the size of the regular oocyte on the right-hand side. During oogenesis, a giant oocyte forms when two oogonia fuse, resulting in a tetraploid cell. Such giant oocytes must be discarded and never used for ICSI due to their aneuploid status.

Beyond visible signs of maturity, human oocytes come in a wide variety of shapes and sizes (**Figures 9.6** and **9.7**). Different oocytes exhibit variations in these visible features, such as size, shape, colour, and cytoplasmic homogeneity. Embryologists grade oocytes according to various criteria, to attempt to predict the most competent oocytes. Oocyte grading has received additional attention by embryologists in countries where legislative restrictions limit the number of oocytes that can be inseminated. In these situations, oocyte grading has become a critical tool to optimize selection of those oocytes that are most likely to result in normal fertilization and formation of a viable embryo.

For a detailed description of the criteria for assessing oocyte quality, readers are directed to the Istanbul consensus on embryo assessment (Alpha Scientists in Reproductive Medicine & ESHRE Embryology Special Interest Group 2011), which describes both oocyte and embryo assessment. An excellent review of different features of oocyte morphology relating to competence has also been provided by Rienzi and her team (2011). General features included overall oocyte shape, ZP thickness, the PVS size and polar body shape. Within the ooplasm, dysmorphisms included areas of cytoplasmic granulation or the presence of vacuoles or refractile bodies. If oocytes could be imaged using polarized light microscopy, then the level of MII spindle birefringence correlated to competence. Finally, at the time of ICSI, the membrane resistance characteristics to the microinjection needle insertion and the ooplasmic viscosity within the injection pipette could also be related to oocyte quality. However, no feature was unanimously evaluated to have prognostic value for the further developmental competence of oocytes (Rienzi et al. 2011).

Beyond the standard microscopic evaluation, new methods for assessing oocyte quality are being proposed. These include noninvasive methods such as metabolomics (Siristatidis et al. 2017) and use of polarized light microscopy to determine ZP birefringence, as better-quality oocytes have been reported to exhibit a higher ZP birefringence (Omidi et al. 2017). More invasive assessment methods include genomic analysis of the polar body and cumulus cells, and also analysis of mitochondria distribution within the ooplasm. However, access to the technologies supporting these methods restricts their use for most IVF laboratories.

OOCYTE COLLECTION

Preparing for the oocyte collection

Following controlled superovulation, when the follicles are judged to be at their optimal size, the patient is given a trigger injection to induce ovulation 40 hours later (see Chapter 8). Oocyte retrieval is usually planned to take place 36 hours after the trigger injection, as the oocytes should be at a mature stage and free-floating in the follicles.

The day before oocyte collection

The whole clinical team should be notified of the proposed theater list on the eve before the planned collection, so that they can familiarize themselves with each patients' case-notes to ensure all required consents are signed and all aspects of the treatment have been considered. Most women will be scheduled for a transvaginal oocyte collection, but other options may need to be considered (**Table 9.1**).

The case notes should document the number of follicles (and expected number of oocytes), the insemination technique (IVF or ICSI) and whether the patient is scheduled for PGD or PGS. The laboratory should check the details of any previous ART treatment to see if any changes to the treatment strategy are needed, e.g. if the IVF fertilization rate was low in a previous cycle, ICSI might have been recommended for future cycles; or if donor sperm is to be used, the embryologists should ensure the correct donor sperm has been ordered and sufficient supplies are present in the cryo-store.

The screening results for patients should also be confirmed for any viruses that could present a health risk to others, including HIV (HIV 1 and 2), hepatitis B (anti-HBC and HBsAg) and hepatitis C (anti-HCV-Ab) (Jindal et al. 2016). Additional tests should be considered depending on the patient history, e.g. for HTLV-1, malaria *Trypanosoma cruzi*, Zika virus, or other similar exposures.

The team can then set up their respective areas accordingly: the clinical team can prepare the treatment room, whilst the embryologists can prepare the embryology laboratory to make up and equilibrate all media and plasticware for laboratory manipulations.

The number of items of plasticware prepared should be sufficient to safely culture the maximum number of oocytes that are anticipated to be collected. Dish and tube preparation should take place in a sterile environment, most commonly provided by a class II vertical air flow hood. Plasticware should be pre-labelled to ensure unequivocal patient identification, e.g. with the patient's full name, date of birth and clinic number. Media should be equilibrated in 37°C incubators overnight, with

Table 9.1 Different oocyte collection methods. Laparoscopic oocyte collection was the original technique used, followed by ultrasound guided oocyte collections. Nowadays, most clinicians use the trans-vaginal route as it is the simplest

Method of oocyte retrieval	Description
Laparoscopic oocyte recovery	Following incision to the inferior rim of the umbilicus and gaseous inflation of the abdomen, the ovaries are directly visualised using a laparoscope and held in place by the forceps. A needle is then inserted into the abdomen to aspirate the follicles. This was the method originally used by Steptoe and Edwards, resulting in the world's first successful IVF baby The method is also used for patients undergoing gamete intrafallopian transfer (GIFT), whereby oocytes are collected laparoscopically, and then one or two oocytes are transferred into the Fallopian tube, alongside a separate sample of prepared sperm
Ultrasound-guided follicle aspiration	
Trans-abdominal	Follicles are imaged using an abdominal ultrasound probe and the needle is introduced abdominally However, problems can occur with abdominal scanning, e.g. due to obesity, bowel gas, or a retroverted uterus. This method can also incorporate passing the needle through the bladder to help visualisation (whereby the bladder is drained and the artificially inflated with a neutral solution such as saline
Trans-vaginal	Follicles are imaged using an ultrasound scan and probe as a vaginal transducer. A needle guide is attached to the probe and is directed towards the ovaries to aspirate each follicle This method is most common as it provides the simplest and shortest route to the ovaries. However, some gynecological issues may preclude the use, e.g. ovaries are inaccessible vaginally due to adhesions and or the patient has Mayer-Rokitansky-Küster-Hauser (MRKH) syndrome, a congenital abnormality whereby the vagina, cervix and uterus are absent

TO FLUSH OR NOT TO FLUSH?

The clinician performing the oocyte collection can either use a single lumen or a double lumen needle. A single lumen needle allows the clinician to pierce a follicle and aspirate the contents once only. This has an advantage of allowing multiple follicles to be aspirated at the same time, which can reduce the duration of the oocyte collection procedure. A single collection tube can frequently contain fluid from several follicles, hence several COCs may identified per tube with this technique.

By contrast, use of a double lumen needle allows a clinician to aspirate the follicle, and then refill it with flush medium which can then be aspirated. If the oocyte is not collected in the initial aspirate, then flushing provides a second opportunity to retrieve the oocyte. The flush medium can either be a culture medium or a simpler solution such as lactate Ringer's or saline. Using saline rather than culture medium has been shown to significantly reduce oocyte-retrieval costs without adversely affecting reproductive outcomes (Loktionov et al. 2017). Provided the COC can be quickly identified, washed and transferred into the preinsemination medium, then the COC should not be compromised.

A disadvantage of flushing is that the procedure tends to increase the operating time and the analgesic requirement; furthermore, a meta-analysis has shown that flushing does not improve the oocyte yield or pregnancy outcomes (Roque et al. 2012). However, flushing has been shown to be effective if there is only a single follicle to aspirate, such as in the natural menstrual cycle (Wolff et al. 2013).

or without CO_2 supply, depending on the type of media used. Mineral oil is commonly used as an overlay for all culture media to prevent evaporation, maintain temperature and pH, and reduce infection risk.

If possible, it can be helpful to dedicate one incubator for oocyte collection. This can be without a gas supply and used to pre-warm the oocyte collection needles, media to flush follicles, and oocyte collection dishes (provided they are made with either HEPES- or MOPS-buffered medium) to maintain the correct pH during the actual collection process.

FOLLICULAR FLUID

Follicular fluid (FF) is the main constituent of the antrum of a growing follicle, alongside the COC and granulosa cells. FF is uniquely composed of polysaccharides, proteins, hormones, metabolites, reactive oxygen species and antioxidant enzymes that regulate the growth and quality of the oocyte and follicle. The high metabolic activity of the growing follicle is reflected in the high concentration of enzymes present in FF.

Healthy follicles are surrounded by a rich vascular network, which promotes movement of plasma proteins into the FF, such that over half the FF proteins are thought to be derived from plasma, with the remainder coming from the COC and granulosa cells.

Many FF constituents have been proposed as indicators of oocyte health, with suboptimal levels found in the FF from women with PCOS and endometriosis, indicating poorer oocyte quality (see Chapter 6 and Chapter 7).

In vitro processing of the oocytes in the IVF laboratory

At the oocyte collection procedure, the follicles are aspirated by a member of the clinical team. This procedure depends on the skill of the aspirating clinician, the type of equipment used and the aspirating pressure. If the aspirating pressure is too high, the oocyte ZP may fracture; although a ZP may break due to an inherent weakness unique to the oocyte regardless of the pressure (**Figure 9.8**).

Tubes containing follicular fluid are passed to the embryologist, to perform the oocyte identification in a class II vertical air flow hood. The tubes are placed in a hot-block to maintain them at 37°C. The embryologist then pours the fluid from each tube into a sterile petri dish (either 60 mm or 100 mm diameter) to examine the fluid via a stereomicroscope fitted with a heated stage to maintain the fluid at 37°C throughout this process. The fluid is thoroughly scanned to identify any COCs.

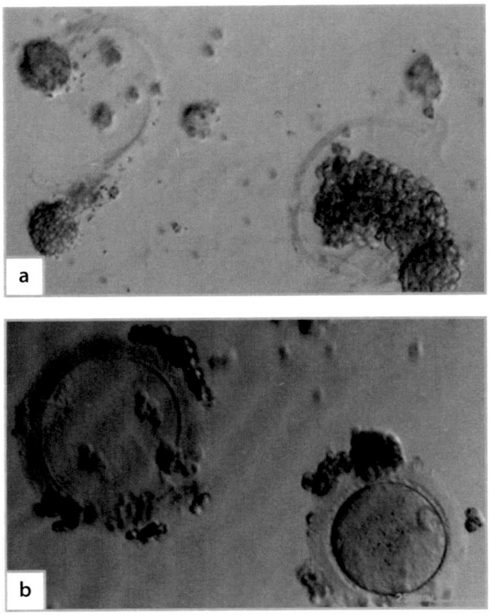

Figure 9.8 If an oocyte is subjected to high aspiration pressure during oocyte collection, its zona pellucida may fracture, such that the oocyte is no longer viable. Some women are also prone to producing oocytes with 'fragile zonae'. (a) Two fractured zonae devoid of ooplasm. (b) A single fractured zona on the left and intact oocyte on the right.

As COCs are identified, they are aspirated using a sterile Pasteur pipette and washed in buffered media to remove any blood cells. The 'cleaned' COCs are then either maintained in the fresh buffered media or transferred to pre-gassed dishes for further culture. Some laboratories prefer to collect into tubes at this stage, accepting that the COCs cannot be observed in the tubes as easily as they can in dishes.

The efficiency of the embryologist is paramount at the oocyte collection, as the procedure can be fast-pace. Multiple follicles may be aspirated at a quick pace, and several tubes of aspirate and flush can be placed into the hot-block. The embryologist should note the order of the tubes, to ensure each tube is systematically examined. Heparin can be added to the flush (2 Ul/mL) to prevent any blood clotting (**Figure 9.9c**), and heparin-supplemented aspiration media is also available commercially from some media manufacturers. However, an efficient embryologist can usually check all aspirates before any clotting taking place, without the use of heparin.

When the oocyte collection is finished, all collected COCs should be transferred to a pre-insemination dish(es) containing a bicarbonate-buffered medium, without HEPES/MOPS, and incubated in a 37°C incubator gassed with 5% CO_2 and 5% O_2. The total COC number in respective dishes and wells should be labelled on the relevant plasticware to identify the location. The clinical team should be informed of the COC number, so that the patient can be made aware of the potential oocyte number, and the clinical team can record the number of oocytes collected from the number of follicles imaged at the last ultrasound scan.

The embryologist should grade the retrieved COCs according to maturity: as immature, mature or postmature. If no pre-ovulatory COCs are observed at the collection, the clinician should be informed, so that the ovarian stimulation response can be checked, to see if this was indicated. It may be useful for the patients to be advised of the COC maturity at this point of their cycle, to pre-warn them in case of low fertilization or poor fertilization results.

In the laboratory, if there are sufficient media droplets/wells, then COCs can be segregated according to maturity at this stage (**Figure 9.9**). The culture of immature COCs can be prolonged, prior to insemination, or subjected to in vitro maturation. However, this should be in accordance with standard protocols. If conventional IVF is planned, it may be that the oocytes within the COCs mature over the insemination period.

FERTILIZATION TECHNIQUES

Conventional IVF insemination

For conventional IVF insemination, the prepared sperm sample should have a high number of fast-moving capacitated sperm, which should be maintained at room temperature. Immediately prior to insemination, this sample should be incubated under the same conditions as the COCs. The same media type can be used for culturing the prepared sperm sample and the COCs, to minimize any differences in media constituents, pH and osmolality.

The number of sperm to be added, and corresponding insemination volume, should be calculated to maximize the chance of fertilization. Care should be taken to avoid an excessively high sperm concentration, as this increases the risk of polyspermy and may compromise embryo development due to the high levels of free radicals introduced with high sperm numbers. A sperm concentration of 100×10^6/mL is recommended, although this can be as low as 20×10^6/mL or as high as 300×10^6/mL, depending on clinical policy (see **Box**).

For the actual insemination process, the sperm sample should be removed from the incubator, and placed in a hot-block at 37°C. After fitting a sterile tip to a micropipetter, set to the required insemination volume, the COC dish should be removed from the incubator and placed on a heated stage in a class II flow hood.

A double identity check should take place at this point, involving both the embryologist performing the insemination and a witness. This ensures that the identity of the oocytes and sperm unequivocally belong to the correct patients. Developing fail-safe mechanisms to prevent patient mix-ups is critical (de los Santos & Ruiz 2013).

The required insemination volume of sperm should then be gently dispensed into the medium containing the COCs (**Figure 9.10**). The insemination should be directed away from the COCs to allow the dispensed sperm to then swim toward the oocytes. In theory, this allows the better swimming sperm to reach the oocyte first.

Once all COCs in a dish have been inseminated, the medium around the COCs should be observed under a higher magnification (e.g. ×400), to check that the sperm are swimming optimally and starting to penetrate the cumulus cells. The dish should then be returned to the incubator where it should remain until the time of the fertilization check, which should take place 16–18 hours later. The insemination time, the concentration of progressively motile sperm inseminated, and the names of the embryologist and witness should be recorded in the embryology notes.

CALCULATING NUMBER OF SPERM FOR IVF

For a post-preparation sample, with a concentration of C (million/mL), a motility of M (% progressively motile), the insemination volume can be calculated using the equation:

$$\text{Volume to inseminate } (\mu L) = 100/C \times M$$

Adding this volume will give an insemination concentration of 100,000 progressively motile sperm if added to a volume of 1 mL culture medium. This volume would need to be reduced for smaller volumes of culture medium

Note: the number of motile sperm inseminated will be approximate, since the medium volume will have changed due to the addition of the COCs to the original volume, and the addition of the insemination volume

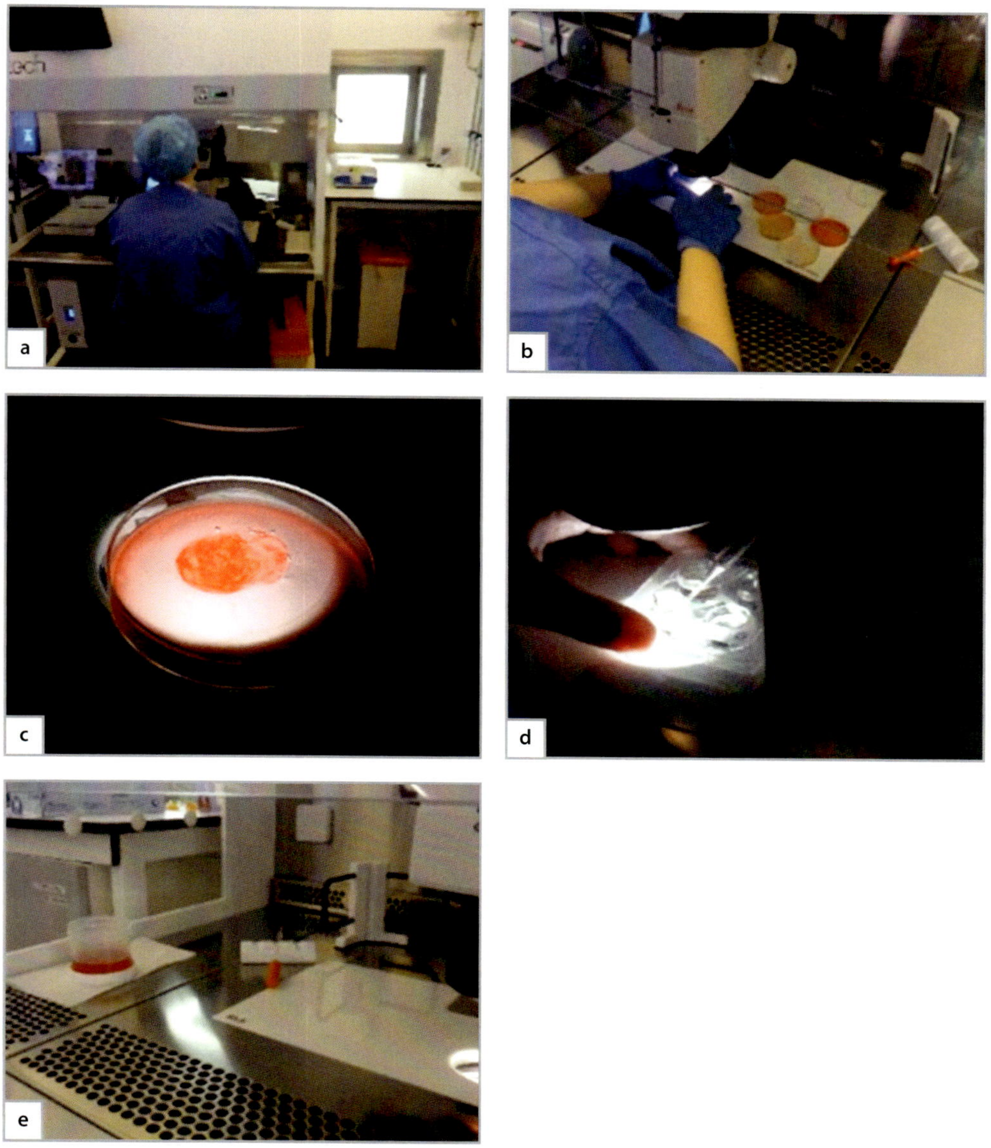

Figure 9.9 An embryologist performing oocyte collection. (a) Setting up for an oocyte collection, with the hatch to the procedure room on the right, where tubes of aspirated follicular fluid will be passed into the hot-block; (b) Checking fluid to identify cumulus-oocyte complexes (COCs); (c) A follicular fluid with a blood clot; (d) Transfer of the COC from the fluid into culture; (e) At the end of the oocyte collection, the fluid without COCs has been collected into a discard container, thus reducing the risk of infection from this biological fluid. Courtesy of the Assisted Conception Services, Glasgow Royal Infirmary, Glasgow, UK.

Different laboratories have variations on the conventional IVF insemination technique. These may include adding the sperm to a separate insemination dish and then adding the COCs; inseminating in large volumes or droplets; and adjusting the time of co-incubation of gametes, such that the COCs are removed to a fresh dish a short time after insemination (Guo et al. 2012). However, use of short insemination times remains controversial, as a 1-hour gamete exposure has been reported to decrease the fertilization rate compared to a standard 18-hour insemination procedure (Barraud-Lange et al. 2008).

Intracytoplasmic sperm injection

The ICSI is used to bypass the physiological barriers of the COC and ZP to deliver a sperm directly into the ooplasm. This method of fertilization was originally developed to help couples where the male had severe infertility, e.g. due to low sperm numbers or poor function. However, ICSI is commonly used as the treatment of choice by fertility clinics for patients without a male factor, such that some clinics have resorted to using ICSI for all inseminations.

Preparation of oocytes for ICSI

In order to perform ICSI, oocytes need to be denuded from their surrounding cumulus cells. Within the COC, cumulus cells are bound by a matrix of hyaluronan oligosaccharide chains cross-linked by hyaluronan-binding proteins and proteoglycans. Denudation is usually facilitated by briefly exposing the COCs to a solution containing a recombinant version of the enzyme hyaluronidase (Hyase), maintained at 37°C. This allows for the enzymatic digestion of the cumulus cells. Since over-exposure to Hyase may harm oocytes, embryologists are recommended to decrease the concentration and duration of oocyte exposure to the enzyme. The Hyase concentration in commercially available media is usually 80 IU/mL, but a diluted concentration of 30–40 IU/mL may be preferred, with a maximum exposure of 30 seconds.

Interestingly, where conventional IVF is preferred, some embryologists prefer to reduce the size of the COC prior to insemination. This can be performed by mechanically 'cutting off' supernumerous cumulus cells or by exposing the COCs to a highly diluted Hyase concentration of approximately 7 IU/mL throughout the insemination period (Ebner et al. 2011).

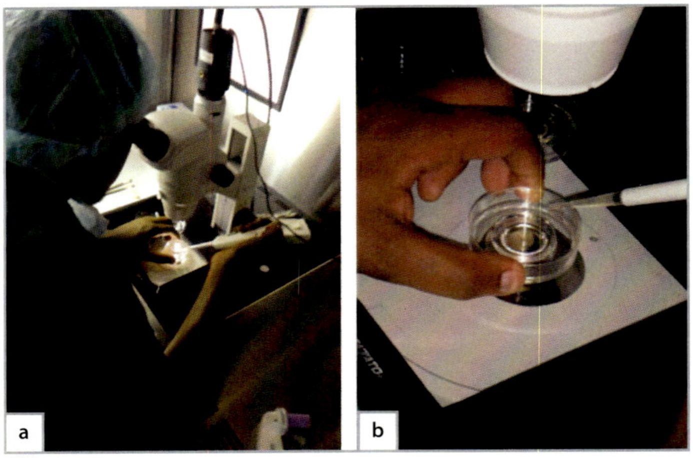

Figure 9.10 Conventional IVF. (a) An embryologist adds a specific volume of highly motile washed sperm to a culture dish containing cumulus-oocyte complexes (COCs). (b) The culture dish with the COCs in the inner well, where the sperm will be deposited. Courtesy of the Mwanza Women's Hospital, Tanzania.

HYALURONAN

Hyaluronan (HA), also termed hyaluronic acid, is found in the extracellular matrices of cells. The human body (estimated for a 70-kg adult) has approximately 15 g of HA, with about 5 g being continuously synthesised and degraded daily. For oocytes, HA is produced by cumulus cells to bind them together in the COC.

Hyaluronidases (Hyases) are enzymes that degrade HA, to lower viscosity and increase tissue permeability. At ovulation, Hyases promote COC expansion, which aids detachment from the follicle wall to enable the COC to be free-floating in the follicular fluid. Hyases also interrupts the gap junctions between the cumulus cells and the oocyte.

To assist oocyte denudation prior to ICSI, COCs are exposed to a medium containing recombinant Hyase. This promotes loosening of HA binding the cumulus cells, to allow access to the oocyte.

Regarding the time when oocytes should be denuded before ICSI, many embryologists prefer to wait until the theoretical time of ovulation (usually 4 hours after collection, if the collection is performed 36 hours after the ovulation trigger injection). However, others suggest that denudation can take place closer to the time of oocyte collection without detriment to maturity (Bárcena et al. 2016).

Denudation pipettes are commonly used to aid mechanical removal of cumulus cells from the ZP following exposure to Hyase. Physically 'loosening off' the cumulus cells should be performed carefully, as oocytes are susceptible to damage from the mechanical stress created by repeated movement up and down the denudation pipette. The lumen diameter of the denudation pipette should be slightly larger than the diameter of the oocyte to minimize the risk of oocyte damage, whilst enabling full cumulus cell denudation. Some embryologists use a series of pipettes of decreasing lumen size, such as Pasteur pipettes, followed by denudation pipettes with lumen diameters of 200 μm, 155 μm and 135 μm.

Once denuded, oocytes should then be washed in buffered media to remove any residual Hyase, and then washed through pre-equilibrated culture media. Oocytes can then be assessed for maturation status and segregated accordingly. It is recommended that ICSI is then performed without delay.

Injection procedure

The ICSI practitioners should be familiar with the micromanipulation equipment to be used. Whilst an inverted microscope with modulation contrast and a heated stage are usually fitted as standard, different manufacturers of micromanipulation equipment may have different joysticks (e.g. electronic, hydraulic or mechanical) and syringes (e.g. air- or oil-accentuated).

TOP TEN CONSIDERATIONS WHEN PERFORMING ICSI

1. Equipment – all ICSI practitioners should be fully familiar with the working of the micromanipulation rig to be used. If a laboratory has more than one rig, a record of which equipment was used should be made, as they may vary in performance, even if the rigs are the same make/model.
2. Operator – not all ICSI practitioners perform ICSI at the same efficiency and speed. According to the ESHRE guidelines for best practice (2015), the duration of sperm localization, immobilization and microinjection should be minimal.
3. Environment – all oocytes should be maintained in vitro at optimal temperature, pH and osmolality throughout the ICSI procedure. This may necessitate lowering the number of oocytes transferred into each ICSI dish, according to the skill level of the embryologist (see point 1) and the difficulty of the case.
4. Stability – each oocyte must be safely secured throughout each ICSI using a holding pipette. This reduces the risk of oocyte movement and damage.
5. Sperm quality – if sperm is not easy to locate then this will add time to the capture problems (see point 3). Records should be kept if there are problems with sperm immobilization or morphology (sometimes sperm are not easily immobilized, or only grossly abnormal-shaped sperm are available).
6. Oocyte quality – oocyte dysmorphisms may exist, e.g. irregularities in ZP thickness, PVS size, oolemma flexibility, cytoplasmic granularity, presence of SER discs, etc. Fully traceable records should be kept, so that each oocyte can be traced from ICSI to fertilization and embryonic development.
7. Oocyte maturity – segregating the MII oocytes prior to transfer to the ICSI dish can save time during the ICSI procedure, rather than assessing maturity of all oocytes at the time of ICSI. Immature oocytes can be re-assessed once all MII oocytes have been microinjected and placed in post-ICSI culture.
8. Oocyte position – the PB should be positioned away from the direct pathway of injection pipette, but the precise PB position, e.g. at 6 o'clock or 12 o'clock, is less relevant.
9. Sperm direction of injection – whilst head-first sperm microinjection may be simpler to visualize, tail-first sperm microinjection is permissible.
10. Failed injection – if a sperm is observed to clearly not enter the ooplasm, this oocyte should be re-injected at the end of the ICSI procedure, when all other MII oocytes have been microinjected. Selecting a different position for penetration also allows the oolemma time to recover prior to another physical breach.

For ICSI, a single sperm must be selected, immobilized and microinjected into an oocyte (**Figure 9.11**). Detailed sperm selection at very high magnification (×6600, compared to standard ×400) can be used to enable motile sperm organelle morphology examination (MSOME) and intracytoplasmic morphologically-selected sperm injection (IMSI). In theory, the extra scrutiny involved in selecting a sperm with optimal morphology should optimize the outcome of

ICSI. However, a decade after the introduction of MSOME and IMSI, the benefit over standard ICSI remains questionable (Setti et al. 2013).

All microinjected oocytes should be washed post-ICSI in pre-equilibrated media, prior to transfer to a culture dish. The dish should then be returned to the incubator until the time of when the oocytes need to be checked to see if they have fertilized. The insemination time should be recorded, including the start and end of the procedure. The timing is critical, as an unnecessary delay may negatively affect the chances of fertilization. The name of the practitioner and the witness, and the micromanipulation rig (if more than one) should also be recorded in the embryology notes. At the end of the ICSI procedure, both the holding and injection micropipettes should be discarded into a clinical waste sharps bin, before setting up fresh sterile pipettes for the next ICSI procedure.

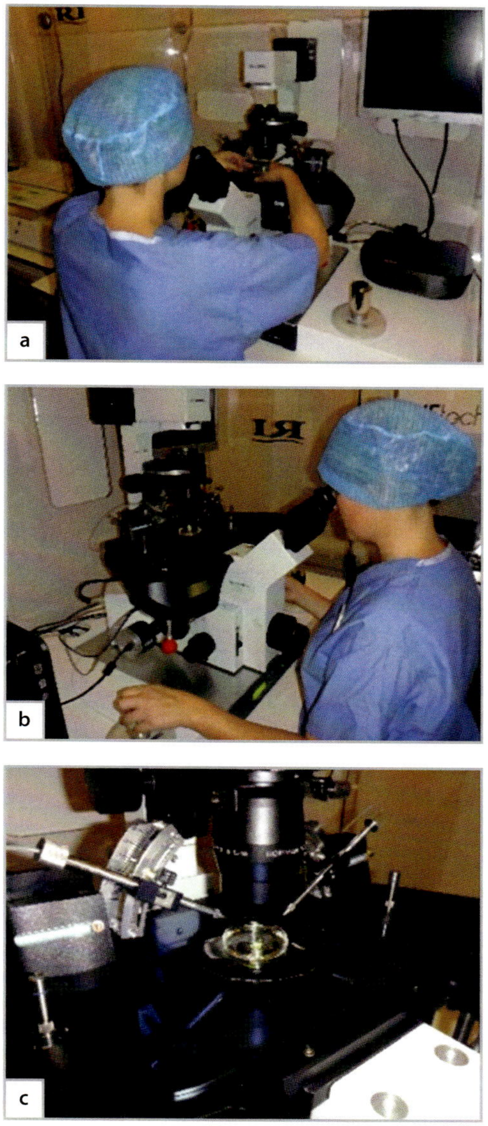

Figure 9.11 An embryologist performing ICSI. (a) Setting up the micromanipulation equipment and moving a dish containing oocytes and sperm ready for ICSI; (b) Performing ICSI, the left-hand syringe controls manipulation of the sperm, whilst the right-hand controls manipulation of the oocyte; (c) the ICSI set-up, with the holding pipette on the left to secure the oocyte in position, and the injection pipette on the right, to inject the sperm into the oocyte. Courtesy of the Assisted Conception Services, Glasgow Royal Infirmary, Glasgow, UK.

ICSI: SHOULD POLYVINYLPYRROLIDONE BE USED?

Since motile sperm may be difficult to capture, immobilize and control in the microinjection pipette, many embryologists transfer the sperm to a viscous solution, such as polyvinylpyrrolidone (PVP). Whilst PVP can aid micromanipulation, the chemical can damage sperm membranes and also remain within the microinjected oocyte and subsequent embryo (Kato & Nagao 2012). Alternative ways to immobilize and handle sperm have been proposed, such as diluting the concentration of PVP solution or using PVP-free media, such as hyaluronic acid-based media (Liu et al. 2017).

CHECKING FOR FERTILIZATION

Following conventional IVF, the oocytes need to first be removed from the insemination dish (**Figure 9.12**). This procedure is similar to oocyte denudation prior to ICSI, but without the need for Hyase, since the motile sperm have usually dispersed much of the cumulus. A 135 µm lumen diameter denudation pipette may be required to dislodge any cumulus cells which remain tightly bound to the ZP. Once denuded, these oocytes should be thoroughly washed through media droplets to remove any residual moving sperm.

Oocytes can then be assessed for visual signs of normal fertilization, such as the presence of 2PN in the ooplasm and two polar bodies in the PVS. An oocyte exhibiting PN is termed a zygote. 2PN zygotes should be segregated for further culture. If a fresh embryo transfer is proposed, then the morphologically 'best' embryo can then be selected for transfer a few days later, whilst other embryos can be cryopreserved for future use.

If 3PN are observed in the ooplasm, this indicates abnormal fertilization has taken place, either from two sperm entering an oocyte (diandric triploidy), or a failure of the extrusion of the second polar body from the oocyte (digynic triploidy). 3PN zygotes should be removed from culture, as they have an abnormal chromosome number and resultant fetuses have highly unfavorable outcomes.

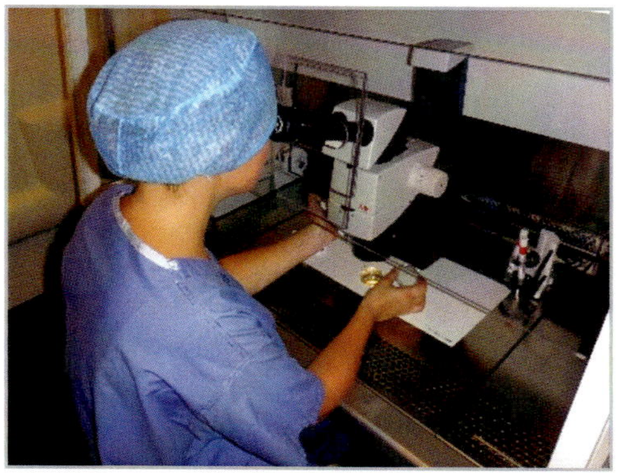

Figure 9.12 An embryologist checking for fertilization. The denuded oocytes are carefully transferred through wash droplets before assessing the oocytes in detail to check if any pronuclei are visible. Courtesy of the Assisted Conception Services, Glasgow Royal Infirmary, Glasgow, UK.

SUMMARY

This chapter has outlined the biological structure of the human oocyte, and how oocyte quality is assessed. A basic description of how oocytes are dealt with in vitro in the IVF laboratory, from the point of oocyte retrieval to the point of insemination, has been given. For further information, it is recommended that readers access atlases on embryology such as the *Atlas of Oocytes, Zygotes and Embryos in Reproductive Medicine* (Elder et al. 2012). Such an atlas provided numerous images of oocytes, demonstrating various dysmorphisms and the types of zygotes and embryos that result.

REFERENCES

Albertini D. The mammalian oocyte. In: Plant TM, Zeleznik A (eds). Knobil and Neill's Physiology of Reproduction (4th edn). New York: Elsevier, 2014.

Alpha Scientists in Reproductive Medicine and ESHRE Special Interest Group of Embryology. The Istanbul consensus workshop on embryo assessment: proceedings of an expert meeting. Hum Reprod 2011; 26:1270–1283.

Bárcena P, Rodríguez M, Obradors A, Vernaeve V, Vassena R. Should we worry about the clock? Relationship between time to ICSI and reproductive outcomes in cycles with fresh and vitrified oocytes. Hum Reprod 2016; 31:1182–1191.

de los Santos MJ, Ruiz A. Protocols for tracking and witnessing samples and patients in assisted reproductive technology. Fertil Steril 2013; 100:1499–502.

Ebner T, Moser M, Shebl O, et al. Blood clots in the cumulus-oocyte complex predict poor oocyte quality and post-fertilization development. RBM Online 2008; 16:801–807.

Ebner T, Moser M, Shebl O, Mayer R, Tews G . Assisting in vitro fertilization by manipulating cumulus-oocyte-complexes either mechanically or enzymatically does not prevent IVF failure. J Turk Ger Gynecol Assoc 2011; 12:135–139.

Eichenlaub-Ritter U. Oocyte ageing and its cellular basis. Int J Dev Biol 2012; 56:841–852.

Elder K, Van den Bergh M, Ebner T (eds). Atlas of Oocytes, Zygotes and Embryos in Reproductive Medicine. Cambridge: Cambridge University Press, 2012.

Freitas C, Neto AC, Matos L, et al. Follicular Fluid redox involvement for ovarian follicle growth. J Ovarian Res 2017; 10:44.

Gook DA, Edgar DH, Borg J, Martic M. Detection of zona pellucida proteins during human folliculogenesis. Hum Reprod 2008; 23:394–402.

Hornak M, Oracova E, Hulinska P, Urbankova L, Rubes J. Aneuploidy detection in pigs using comparative genomic hybridization from the oocytes to blastocysts. PLoS One 2012; 7:e30335.

Jindal SK, Rawlins RG, Muller CH, Drobnis EZ. Guidelines for risk reduction when handling gametes from infectious patients seeking assisted reproductive technologies. Reprod Biomed Online 2016; 33:121–130.

Kato Y, Nagao Y. Effect of polyvinylpyrrolidone on sperm function and early embryonic development following intracytoplasmic sperm injection in human assisted reproduction. Reprod Med Biol 2012; 11:165–176.

Liu M. The biology and dynamics of mammalian cortical granules. Reprod Biol Endocrinol 2011; 9:149.

Liu Y, Feenan K, Chapple V, Roberts P, Matson P. Intracytoplasmic sperm injection using hyaluronic acid or polyvinylpyrrolidone: a time-lapse sibling oocyte study. Hum Fertil (Camb) 2017:1–8.

Loktionov D, Oduola O, Cloherty J, Warner SM, Purandare N. Comparison of costs associated with substituting culture medium with saline solution for follicular flushing during oocyte retrieval. Int J Gynaecol Obstet, 2017; 139:180–184.

Lord T, Aitken RJ. Oxidative stress and ageing of the post-ovulatory oocyte. Reproduction 2013; 146:R217–227.

MacLennan M, Crichton JH, Playfoot CJ, Adams IR. Oocyte development, meiosis and aneuploidy. Semin Cell Dev Biol 2015; 45:68–76.

Mann JS, Lowther KM, Mehlmann LM. Reorganization of the endoplasmic reticulum and development of Ca2+ release mechanisms during meiotic maturation of human oocytes. Biol Reprod 2010; 83:578–583.

Omidi M, Faramarzi A, Agharahimi A, Khalili MA. Noninvasive imaging systems for gametes and embryo selection in IVF programs: a review. J Microsc 2017; 267:253–264.

Petit FM, Serres C, Auer J. Moonlighting proteins in sperm-egg interactions. Biochem Soc Trans 2014; 42:1740–1743.

Rienzi L, Vajta G, Ubaldi F. Predictive value of oocyte morphology in human IVF: a systematic review of the literature. Hum Reprod Update 2011; 17:34–45.

Roque M, Sampaio M, Geber S. Follicular flushing during oocyte retrieval: A systematic review and meta-analysis. J Assist Reprod Genet 2012; 29:1249–1254.

Setti AS, Paes de Almeida Ferreira Braga D. Twelve years of MSOME and IMSI: a review. Reprod Biomed Online 2013; 27:338–352.

Shaw-Jackson C, Van Beirs N, Thomas AL, Rozenberg S, Autin C. Can healthy babies originate from oocytes with smooth endoplasmic reticulum aggregates? A systematic mini-review. Hum Reprod 2014; 29:1380–1386.

Siristatidis CS, Sertedaki E, Vaidakis D. Metabolomics for improving pregnancy outcomes in women undergoing assisted reproductive technologies. Cochrane Database Syst Rev 2017; 5:CD011872.

Wolff M, Hua YZ, Santi A, Ocon E, Weiss B. Follicle flushing in monofollicular in vitro fertilization almost doubles the number of transferable embryos. Acta Obstet Gynecol Scand 2013; 92:346–348.

Chapter 10 Oocyte donation

Maria Jesus López, Juan José Guillén, Rita Vassena, Amelia Rodriguez Aranda

INDICATIONS FOR USE OF DONATED OOCYTES

The use of donated oocytes was initially indicated for cases of premature ovarian failure or in order to avoid the transmission to the offspring of severe genetic diseases. However, the clinical characteristics of women undergoing assisted reproduction technologies (ART) have changed significantly since the first reported oocyte donation cycle in the 1980s (Lutjen et al. 1984). This change has been brought about by socio-demographic modifications, resulting in women delaying the decision to conceive until an older age. This has resulted in more women reaching menopause without having children, and in an increase in the number of women who want children but have age-related qualitatively diminished ovarian reserve.

According to the European Society of Human Reproduction and Embryology (ESHRE) registry, oocyte donation cycles in Europe have doubled in recent years, from 15,028 in 2007 to 30,198 in 2011 (Kupka et al. 2016). This reflects the use of oocyte donation for various reasons.

Premature ovarian failure or premature ovarian insufficiency

Quantitative ovarian reserve can be predicted to a certain extent by evaluating the three classic ovarian markers: follicle-stimulating hormone (FSH), anti-Müllerian hormone (AMH) and antral follicle count (AFC) (Hsieh et al. 2001, Gomez et al. 2016). In cases of low ovarian response, cancellation rates for in-vitro fertilization (IVF) cycles are higher and the pregnancy and 'take home baby' rates are lower.

Advanced reproductive age

Women's fertility declines progressively with age because of the depletion of the oocyte reserve and poorer oocyte quality. Studies have reported clinical pregnancy rates per initiated cycle, at 7.7%, 5.4% and 1.9% for women aged 42, 43 and 44 years old (Hourvitz et al. 2009), and 8.3% and 5.3% for women aged 43 and 44 years, while 2119 babies were born to mothers over the age of 45 in 2015, according to National Statistics (UK) (Cetinkaya et al. 2013).

Whilst donor oocyte treatment can help, the use of oocyte donation for older women raises ethical issues. Arguments in favor are based on societal practices, gender equality and reproductive freedom. Arguments against are based on the observation that oocyte donation for older women is not 'natural' due to the natural limit in reproductive fitness, and the greater (but unproven) likelihood that children from older patients will suffer parental loss (one or both) before they reach adulthood (American Society for Reproductive Medicine 2013).

Previous failed ART attempts with own oocytes

Treatment failure with a woman's own oocytes has been defined as three unsuccessful IVF cycles, including fresh and frozen embryo transfers (Tan et al. 2005). In these cases, and after ruling out other causes of IVF failure (e.g. severe male factor, male karyotype problems, uterine cavity problems, and thrombophilia), a medical strategy could be to improve oocyte quality through oocyte donation.

Genetic problems

This category of patient comprises women who are carriers, or are affected by a known genetic disease, or have a family history or significant genetic defect. In dominant hereditary diseases, the risk of having affected descendants is 50%. If both parents are carriers of a recessive hereditary disease, the risk of having affected descendants is 25%.

In cases of karyotype alterations (e.g. chromosome translocations or aneuploidies), there can be a higher risk of miscarriage and affected offspring. In these cases, when the genetic cause of the disease is known, preimplantation genetic diagnosis (PGD) can be performed to help select a healthy embryo for transfer (see Chapter 15). However, for PGD to be efficient, a relatively high number of embryos in autologous IVF cycles is needed in order to improve the chances of selecting a healthy embryo. In cases where there is a bad prognosis of PGD or the patient objects to PGD, gamete donation could be considered.

In cases where there is no known mutation but there is a family history of genetic disease, PGD will most likely not be possible, and gamete donation can also be considered to decrease the genetic risk to the offspring.

Gonadal dysgenesis

This is indicated for women whose ovaries have fibrotic stroma and an absence of oocytes, due to alterations in chromosome X (e.g. in Turner syndrome) or an absence of karyotype alterations (e.g. X pure gonadal dysgenesis).

SELECTION CRITERIA FOR POTENTIAL OOCYTE DONORS

Oocyte donors should have a satisfying experience, feel accompanied throughout the process, and complete the donation without medical complications. Meanwhile, the medical center should ensure satisfaction, safety and confidentiality, in strict compliance with the law, and all within the framework of a quality management system.

The first step for selecting an oocyte donor candidate is to inform the woman verbally and in writing about the process, possible side-effects and complications. Once the candidate donor understands, accepts and signs the documentation to continue, selection can begin.

All potential donors should be of legal age, be in good psycho-physical health and sound mind. In Spain and the UK, oocyte donation is allowed between the ages of 18 and 35 years. Candidates must meet certain requirements including phenotypic and psychological characteristics, clinical conditions, and analytical determinations to demonstrate that they do not suffer from genetic, hereditary or infectious diseases which could be transmitted to the recipient or the offspring. These factors must be assessed in accordance with the state of knowledge of science and technology at the time of the donation.

Throughout this section we will analyze the medical tests which should be performed, according to Spanish guidelines, UK law, and guidelines published by the American Society for Reproductive Medicine (ASRM).

Medical interview

Donors should be selected on the basis of their medical history, obtained in a face-to-face interview by a physician. Every effort should be made to identify and select those women who, based on their relevant personal and familial medical history, will not transmit a genetic, hereditary or infectious disease.

Moreover, if the physician discovers any information that may present a risk to the health of the oocyte recipient, or to the future offspring, or to the donor herself, further scrutiny is warranted, such that the donor might need to be excluded. It is also important to remember that all candidates must undergo a psychological evaluation by an accredited professional.

UK guidelines recommend that the ideal oocyte donor has proven fertility and has completed their family (UK guidelines 2008). These criteria are beneficial since such women will already have proven they can produce viable oocytes. However, donors without proven fertility do not provide lower pregnancy rates to a recipient, and hence, applying such restrictive criteria may reduce further an already acute shortage of donors (Faber et al. 1997).

Physical examination

All candidates must first undergo a complete physical and gynecological examination. The latter must include a breast and pelvic examination, cytology and transvaginal ultrasound to exclude gynecological conditions that would contraindicate ovarian stimulation and oocyte collection. There should be an appraisal of the ovarian reserve, to exclude predicted poor responders from the program.

Sexually transmitted infections (STIs) such as a chlamydia, gonorrhea and trichomoniasis should be screened for. Furthermore, a history of acute or chronic pelvic inflammatory disease (PID) may also be grounds for exclusion since PID increases the risk of complications following oocyte collection.

SCREENING TESTS

All donors should undergo basic blood typing, Rhesus (Rh) status, blood count, basic biochemistry, coagulation tests and screening for blood-borne viruses (BBVs). This allows for matching of donors for both blood type and Rh factor. Further screening is performed for rubella, syphilis, human cytomegalovirus (CMV), HIV (anti-HIV 1 and 2), hepatitis B virus (HBsAg and anti-HBc), hepatitis C virus (anti-HCV-Ab), and in certain circumstances HTLV 1 and 2 (HTLV-1 and -2 antibody testing). If any of the BBV tests prove positive and the result is confirmed via a repeat test, then the candidate donor should be excluded from the program, and referred to a specialist for advice and clinical management.

Additional carrier screening for oocyte donors

One of the goals of an oocyte donation program is to protect the child conceived through donation from acquiring a serious heritable disorder. To improve detection of genetic risk beyond the donor's medical history, a genetic carrier screen can be performed to rule out the most prevalent autosomal recessive diseases relating to the donor's ethnicity.

However, this limited approach has two fundamental flaws. Firstly, candidates for oocyte donation might not have data on their ancestors, or the information they provide may be inaccurate. Secondly, there is a worldwide trend toward multiethnic societies, based on the mix of different ethnicities. This makes it increasingly difficult to establish what ethnic group an individual belongs to, and therefore to assign a risk to the individual.

One solution to this is to implement a pan-ethnic, expanded carrier screening test. Current array or sequencing technology allows us to screen simultaneously for thousands of mutations in hundreds of related serious genetic disease genes (Lindheim et al. 2015, Edwards et al. 2015).

According to recent data, most individuals carry at least one mutation associated with a serious genetic disease. It has been calculated that the probability of a couple from the general population having a mutation, leading to the same disease is ~4% (Martin et al 2015). In such circumstances, the risk of having a child affected by a serious genetic disease would be ~1%.

The inclusion of expanded carrier screening in our daily clinical practice aims to detect couples at an increased risk of transmitting a genetic disease to their offspring. For oocyte recipients, this offers the option of assigning a genetically matched and compatible donor, i.e. a donor who will not carry mutations in the same gene as the partner of the couple.

Genetic screening

When deciding what genetic diseases to screen for, certain criteria have been proposed (Grody et al. 2013, Edwards et al. 2015). These state that the disease must:

- Be severe enough to warrant testing for prenatal diagnosis
- Be considered serious enough to cause cognitive deficits, or the need for medical or surgical treatment, or affect the quality of life of the individual in the future
- Have high penetrance and stable expressivity

These currently include diseases in which different mutations cause different phenotypic expressions, e.g. Fragile X syndrome (FXS), or rare diseases (carrier frequency 1:100 to 1:250).

Although being a carrier for an autosomal recessive disease is by no means ground for exclusion from the donation program, a donor found to carry an X-linked disease should be excluded from donating.

All patients and potential donors who are offered expanded carrier screening (ECS) should be informed and advised by a professional before and after its completion (via genetic counseling). Furthermore, they have the right to not be informed of genetic data available after the test. This information is always kept confidential and subject to data protection laws.

In order for ECS to be effective at decreasing the reproductive risk, the male partner of the recipient should also be tested, and a genetic match attempted with a possible donor. All patients must be informed that there is always a residual risk even when the ECS indicates that both individuals are not carriers of any of the tested mutations. The residual risk should be calculated and options discussed to decrease the risk further.

The individual being tested should also understand that being a carrier in one of the alleles of a mutation linked to a genetic autosomal recessive disease does not usually carry any clinical significance, i.e. the person will not develop the disease. In the same way, couples who use donor gametes should understand that donors, just like themselves, might be carriers of autosomal recessive conditions. If the individual or a relative is affected by a specific genetic disease, an ECS should not be the preferred preventive approach. Instead, other tests might be necessary, such as gene sequencing with a family study.

It should be noted that performing an ECS does not replace prenatal diagnostic test or the newborn screening.

Karyotyping

Guidelines from the Spanish Fertility Society (SEF), the UK professional bodies and the ASRM recommend that all donors are screened for chromosomal abnormalities (Matorras & Hernández 2007, Alonso et al 2012 [Spanish guidelines], Association of Biomedical Andrologists, 2008 [UK guidelines], American Society for Reproductive Medicine 2013 [US guidelines]). These recommendations take into account the low frequency of such abnormalities (<1% of the general population) and that only around two people per 1000 have a balanced translocation. Any donor found to have a significant chromosomal abnormality should be excluded from the program and offered genetic counseling.

Cystic fibrosis

Cystic fibrosis (CF) is the most common serious genetic disease among Caucasians, with an autosomal recessive inheritance pattern. The incidence of carriers in northern European populations is about 1 in 25. CF is a multisystemic disorder that affects the digestive tract, sweat glands, reproductive system and respiratory tract.

CF is determined by the presence of one or more mutations in both alleles of a gene located on chromosome 7, called the CF transmembrane conductance regulator (CFTR) gene. CFTR encodes for the CFTR protein, which is responsible for regulating the transport of chloride and sodium ions through the cell membranes of the glandular epithelium. Malfunction of this transport protein causes secretions to have a lower water content, being more viscous, and therefore more difficult to remove.

Spinal muscular atrophy

Spinal muscular atrophy (SMA) is a hereditary neuromuscular disease characterized by progressive symmetrical proximal weakness and atrophy of muscle groups. It is caused by a loss of motor neurons in the spinal cord and brainstem. The autosomal recessive disorder is caused by mutations in the SMN1 (survival of motor neuron 1) gene, while the SMN2 gene is considered to be a genotypic modifier. There are four clinical forms of SMA (type I–IV) distinguished by the pattern of features, severity of symptoms and the age of onset (see **Table 10.1**). The ASRM recommends SMA screening for all prospective donors (American Society for Reproductive Medicine 2013).

Sickle-cell anemia and thalassemia syndromes

Sickle-cell disease (SCD) describes a group of inherited blood disorders, the most common type being sickle-cell anemia (SCA). In SCA, a mutation in the gene for the oxygen-carrying protein hemaglobin A (HbA) results in production of a mutated form, called hemoglobin S (HbS), instead of HbA. Red blood cells containing HbS are rigid and sickle-like in shape (instead of being flexible and disc-shaped). As of 2013, about 3.2 million people have SCD while an additional 43 million have the sickle-cell trait (Global Burden of Disease Study 2013) (**Figure 10.1**).

UK and ASRM guidelines recommend screening for SCA in African, Afro-Caribbean or African-American women, since they have a high prevalence of HbS (SCD) (UK Guidelines 2008, Ethics Committee of the ASRM 2013).

Thalassemias are inherited blood disorders that reduce the production of normal hemoglobin. There are two main types of thalassemia:

1. Alpha thalassemia occurs when a gene or genes related to the alpha globin protein are missing or mutated
2. Beta thalassemia occurs when similar gene defects affect production of the beta globin protein

People with thalassemia have low levels of hemoglobin, leading to a lack of oxygen in many parts of the body. Affected individuals also have a shortage of red blood cells which can cause pale skin, weakness, fatigue, and more serious complications.

Alpha thalassemia occurs most often in people from Southeast Asia, the Middle East, China, and in those of African descent. Beta thalassemia is a fairly common blood disorder worldwide, occurring most frequently in people from Mediterranean countries, North Africa, the Middle East, India, Central and Southeast Asia.

It is recommended that Mediterranean women are screened for beta thalassemia and women from China or South-East Asia for alpha thalassemia, if the mean corpuscular volume of blood count is <80 fL.

Table 10.1 Spinal muscular atrophy: the four clinical forms. Spinal muscular atrophy is a genetic disorder that affects the control of muscle movement and is graded into four types accoridng to severity

Type	Symptoms and onset
I (also called Werdnig-Hoffman disease)	• Severe form • Evident at birth or within the first few months • Affected infants are developmentally delayed • Most are unable to support their head, or sit unassisted • Children have breathing and swallowing problems that may lead to choking or gagging
II	• Characterized by muscle weakness that develops in children between 6 and 12 months • Children can sit without support, but may need help getting to a seated position • Individuals cannot stand or walk unaided
III (also called Kugelberg-Welander disease or juvenile type)	• Milder features • Onset between early childhood and adolescence • Individuals can stand and walk unaided, but walking and climbing stairs may become increasingly difficult • Many affected individuals will require wheelchair assistance later in life
IV	• Onset is usually after 30 years • Mild to moderate muscle weakness, tremor, twitching, or mild breathing problems • Typically, only muscles close to the core, such as the upper arms and legs, are affected

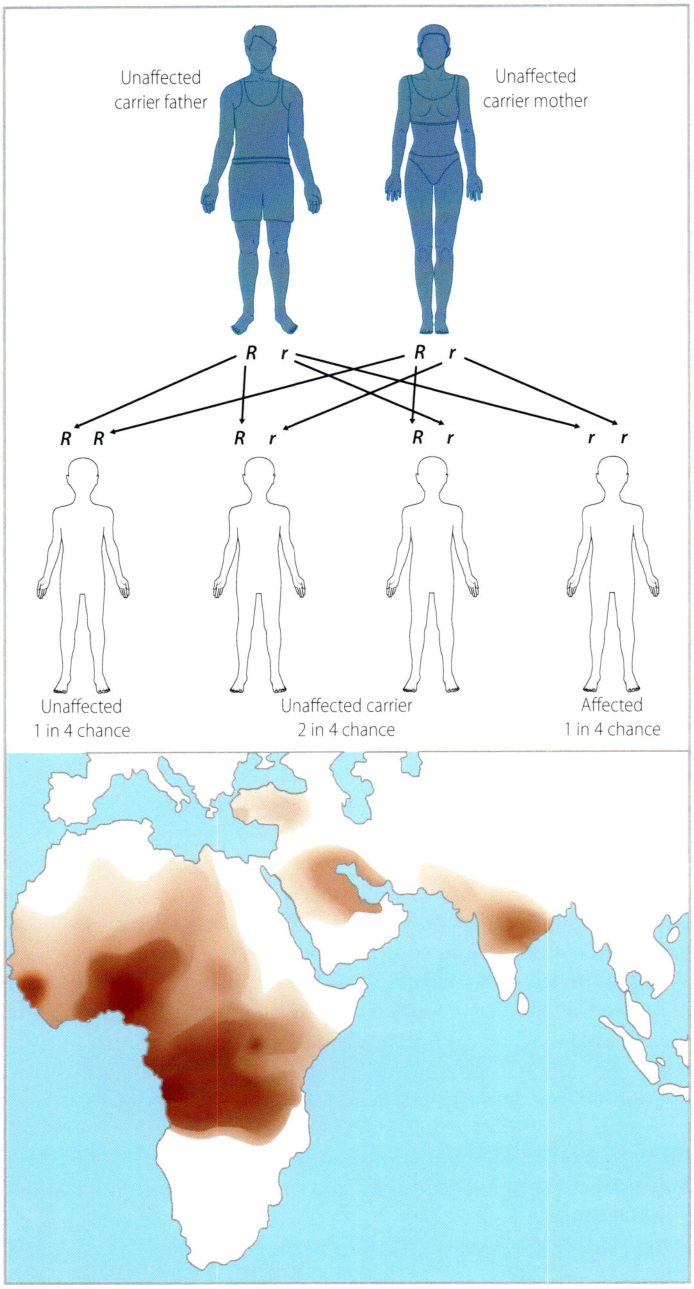

Figure 10.1 Inheritance of sickle cell disease (SCD) is autosomal recessive at a single gene locus. People who are heterozygous are carrier: they carry one allele for normal hemoglobin A (R) and one allele for hemoglobin S (r). They are largely unaffected by SCD but because they produce both types of hemoglobin they may suffer some SCD-related problems. They are said to have the sickle cell trait. If two such unaffected carriers have a child, there is a 1 in 4 chance that the child will be homozygous for HbS (rr). This child would only have HbS and therefore have full SCD. The map shows the African, European and Asian areas with high frequency of sickle cell trait and SCD. The intensity of dark brown color indicates a higher frequency of SCD in that region.

MEAN CORPUSCULAR VOLUME

The mean corpuscular volume (MCV) is a measure of the average number of red blood cells in a specimen of blood. The value is obtained by multiplying blood volume by the percentage of blood that is cellular (i.e. the hematocrit), and dividing this figure by the number of red blood cells in that volume.

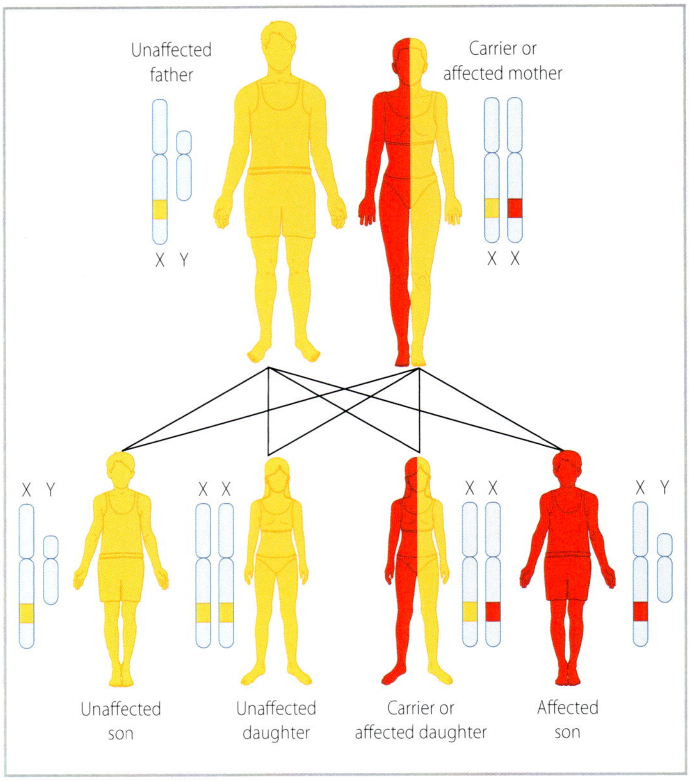

Figure 10.2 A pedigree illustration of X-linked disease inherited from an unaffected carrier female and unaffected male.

Fragile X syndrome

Fragile X syndrome (FXS) is one of the most frequent causes of hereditary mental retardation. However, figures differ according to different studies and some researchers consider the prevalence to be underestimated (Hagerman 2008).

Whilst more males are affected (around 1 in 4000), when X-linked and dominantly transmitted, females are also affected (around 1 in 6000) (**Figure 10.2**).

FXS is caused by a mutation in a single gene, the fragile X mental retardation 1 (*FMR1*) gene. Affected males usually have moderate to severe mental retardation and physical features such as long face, prominent chin, large and winged ears. During childhood, the disease usually manifests itself with attention deficit, hyperactivity, distractibility, impulsiveness, restlessness, over activity and sensory problems. In fact, 40% of women come to show signs of the disease in the form of intellectual disability and facial dysmorphia (see **Table 10.2**).

SAFETY AND COMFORT OF OVARIAN STIMULATION FOR OOCYTE DONORS

Controlled ovarian stimulation (COS) in oocyte donors should maximize donor safety and comfort, whilst guaranteeing good quality oocytes at the time of collection. Since oocyte donors are often young women with a high ovarian reserve, significant efforts have been placed to develop protocols which minimize the risk of early ovarian hyperstimulation syndrome (OHSS) (Bodri et al. 2008).

Two different gonadotropin-releasing hormone (GnRH) analogs are generally used in superovulation IVF cycles: the more recent GnRH antagonist and the classical GnRH agonist (see Chapter 8). GnRH

Table 10.2 Physical features associated with fragile X syndrome

Body area	Feature
Head	Normal structure Broad forehead Elongated face Large prominent ears Strabismus (crossed eyes) Highly arched palate
Arms/hands	Hyperextendible joints Hand calluses (from self-abuse) Pectus excavatum (indentation of chest) Mitral valve prolapse (benign heart condition
Lower abdomen/ upper thighs	Enlarged testicles Hypotonia (low muscle tone) Soft, fleshy skin
Feet	Flat feet

analogues are used in IVF cycles to prevent a luteinizing hormone (LH) surge during COS. The GnRH antagonists appeared on the market in the early 1990s, and have proven to be an effective alternative to GnRH agonists in preventing LH surges. The GnRH agonist is classically introduced in the menstrual cycle preceding the COS, which results in the superovulation phase of the IVF cycle being longer in duration (hence the term 'long protocol'). By contrast, GnRH antagonists are introduced once the COS has started, which has advantages for donor convenience, treatment simplification and less superovulation (hence the term 'short protocol').

GnRH antagonist (short) protocols are often used for oocyte donors. Furthermore, a meta-analysis has shown no significant difference in ongoing pregnancy rate between the GnRH agonist and antagonist cycles in oocyte donation programs (risk ratio [RR] 1.15, 95% confidence interval [CI] 0.97 to 1.36). The duration of stimulation was confirmed to be significantly lower with the GnRH antagonist protocol, and no significant differences were observed in the number or quality of oocytes retrieved (Bodri et al. 2011).

In addition, their use allows the triggering of ovulation with GnRH agonists instead of human chorionic gonadotropin (hCG). This results in a much lower incidence of OHSS, without any drawback for the donor, since her temporary endometrial receptivity state is not an issue in this case. The introduction of this kind of ovulation trigger has shown comparable live birth rates to hCG trigger cycles from oocyte donation (Youssef et al. 2014).

COS for oocyte donation is usually started on the 2nd day of menstruation with daily gonadotropins injections (recombinant FSH or high purified menotropin) or a single dose of long-acting FSH agonist (e.g. corifollitropin alfa). This latter option increases the comfort of the injection schedule for donors. In the first COS cycle, the dose of gonadotropin is usually chosen based on ovarian reserve markers, while in subsequent cycles, it can be modified according to previous ovarian response. The GnRH antagonist can be introduced fixedly on day 7 of stimulation, or alternatively when a follicle of 14 mm in diameter or an estradiol level of 400 pg/mL is observed. The administration of both gonadotropin and GnRH antagonist is continued until the ovulation trigger: the criteria for triggering ovulation can vary, but is usually planned when three or more follicles with a diameter ≥18 mm are observed by transvaginal ultrasound.

Follicular scans during COS can be performed either by three-dimensional (3D) sonography or more classical two-dimensional (2D) sonography. Both are comparable in accuracy and in predicting the number of mature oocytes retrieved. However, 3D sonography allows for shorter exploration times, which translates into higher patient comfort and less operator time. Moreover, 3D sonography provides a higher correlation with the real follicle volume and with the number of expected mature oocytes collected (Rodríguez 2014).

OOCYTE RECIPIENTS

Medical tests

Medical tests should evaluate the recipient's health in order to minimize side-effects of the hormone treatment, obstetric complications in case of pregnancy, and to evaluate the partner's health status (**Table 10.3**). If the recipient is found to be infectious for any test before treatment, she should be referred to an appropriate infectious disease specialist, but positivity should not be used as a criterion for exclusion from reproductive treatment.

In cases of women ≥45 years, an electrocardiogram, a mammography, glycemic level and a medical certification of general good health are recommended. In cases of failure of prior IVF cycles with the recipient's own oocytes, tests such as hysteroscopy to evaluate uterine cavity, and a thrombophilia disease panel are also recommended.

Table 10.3 Health evaluation of oocyte donors and male partner recipients. Medical tests are needed to evaluate the health of both the oocyte donor and the recipient, in order to minimize side-effects of the hormone treatment, obstetric complications in case of pregnancy, and to evaluate the recipient partner's health status

Test	Reason
Gynecological evaluation, cervical smear, transvaginal pelvic ultrasound	To rule out gynecological diseases and syphilis
Full blood screen, including liver function and coagulation tests	To rule out hereditary anemias (e.g. thalassemia or sickle cells anemia)
Blood type, Rhesus factor	To match it with donor and partner's blood group
Indirect Coombs test	In case of Rh negative, to minimize and prevent the risk of hemolytic fetal anemia
Rubella	In case of negative rubella antibodies, recipients should be offered immunization to avoid infection during pregnancy
Cytomegalovirus (CMV)	To rule out the current infection of CMV; if positive, it is recommended that treatment is postponed
Treponema	If positive, penicillin treatment would be indicated if the infection had not been treated before
p24 antigen	To address potential medical or legal complications if the recipients seroconverts during or after the ART treatment
Blood-borne viruses (HIV, hepatitis B & C)	To ensure no transmission of any infection between the donor and recipient.

Semen analysis is needed to evaluate sperm parameters and rule out a severe male factor. In cases of failure of prior IVF autologs cycles of the recipient, a male karyotype test can also be considered.

Endometrial preparation in the oocyte recipient

To optimize pregnancy rates, the embryo and the endometrium should be synchronized. There are two options to achieve this synchronization: (1) exogenous hormone therapy can be used to create an 'artificial endometrial cycle'; or, (2) endogenous hormone production from developing follicles can be used in a 'natural or modified natural cycle'.

An artificial endometrial cycle

The artificial endometrial cycle consists of three steps:

1. **Hypophysis desensitization**
   This is usually produced by GnRH agonists. There are different drugs and manners of administration [e.g. triptorelin 3 mg or 3.75 mg intramuscularly (IM); or leuprorelin 3.75 mg IM or subcutaneous (SC); or goserelin 3.6 mg SC]. This phase is necessary if the recipient has menstrual cycles (regular or irregular). In case of regular cycles, the GnRH agonist should be administered in the middle of the luteal phase; in cases of irregular cycles, oral contraceptive pills are recommended to control the cycle and allow GnRH agonist administration in the correct moment. In cases of recipients whom have experienced at least 12 months of amenorrhea, its administration is not necessary.
2. **Estrogen treatment prior to donor oocyte retrieval**
   The estrogen phase is based on the administration of estrogens to thicken the endometrium. It starts on the onset of menstruation after hypophysis desensitization. Estrogen can be administered through different routes:
   - Orally with either an increasing (2 mg/day from day 1 to day 4, 4 mg/day from day 5 to day 9, 6 mg/day from the day 10) or a constant dose (6 mg/day)
   - Transdermally with an increasing (75 μg every 3 days for the 1st week and 150 μg every 3 days from the 2nd week) or a constant dose (150 μg per 3 days) from the beginning.

   There are no differences concerning reproductive outcomes in the recipient with either administration routes or dose protocols (Madero et al. 2016).
3. **Estrogen and progesterone treatment after donor oocyte retrieval**
   Progesterone is the natural hormone produced by the corpus luteum that helps to prepare the endometrium for embryo implantation and the maintenance of pregnancy. Thereafter, the trophoblast increases progesterone production, becoming its main source after the 12th week of pregnancy.

   Due to GnRH agonist action, there is no functioning corpus luteum during exogenous hormone therapy for endometrium preparation, so there is a luteal progesterone deficiency. Since progesterone supplementation has an important impact success, progesterone is started on the oocyte retrieval day in the 80% of centers and 15% on the day of embryo transfer (Vaisbuch et al. 2014). The introduction of progesterone supplementation before oocyte retrieval has been shown to decrease the success rate (Sohn et al. 1999).

   Several routes for progesterone administration are used: intramuscular injection, vaginal pessaries or creams, oral pills and more recently subcutaneous injections. In 77% of cases, vaginal progesterone is used and in the remaining cases oral or intramuscular progesterone are used (Vaisbuch et al. 2014).

   The most commonly used dose for intramuscular progesterone is 50–100 mg/day, while vaginal and oral doses are 400–600 mg/day; doses lower than 300 mg/day are inferior in efficacy to intramuscular progesterone (Smitz et al. 1992); vaginal gels are applied once or twice per day (Dal Prato et al. 2008), and the subcutaneous dosage is one injection of 25 mg/day. The choice of progesterone supplementation should be based on patient convenience and availability, since no differences in the ability of supporting the luteal phase have been shown among different routes of administration (Yanushpolsky 2015).

   There are still limited data and little consensus on the necessary duration for progesterone supplementation in early pregnancy, beyond first positive pregnancy test. A meta-analysis has indicated that progesterone supplementation beyond the first positive hCG test after IVF/ICSI might generally be unnecessary (Liu et al. 2012). However, large prospective randomized trials are still needed in order to settle the issue of duration of progesterone support in early IVF pregnancies. In most cases, progesterone supplementation is continued up to 8–12 weeks of gestation, possibly due to patient's and doctor's anxiety (Vaisbuch et al. 2014).

Natural or modified natural cycle

In this type of cycle, endometrial preparation is achieved by taking advantage of endogenous hormone production from the developing follicle. Fertilization of the donated oocytes is carried out when the spontaneous LH surge is detected in the recipient, or after administering hCG to initiate luteinization. To carry out this protocol, follicular development in the recipient is monitored every 2–3 days from day 7–8 of the menstrual cycle. In each one, estradiol, LH and progesterone levels have to be tested and an ultrasound scan has to be performed to measure the follicle size.

When a follicle of 17 mm in diameter is achieved, or when a LH surge is naturally started, hCG is administered. Two days later, IVF/ICSI is performed on the donated oocytes. Where a natural LH surge is utilized, it is important to control hormones daily in order to identify the LH surge and time exactly the day of fertilization. When transferring embryos from donated oocytes to a recipient during a natural cycle, the luteal support can be optional, since the ovarian progesterone production is not compromised by the COS.

When considering a natural cycle for oocyte reception, it can be difficult to synchronize the timing of the donor's oocyte retrieval with the recipient's LH surge. Thus, this type of protocol is practically feasible only if cryopreserved donor oocytes are used, or cryopreserved embryos using donated oocytes. Recently, a randomized controlled trial (RCT) has indicated that reproductive outcomes are the same regardless of endometrial preparation protocol (Groenewoud et al. 2016).

The choice of endometrium preparation will depend on the recipient's availability, her menstrual cycle pattern and presence, and how well the recipient tolerates hormonal treatment. Moreover, the clinic's access to banked oocytes will greatly influence the timing and flexibility of treatment.

OBSTETRICAL RISKS IN OOCYTE RECIPIENTS

Pregnancy complications increase with maternal age, even when women are known to be healthy. Advanced maternal age is related to an increased risk of a variety of adverse pregnancy outcomes which are independent of body mass index (BMI), parity and socioeconomic status (Kenny et al. 2013). Furthermore, an increased incidence of pathologies has been reported for oocyte recipients compared to women who conceive naturally or via ART with their own oocytes, including gestational diabetes, hypertensive disorders, placental abnormalities and pre-term delivery (Sheffer-Mimouni et al. 2002).

For oocyte recipients, the most frequently observed obstetric complication is bleeding in the 1st and 2nd trimester, which is associated with adverse fetal outcomes even when of short duration (Sheffer-Mimouni et al. 2002).

Additional obstetric complications are hypertensive disorders such as chronic hypertension, gestational hypertension, pre-eclampsia, severe pre-eclampsia and eclampsia. Despite the multifactorial pathophysiology, recent reports support the hypothesis that hypertensive disorders may result from altered or inadequate immune-protection of the fetoplacental unit, due to the immunologically unrelated embryo which originated from a donor oocyte (Gundogan et al. 2010, van der Hoorn et al. 2011). Its prevalence in women after oocyte donation is 2.5-fold higher than in women who spontaneously conceive (Elenis et al. 2015) with the difference mainly observed for severe forms: pre-eclampsia and eclampsia. In a multivariate analysis, the only variables significantly associated with hypertensive disorders risk were oocyte donation and woman's age (Letur et al. 2016).

Moreover, a recent systematic review observed oocyte donation is a risk factor for the development of pre-eclampsia compared to autologous oocyte cycles (with a weighted OR of 3.12) and neither multiple pregnancies nor patient age significantly explained the variability of the effect of oocyte donation on pre-eclampsia (Blazquez et al. 2016).

The incidence of gestational diabetes is reported to be 3% in non-donor conceptions (Xiong et al. 2001). However, this incidence has been shown to rise almost ten-fold to 24% for oocyte recipients, regardless of maternal age, and with many requiring insulin for adequate glycemic control (Sheffer-Mimouni et al. 2002).

In addition, non-emergency cesarean section is performed more often for oocyte recipients (55%) versus pregnant women with autologous oocytes (26%) (Elenis et al. 2015). As a consequence, adverse perinatal outcomes are associated with these pathologies and a greater rate of admissions to the neonatal intensive care unit.

Oocyte recipients and medical staff should be aware of these increased risks. Counseling should be given to make potential recipients aware of the possible obstetric complications so they can be prepared for them.

INTERNATIONAL LEGISLATION AND LEGAL FRAMEWORK

Oocyte donation seems to be the ART with the most heterogeneous regulation, not only globally, but also between neighboring or culturally similar countries. Differences relate to religious, social and economic history.

Some countries forbid oocyte donation, whilst others regulate practice in two different ways: either by guidelines (proposed by professional or scientific organizations, which set rules to be followed by practitioners) or by laws.

An example of guidelines comes from the UK, where several professional bodies from reproductive science came together to create national guidelines for the medical and laboratory screening of sperm, egg and embryo donors (UK guidelines, 2008). At the time of writing these guidelines are being updated, with a revised version due to be published in 2019.

An example of law came from the European Parliament and the European Council who published three Directives between 2004 and 2006, establishing quality standards and safety requirements to be transferred to the member states legislation where gamete donation is allowed. These are commonly known as the European Union Tissues and Cells Directives (EUTCDs).

The objectives of the EUTCDs were to:

- Unify criteria, due to the diversity of standards in handling human tissues in different member states
- Promote the implementation of quality systems and safety regarding the transmission of infectious diseases
- Improve traceability and accurate identification of samples

In Europe, the legality of oocyte donation continues to differ greatly between countries (**Table 10.4**).

Table 10.4 Examples of international differences in the legality of oocyte donation (correct at the time of writing, but note these may change due to the dynamic nature of the law in this area)

Banned	Legally permitted and regulated	Carried out without a legal framework
Germany	Spain	Poland
Austria	Czech Republic	India
Switzerland	Belgium	
Italy	Greece	
Japan	France (if anonymous and no compensation paid)	
	UK	
	Slovakia	
	Denmark	
	Canada (if non-anonymous and no compensation paid)	
	USA	
	South Africa	

ALTRUISM, COMPLIANCE AND CONFIDENTIALITY

The three ethical pillars on which oocyte donation can be considered to be based are altruism, compliance and confidentiality.

Altruism

The European Parliament in Article 12 of 2004/23/EC states that: 'Donors may receive compensation strictly limited to expenses and inconveniences related to the donation. In that case, member states define the conditions under which compensation may be granted.'

This compensation is designed to cover any financial losses reasonably incurred by the donor in connection with her donation and the inconvenience to which she will be subjected during the process. In the UK, an oocyte donor can receive compensation of up to £750 for each donation cycle, with the possibility of claiming additional expenses to cover incidental expenses (e.g. travel, accommodation, and childcare) provided the donor is a permanent UK resident.

In Spain, a similar level of compensation has been agreed up to 1000€. A donor cannot request a price per donated oocyte, and no difference in compensation is warranted based on the number of oocytes that are collected.

Compliance

It is strongly recommended that the terms of an oocyte donation are formalized in writing by a legally binding document between the donor and the authorized center. Before signing, the donor must be informed of the purposes and consequences of the contract, and also be fully informed about all aspects of the process.

Confidentiality

The European Parliament 2004/23/EC, Article 14, Item 3 states: 'Member States shall take all necessary measures to ensure that the identity of the recipient to the donor or his family and vice versa is not disclosed, subject to the legislation force in member states on the conditions for communication of information, particularly in the case of gamete donation.'

In Spain, gamete donation is completely anonymous, so that both the recipient and the child born from the donation may only have general information about the donor. By contrast, in the UK, the Human Fertilisation and Embryology Authority (HFEA) removed the donor anonymity clause in June 2004. As a result, an oocyte recipient can still request at any time to receive some general non-identifying information about the donor. However, since 31st March 2005, when the donor-conceived offspring reaches the age of 16 years, that person can apply to the HFEA to receive all the non-identifying information that the donor provided at the time of donation. At the age of 18 years, that person can further apply to the HFEA to find all the information provided, including identifying information such as name and surname of the donor, the date of birth and district in which they were born, the appearance, National Health Service (NHS) number and the last-known address. Other European countries, for example, Finland and Sweden have also banned anonymous gamete donation (**Table 10.5**).

Table 10.5 Examples of international differences, regarding anonymity of oocyte donation. (Correct at the time of writing, but note these may change due to the dynamic nature of the law in this area)

Anonymous	Nonanonymous	Both
Spain	UK	US
France	Sweden	Denmark
	Finland	
	Canada	

Number of children born from one donor

A number of European countries have limits. For example, the maximum authorized number of children born in Spain that have been generated with gametes from the same donor is six. In the UK, there is a maximum limit of 10 families that can be formed from the oocytes from a single donor, rather than the number of children.

Whilst donors have the right to perform any number of donations, this is restricted by clinicians for health reasons.

CONCLUSION

This chapter has provided an overview of how donated oocytes may be used in ART, including their indications for use. Whilst different legislations exist in different countries around this area of fertility treatment, the medical side of the treatment remains consistent to optimise success.

For oocyte donors, the selection criteria, screening methods and ovarian stimulation regime have been described. For oocyte recipients, the pre-treatment medical tests and ways in which the endometrium can be prepared to receive embryos created from donor oocytes have been covered. While oocyte donation treatment can have high success rates, it is important that recipients are always made aware of the obstetric risks with this type of treatment.

REFERENCES

Alonso J, Boada M, Bou C, Gómez MJ, Gris JM, Ramírez JP. Recommendations for the application of RD 1301/2006. Paper prepared by the joint working group of the Spanish Fertility Society (SEF) and the Association for the Study of Reproductive Biology (ASEBIR) for the analysis of RD 1301/2006. Madrid: Spanish Fertility Society, 2012.

American Society for Reproductive Medicine (Ethics Committee). Oocyte or embryo donation to women of advanced age: a committee opinion. Fertil Steril 2013; 100:337–340.

Association of Biomedical Andrologists, Association of Clinical Embryologists, British Andrology Society, British Fertility Society, Royal College of Obstetricians and Gynaecologists. UK guidelines for the medical and laboratory screening of sperm, egg and embryo donors. Hum Fertil (Camb) 2008; 11:201–210.

Blazquez A, Garcia D, Rodriguez A, et al. Is oocyte donation a risk factor for preeclampsia? A systematic review and meta-analysis. J Assist Reprod Genet 2016; 33:855–863.

Bodri D, Sunkara SK, Coomarasamy A. Gonadotropin-releasing hormone agonists versus antagonists for controlled ovarian hyperstimulation in oocyte donors: a systematic review and meta-analysis. Fertil Steril 2011; 95:164–169.

Bodri D, Guillen JJ, Polo A, et al. Complications related to ovarian stimulation and oocyte retrieval in 4052 oocyte donor cycles. Reprod Biomed Online 2008; 17:237–243.

Cetinkaya MB, Siano LJ, Benadiva C, et al. Reproductive outcome of women 43 years and beyond undergoing ART treatment with their own oocytes in two Connecticut university programs. J Assist Reprod Genet 2013; 30:673–678.

Dal Prato L, Bianchi L, Cattoli M, et al. Vaginal gel versus intramuscular progesterone for luteal phase supplementation: a prospective randomized trial. Reprod Biomed Online 2008; 16:361–367.

Edwards JG, Feldman G, Goldberg J, et al. Expanded carrier screening in reproductive medicine-points to consider: a joint statement of the American College of Medical Genetics and Genomics, American College of Obstetricians and Gynecologists, National Society of Genetic Counselors, Perinatal Quality Foundation, and Society for Maternal-Fetal Medicine. Obstet Gynecol 2015; 125:653–662.

Elenis E, Svanberg AS, Lampic C, et al. Adverse obstetric outcomes in pregnancies resulting from oocyte donation: a retrospective cohort case study in Sweden. BMC Pregnancy Childbirth 2015; 15:247.

Faber BM, Mercan R, Hamacher P, et al. The impact of an egg donor's age and her prior fertility on recipient pregnancy outcome. Fertil Steril 1997; 68:370–372.

Global Burden of Disease Study 2013 Collaborators. Global, regional, and national incidence, prevalence, and years lived with disability for 301 acute and chronic diseases and injuries in 188 countries, 1990-2013: a systematic analysis for the Global Burden of Disease Study 2013. Lancet 2015; 386:743–800.

Gomez R, Schorsch M, Hahn T, et al. The influence of AMH on IVF success. Arch Gynecol Obstet 2016; 293:667–673.

Grody WW, Thompson BH, Gregg AR, et al. ACMG position statement on prenatal/preconception expanded carrier screening. Genet Med 2013; 15:482–483.

Groenewoud ER, Cohlen BJ, Al-Oraiby A, et al. A randomized controlled, non-inferiority trial of modified natural versus artificial cycle for cryo-thawed embryo transfer. Hum Reprod 2016; 31:1483–1492.
Gundogan F, Bianchi DW, Scherjon SA, Roberts DJ. Placental pathology in egg donor pregnancies. Fertil Steril 2010; 93:397–404.
Hagerman PJ. The fragile X prevalence paradox. J Med Genet 2008; 45:498–499.
Hourvitz A, Machtinger R, Maman E, et al. Assisted reproduction in women over 40 years of age: how old is too old? Reprod Biomed Online 2009; 19:599–603.
Hsieh YY, Chang CC, Tsai HD. Antral follicle counting in predicting the retrieved oocyte number after ovarian hyperstimulation. J Assist Reprod Genet 2001; 18:320–324.
Kenny LC, Lavender T, McNamee R, et al. Advanced maternal age and adverse pregnancy outcome: evidence from a large contemporary cohort. PLoS One 2013; 8:e56583.
Kupka MS, D'Hooghe T, Ferraretti AP, et al. Assisted reproductive technology in Europe, 2011: results generated from European registers by ESHRE. Hum Reprod 2016; 31:233–248.
Letur H, Peigne M, Ohl J, et al. Hypertensive pathologies and egg donation pregnancies: Results of a large comparative cohort study. Fertil Steril 2016; 106:284–290.
Lindheim SR, Jaeger AS. Expanded preconception carrier screening in clinical practice: cutting the Gordian Knot. Fertil Steril 2015; 104:281–282.
Liu XR, Mu HQ, Shi Q, et al. The optimal duration of progesterone supplementation in pregnant women after IVF/ICSI: a meta-analysis. Reprod Biol Endocrinol 2012; 10:107.
Lutjen P, Trounson A, Leeton J, et al. The establishment and maintenance of pregnancy using in vitro fertilization and embryo donation in a patient with primary ovarian failure. Nature 1984; 307:174–175.
Madero S, Rodriguez A, Vassena R, Vernaeve V. Endometrial preparation: effect of estrogen dose and administration route on reproductive outcomes in oocyte donation cycles with fresh embryo transfer. Hum Reprod 2016; 31:1755–1764.
Martin J, Asan, Yi Y, et al. Comprehensive carrier genetic test using next-generation deoxyribonucleic acid sequencing in infertile couples wishing to conceive through assisted reproductive technology. Fertil Steril 2015; 104:1286–1293.
Matorras R, Hernández J (eds). Guidelines. Study and treatment of the sterile couple: Recommendations of the Spanish Fertility Society, with the collaboration of the Spanish Association for the Study of Reproductive Biology, Spanish Association of Andrology and the Spanish Society of Contraception. Madrid: Spanish Fertility Society, 2007.
Rodríguez A. Learning curves in 3-dimensional sonographic follicle monitoring during controlled ovarian stimulation. J Ultrasound Med 2014; 33:649–655.
Sheffer-Mimouni G, Mashiach S, Dor J, et al, Factors influencing the obstetric and perinatal outcome after oocyte donation. Hum Reprod 2002; 17:2636–2640.
Smitz J, Devroey P, Faguer B et al. A prospective randomized comparison of intramuscular or intravaginal natural progesterone as a luteal phase and early pregnancy supplement. Hum Reprod 1992; 7:168–175.
Sohn SH, Penzias AS, Emmi AM, et al. Administration of progesterone before oocyte retrieval negatively affects the implantation rate. Fertil Steril 1999; 71:11–14.
Vaisbuch E, de Ziegler D, Leong M, et al. Luteal-phase support in assisted reproduction treatment: real-life practices reported worldwide by an updated website-based survey. Reprod Biomed Online 2014; 28:330–335.
van der Hoorn ML, Scherjon SA, Claas FH. Egg donation pregnancy as an immunological model for solid organ transplantation. Transpl Immunol 2011; 25:89–95.
Xiong X, Saunders LD, Wang FL, et al. Gestational diabetes mellitus: prevalence, risk factors, maternal and infant outcomes. Int J Gynaecol Obstet 2001; 75:221–228.
Yanushpolsky EH. Luteal phase support in in vitro fertilization. Semin Reprod Med 2015; 33:118–127.
Youssef MA, Van der Veen F, Al-Inany HG, et al. Gonadotropin-releasing hormone agonist versus HCG for oocyte triggering in antagonist-assisted reproductive technology. Cochrane Database Syst Rev 2014; CD008046.
Tan BK, Vandekerckhove P, Kennedy R, et al. Investigation and current management of recurrent IVF treatment failure in the UK. BJOG 2005; 112:773–780.

Chapter 11 Implantation

Mariano Mascarenhas, Mohan S Kamath, Sesh Kamal Sunkara

INTRODUCTION

Embryo implantation is a complex process involving maternal hormonal changes, immune responses and maturational events in the embryo. Successful implantation entails synchronized events between a receptive endometrium and a competent embryo. A pregnancy could fail when the events are not coordinated.

There are several factors that can lead to failed implantation. Until recently, there has been less emphasis on the biological processes involved in human embryo implantation. Researchers have endeavored to unravel the key aspects of implantation by studying the various endometrial, immunological, genomic and embryological facets. Although assisted reproductive technologies (ARTs) have aided our understanding of human implantation to a certain extent, there remain areas which are not yet fully understood. This chapter details the various facets of embryo implantation.

Implantation of the embryo into the endometrium is an essential step for a successful pregnancy. Implantation is defined as the process by which the embryonic trophoblast adheres to the uterine endometrium. A detailed understanding of the pathophysiological processes during implantation is essential to understand the pathway to a successful conception and also, improve the outcome of fertility treatment. Most of the knowledge on implantation in human embryos is derived from studies on animal models.

STAGES OF IMPLANTATION

Implantation involves three sequential stages - apposition, adhesion and invasion (Tabibzadeh & Babaknia 1995) (**Figure 11.1**).

Apposition

The initial phase of apposition occurs approximately at day 5-6 postovulation when the blastocyst enters the uterine environment and hatching from the zona pellucida (ZP) takes place. During this phase, there is progesterone-dependent expression of pinopodes on the endometrial cells which actively reabsorb the secretory fluid. The plasma membrane of the hatched embryonic trophoblast cells makes initial contact with the apical plasma membrane of the surface epithelial cells.

Adhesion

Subsequently, the stage of adhesion takes place at day 6-7 postovulation and involves the formation of a specialized sub-membranous filamentous network consisting of integrins, testin/trophinin, proteoglycans, cadherins, lectin/glycan, and glycan/glycan interactions. This filamentous network causes sufficiently strong binding of the embryo to the endometrium to resist dislodging by uterine flushing.

Invasion

The next stage of implantation occurs between days 7 and 12 postovulation. The invasion stage involves penetration of the embryonic syncytiotrophoblast between the endometrial surface epithelial cells leading to loss of interepithelial cell junctions and formation of cell junctions between the trophoblast and the epithelial cells.

The process of implantation is not just mechanical, whereby the embryo acts as an intruder into the decidualized endometrium, but it is

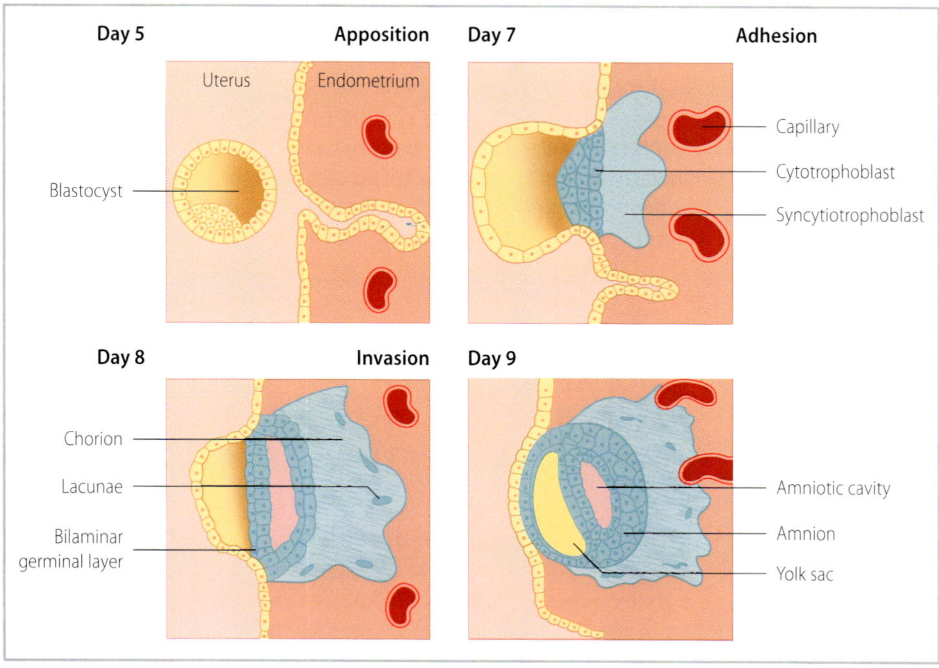

Figure 11.1 Events during apposition (day 5), adhesion (day 7) and final implantation (invasion) of a blastocyst into the endometrial stroma (day 8 and 9).

also a complex interplay of maternal and embryonic factors which regulates the extent and degree of trophoblast invasion. In addition to the embryo and the endometrial cells, the cumulus cells (Benkhalifa et al. 2012) appear to play a role in implantation by being an important source of prostaglandins and angiogenesis factors at the site of implantation.

HORMONAL FACTORS AND THE ROLE OF CYTOKINES

The human endometrium is a highly dynamic structure with a wide spectrum of stage-specific gene expression. The endometrial changes during the menstrual cycle are driven primarily by the fluctuations of the steroid hormones - estrogen and progesterone.

In addition to estrogen and progesterone receptors, the endometrium also expresses androgen receptors and there is some evidence that androgens also play a role in endometrial maturation.

Window of implantation

The timing of the onset of ovulation and the subsequent hormonal changes are key steps to ensure synchronicity of oocyte-embryonic development and endometrial maturation. The endometrium is only receptive to implantation of a viable blastocyst for a short time-span during the menstrual cycle. This period of endometrial receptivity, also known as the 'window of implantation' (WOI), usually starts between day 6–8 postovulation and lasts for 4 days.

The process of implantation involves a wide array of cytokines and growth factors acting in an autocrine and paracrine fashion. Of these, the interleukin (IL) systems (IL-1, IL-11, IL-15), leukemia inhibitory factor (LIF), members of the transforming growth factor (TGF)-β superfamily and the colony-stimulating factors (CSFs) have been the most studied. These cytokines appear to be highly interconnected and have similar and overlapping functions, making the development of specialized therapeutic targeting difficult (Dimitriadis et al. 2005).

Furthermore, it is well established that progesterone, secreted by the corpus luteum, helps to prepare the endometrium for implantation.

In ART, due to down-regulation of the pituitary, progesterone levels may remain low. To support endometrial proliferation to aid implantation, patients can supplement cycles with progesterone (oral, vaginal or intramuscular), or the hormone human chorionic gonadotrophin (hCG), or gonadotropin-releasing hormone (GnRH) agonists (van der Linden et al. 2015).

THE IMMUNE SYSTEM

The immune system also plays a major role in the process of implantation to facilitate the tolerance of the 'foreign' embryonic antigen by the 'native' maternal immune system. The human leukocyte antigen (HLA) compatibility system appears to mediate this immune interaction, with the major players being the extraembryonic trophoblastic cells and the uterine natural killer (uNK) cells.

The embryonic trophoblastic cells appear to express a unique combination of HLA-C, HLA-E and HLA-G molecules. The uNK cells in the endometrium show a different phenotype on cluster differential (CD) stains to the NK cells in the peripheral vascular system with a $CD56_{bright}$, $CD16^-$, $CD3^-$ phenotype and appear to be functionally unique.

The uNK cells, unlike their counterparts in the peripheral vascular system, have lost their cytotoxic effect. This differentiation appears to be mediated by IL-5, secreted by the dendritic cells, and TGF-β1, secreted by the macrophages in the endometrium.

> **TRANSFORMING GROWTH FACTOR BETA**
>
> Transforming growth factor beta 1 (TGF-β1) is a polypeptide member of the transforming growth factor beta superfamily of cytokines. It is a secreted protein that performs many cellular functions, including the control of cell growth, cell proliferation, cell differentiation and apoptosis.

The uNK cells appear to play a role not only in regulating implantation, but also in trophoblast invasion, remodelling of the spiral arteries and placental development. Therefore, the mechanisms involved in immune tolerance play a vital role in acceptance of the fetal graft and the continuation of a successful pregnancy (Croy et al. 2003).

IMPLANTATION AND NATURAL SELECTION

The endometrium plays a role not only in recognizing and allowing growth of a normal embryo, but also in preventing the implantation of abnormal embryos. Derangements of this selective mechanism have been hypothesized to cause the 'super-fertility' seen in women with recurrent miscarriages. In these events, implantation of genetically abnormal embryos occurs, leading to first trimester miscarriages (Teklenburg et al. 2010).

Implantation involves a complex interplay of embryonic and endometrial cross-talk and any of the factors listed below can cause a derangement of this delicately controlled process.

RECURRENT IMPLANTATION FAILURE

Recurrent implantation failure (RIF) is an important cause of repeated in vitro fertilization (IVF) failure. It is estimated that approximately 10% of women seeking IVF treatment will experience this particular problem (Coughlan et al. 2014).

RIF is usually suspected when there has been a failure to reach the stage of a sonographically detectable pregnancy despite multiple attempts at ART. However, there is much debate among experts as to the number, quality and stage of development of embryos transferred and the number of embryo transfer (ET) attempts that must have occurred before a diagnosis of RIF can be made and investigations initiated. A recent review has analyzed this debate and suggested that RIF should be diagnosed when there has been a failure to reach a clinical pregnancy after the ET of at least four good-quality embryos in three ET cycles (fresh or frozen) in a woman under 40 years (Coughlan et al. 2015).

Etiology

Embryonic aspects

Embryonic aspects which can cause implantation failure can be broadly categorized as embryonic genetic aneuploidy, oocyte quality, and sperm quality.

Embryonic genetic aneuploidy

The process of implantation appears to fulfil a role in natural selection, by selecting only normal embryos and de-selecting nonviable embryos. ET at the blastocyst stage appears to improve implantation rates by providing an improved mode of embryo selection. This is also brought out by studies utilizing preimplantation screening (PGS) which show a significantly higher proportion of chromosomally abnormal embryos in couples with recurrent implantation failure than in controls (Rubio et al. 2013).

In addition, implantation rates appear to reduce with increased maternal age, again pointing to the role of embryonic genetic aneuploidy. When embryos are genetically screened using PGS, the implantation rates appear to improve significantly. Franasiak and collegues (2014), reported a predictable increase in aneuploidy after 26 years of age. They observed a rate of >40% aneuploidy in women 23 years and under, while the 'no euploid embryo rate' was up to 6% in women aged 26–37 years, 33% at age 42 years, and 53% at age 44 years. However, the implantation rate does not approach 100% even with ET of only euploid blastocysts. This indicates that factors other than genetic aneuploidy are required for successful implantation.

Oocyte quality

Increased maternal age is correlated with an increased risk of chromosomal nondisjunction in the oocytes, leading to a reduction in implantation rate. The high dose of gonadotropins used during ovarian stimulation for ART has been suggested to have an impact on implantation via detrimental effects on both oocyte quality and the developing endometrium (Collins 2009). A poorly developed endometrium with a high progesterone value on the day of egg collection can contribute to implantation failure. To overcome this situation, some clinics follow the 'freeze-all strategy', whereby all embryos are cryopreserved, and an ET of a warmed/cryopreserved embryo then takes place in a subsequent cycle. This freeze-all strategy has reported encouraging results to date (Blockeel et al. 2016).

The oocyte is the sole source of mitochondria for the embryo and defects in either the number or activity of this mitochondrial complement is also suggested to reduce implantation (Fragouli et al. 2015).

An interesting observation appears to be a role of cumulus cells in implantation as suggested by a trial where co-culture of embryos with cumulus cells appeared to be helpful in RIF patients (Benkhalifa et al. 2012).

Sperm quality

The main contribution of the sperm to the embryo is its DNA. Sperm DNA damage can be induced through excess reactive oxygen species generation. This may be due to poor lifestyle issues such as smoking, infection of the genital tract, varicocele or a defective antioxidant system. Some researchers have suggested that an increased DNA fragmentation index (DFI) impairs fertilization and compromises embryonic viability. This then leads to implantation failure or increased rates of early miscarriage (Zhang et al. 2013).

Strategies such as preferentially using surgically-retrieved testicular sperm (which could have a lower DFI), or improving methods of sperm selection through higher magnification or use of hyaluronic acid expression, have yet to be established (Coughlan et al. 2015).

Infertile men with evidence of exposure to pollutants may benefit from sperm DNA testing as it may help reinforce the importance of lifestyle modifications (e.g. quitting cigarette smoking) (Agarwal et al. 2016). However, the value of DFI in predicting implantation failure remains controversial (Osman et al. 2015) and any meaningful use of DFI as a diagnostic workup needs to be treated with caution.

Endometrial aspects

Altered sex steroids

As noted above, the endometrium is only receptive to the embryo in the WOI. Any disturbance in this WOI can lead to disruption of the delicate and time-dependent cross-talk between the embryo and the endometrium. Endometrial maturation is highly dependent on the cyclic fluctuations of estrogen and progesterone. Ovarian stimulation with gonadotropins leads to supraphysiological levels of estrogen and premature rise of progesterone leading to a premature advancement in the stages of endometrial maturation. This can shorten and displace the WOI, leading to embryo-endometrial dyssynchrony and implantation failure. The effect is especially marked when the progesterone levels on the day of ovulation trigger are >1.5 ng/mL (Mascarenhas et al. 2015). At a cellular level, changes in the timing of endometrial pinopode expression and alterations in genetic expression for cytokine and paracrine molecules and surface receptors can have a detrimental effect on implantation (Fatemi & Popovic-Todorovic 2013).

Thrombophilias

The embryo is dependent on the endometrium for its nutrition, leading to an interest in the role of endometrial blood flow on implantation. Thrombophilias are a particular attractive therapeutic target for improving implantation rates, but the link between thrombophilias and implantation failures have thus far proved elusive. Antiphospholipid syndrome has been shown to increase the risk of first trimester miscarriage, but this could be due to mechanisms other than the increased risk of thrombosis. Such mechanisms could include alterations in the complement mechanism and effects on trophoblast differentiation and invasion. Inherited thrombophilias on the other hand, have not been conclusively linked to implantation failure or first trimester miscarriages (RCOG SAC Opinion 2011).

Immunological aspects

An aberrant maternal immune response at the embryo-endometrial interface leading to a rejection of the fetal graft has been proposed as a hypothesis to explain implantation failure. Alteration in systemic cytokines and T-helper cell type 1: type 2 ratio has been suggested to be associated with RIF. There has been an interest in determining the link between uNK cells and reproductive outcomes especially in women with recurrent miscarriages. At present, there appears to be insufficient evidence to link an elevated uNK cell density in the endometrium to recurrent miscarriages and a meta-analysis has suggested that further research is needed (Seshadri & Sunkara 2014). The extrapolation of uNK cells from recurrent miscarriages to recurrent implantation failure is still tenuous at best.

Gynecological diseases

Polycystic ovary syndrome (PCOS) has also been suggested to have an effect on endometrial receptivity markers such as $\alpha_v\beta_3$ integrin and also altered expression of steroid (androgen and estrogen) receptors and the receptor co-activators (Cakmak & Taylor 2011). For details on PCOS, see Chapter 6.

Uterine cavity abnormalities, whether congenital (e.g. a septate uterus) or acquired (e.g. via fibroids or adenomyosis) can result in distortion of the uterine cavity and a hostile environment for an embryo to attempt to implant into.

INVESTIGATIONS FOR RIF AND POSSIBLE TREATMENTS

Evaluation of uterine cavity

Hysteroscopy is the gold standard for uterine cavity evaluation when there is a suspicion of uterine abnormalities on ultrasound scan. The detection and treatment for congenital or acquired uterine abnormalities such as septum, polyp, adhesions or myomas through hysteroscopy does benefit women with subfertility even when they are not symptomatic (Bosteels et al. 2010). However, the routine use of hysteroscopy in the presence of normal ultrasound findings has not been shown to be useful in RIF in large scale trials (El-Toukhy et al. 2016).

Hydrosalpinx

In cases of RIF, a diligent search by transvaginal ultrasound should be made for visible hydrosalpinges which if seen, should be treated. This was first demonstrated via an RCT in 1999, whereby increased pregnancy rates resulted after salpingectomy of hydrosalpinx (Strandell et al. 1999).

There are concerns that salpingectomy might impact ovarian reserve by affecting ovarian blood flow, but most studies indicate that that this is not the case. When there is significant pelvic scarring with distortion of tubo-ovarian anatomy and a concern for damage to ovarian cortex during salpingectomy, laparoscopic tubal occlusion is an acceptable alternative to salpingectomy with similar improvement to reproductive outcomes. However, ultrasound guided aspiration of hydrosalpinges or hysteroscopic tubal occlusion should be avoided as they have not be shown to be as effective as salpingectomy (Johnson et al. 2010; Dreyer et al. 2016).

Thrombophilias

Though the role of thrombophilia and antiphospholipid antibodies in recurrent pregnancy losses is established, their association with RIF has not been conclusively proven. Some studies have indicated a higher prevalence of acquired and inherited thromobophilias in patients with RIF (Qublan et al. 2006) whilst others have not shown any such association (Martinelli et al. 2003). Some authors argue that thrombophilia testing should be advised only if there are risk factors in personal or family history (Ata & Urman 2016). There appears to be a role of low-molecular-weight heparin in RIF with an identified thrombophilia but further trials are needed before routine use can be recommended (Potdar et al. 2013).

Thin endometrium

A recent meta-analysis of 22 studies reported a halving of clinical pregnancy rates when the endometrial thickness was <7 mm (Kasius et al. 2014). However, the authors concluded that further research was required to understand the mechanism and significance of this finding.

In RIF, a persistent thin endometrium (<7 mm) should be considered as one of the possible causes. Intrauterine adhesions can cause a thin endometrium which can be identified by hysteroscopy. Treatment can be performed via adhesiolysis, but recurrence of adhesions remains a challenge.

Various treatment protocols have been described in the literature to improve an unexplained thin endometrium. These include hormonal manipulation with high doses of estrogen or use of hCG, vasoactive mediators (e.g. aspirin, pentoxifylline, sildenafil and L-arginine), intrauterine infusion of granulocyte colony-stimulating factor (G-CSF), and use of bone marrow stem cells. However, none of these methods have been consistently shown to improve endometrial thickness or clinical outcomes. If all these measures fail, surrogacy has been suggested as a last resort (Lebovitz & Orvieto 2014). See Chapter 12 for detailed coverage of surrogacy.

Immunological factors

Immunological factors have been suggested as possible cause for RIF. Couples sharing HLA alleles are presumably at high risk of RIF and recurrent pregnancy losses (Creus et al. 1998).

HUMAN LEUKOCYTE ANTIGEN SYSTEM

The human leukocyte antigen (HLA) system is a gene complex encoding the major histocompatibility complex (MHC) proteins. These cell-surface proteins are responsible for the regulation of the immune system in humans.

There is lack of clarity regarding the cut-off of abnormal uNK cell density or numbers and correlation between uNK and NK cells in the blood. Hence, NK cell testing and immunotherapy is currently not recommended in routine care apart from the context of clinical studies (Seshadri & Sunkara 2014).

The role of immunomodulatory therapies such as corticosteroids, intravenous immunoglobulins, intravenous lipid infusion or G-CSF is still very much unclear, and given that these therapies (especially parenteral agents) can cause significant side-effects, they should be offered only in the context of a clinical trial and patients should be counselled regarding the lack of evidence for their effectiveness (Moffett & Shreeve 2015).

Genetic factor

There is a role for karyotyping for people who experience recurrent miscarriages, especially in couples with a family history of miscarriage (Franssen et al. 2005). However, the role of genetic testing in RIF is yet to be established. Those studies which have suggested a relationship between RIF and karyotyping utilized a much higher threshold of 10–50 embryos being transferred in more than six ETs before karyotyping was advised (Stern et al. 1999, Raziel et al. 2002).

If chromosomal abnormalities are identified, PGS and ET of only euploid embryos can improve implantation rates (see Figure 15.9 for the biopsy process for PGS). The role of routine PGS in couples who have not been diagnosed with chromosomal abnormalities is still unclear with studies showing that it may have a role in couples with good prognosis (Dahdouh et al. 2015, Paulson 2016).

Endometrial receptivity assessment

Endometrial receptivity array (ERA) is a microarray technique used to analyze the transcriptomic signature of an endometrial biopsy. As previously described, the endometrium expresses a unique genetic profile during the WOI and an ERA can be used to classify the endometrium as receptive or nonreceptive.

Studies using ERA indicate an increased incidence of the displacement of WOI in RIF patients and adjusting the timing of ET accordingly appears to improve implantation rates (Ruiz-Alonso et al. 2013). There have been a few studies to evaluate other markers of endometrial receptivity in RIF, e.g. integrins and nucleolar channel systems, but whether this would be useful in routine clinical practice is still unknown (Coughlan et al. 2013; Nejat et al. 2014).

Endometrial 'scratch'

There has been interest in the role of causing a minor endometrial injury, known as an 'endometrial scratch', in the month before ART to attempt to improve implantation rates.

A meta-analysis has suggested an improvement in live birth rate following endometrial scratch but also acknowledged that the trials included had methodological limitations and low number of study subjects (Nastri et al. 2012). Furthermore, another study concluded that there is insufficient evidence to support the use of endometrial injury in women with RIF undergoing ART, while the procedure-associated complication rate has not been suitably assessed (Panagiotopoulou et al. 2015). Clinical implementation should, thus, be deferred until robust evidence becomes available.

Assisted hatching

Hatching of the blastocyst through the ZP is a vital prerequisite for the trophectoderm cells to make contact with the endometrial cells and initiate the process of implantation. It has been suggested that extended culture in vitro and cryopreservation techniques may harden the ZP causing hatching difficulties. Assisted hatching (AH) has been suggested to overcome this, but there is no evidence on improvement in live birth rates (Carney et al. 2012). An American Society for Reproductive Medicine (ASRM) committee opinion suggested that while AH should not be recommended routinely, it may have a role in selected patients with poor prognosis including previous failed ART cycles. However, there remains a concern of increased monozygotic twinning and multiple pregnancies with AH which may compromise overall clinical outcome (Practice Committee of the ASRM and Practice Committee of the Society for Assisted Reproductive Technology 2014).

CONCLUSION

Recognizing failed implantation as an obstacle to the success of ART, there should be an emphasis towards understanding crucial biological processes involved in the human embryo implantation process. Researchers have endeavored to unravel the key aspects of implantation by studying various endometrial, immunological, genomic and embryological facets. There have been a plethora of interventions that are suggested for improving implantation and more importantly overcoming the challenge of RIF. A firm basic science background and comprehension of the evidence is central to implementing what is right for the patient.

REFERENCES

Agarwal A, Majzoub A, Esteves SC, Ko E, Ramasamy R, Zini A. Clinical utility of sperm DNA fragmentation testing: practice recommendations based on clinical scenarios.Transl Androl Urol 2016; 5:935–950.

Ata B, Urman B. Thrombophilia and assisted reproduction technology-any detrimental impact or unnecessary overuse? J Assist Reprod Genet 2016; 33:1305–1310.

Benkhalifa M, Demirol A, Sari T, Balashova E, et al. Autologous embryo-cumulus cells co-culture and blastocyst transfer in repeated implantation failures: a collaborative prospective randomized study. Zygote Camb Engl 2012; 20:173–180.

Bosteels J, Weyers S, Puttemans P, et al. The effectiveness of hysteroscopy in improving pregnancy rates in subfertile women without other gynaecological symptoms: a systematic review. Hum Reprod Update 2010; 16:1–11.

Blockeel C, Drakopoulos P, Santos-Ribeiro S, Polyzos NP, Tournaye H. A fresh look at the freeze-all protocol: a SWOT analysis. Hum Reprod. 2016; 31:491–497.

Cakmak H, Taylor HS. Implantation failure: molecular mechanisms and clinical treatment. Hum Reprod Update 2011; 17:242–253.

Carney SK, Das S, Blake D, et al. Assisted hatching on assisted conception [in vitro fertilisation (IVF) and intracytoplasmic sperm injection (ICSI)]. Cochrane Database Syst Rev [Internet], 2012.

Collins J. Mild stimulation for in vitro fertilization: making progress downward. Hum Reprod Update 2009; 15:1–3.

Coughlan C, Clarke H, Cutting R, et al. Sperm DNA fragmentation, recurrent implantation failure and recurrent miscarriage. Asian J Androl 2015; 17:681–685.

Coughlan C, Ledger W, Wang Q, et al. Recurrent implantation failure: definition and management. Reprod Biomed Online 2014; 28:14–38.

Coughlan C, Sinagra M, Ledger W, Li TC, Laird S. Endometrial integrin expression in women with recurrent implantation failure after in vitro fertilization and its relationship to pregnancy outcome. Fertil Steril 2013; 100:825–830.

Creus M, Balasch J, Fábregues F, et al. Parental human leukocyte antigens and implantation failure after in-vitro fertilization. Hum Reprod 1998; 13:39–43.

Croy BA, He H, Esadeg S, et al. Uterine natural killer cells: insights into their cellular and molecular biology from mouse modelling. Reprod Camb Engl 2003; 126:149–160.

Dahdouh EM, Balayla J, García-Velasco JA. Impact of blastocyst biopsy and comprehensive chromosome screening technology on preimplantation genetic screening: a systematic review of randomized controlled trials. Reprod Biomed Online 2015; 30:281–289.

Dimitriadis E, White CA, Jones RL, Salamonsen LA. Cytokines, chemokines and growth factors in endometrium related to implantation. Hum Reprod Update 2005; 11:613–630.

Dreyer K, Lier MCI, Emanuel MH, et al. Hysteroscopic proximal tubal occlusion versus laparoscopic salpingectomy as a treatment for hydrosalpinges prior to IVF or ICSI: an RCT. Hum Reprod 2016; 31:2005–2016.

El-Toukhy T, Campo R, Khalaf Y, et al. Hysteroscopy in recurrent in-vitro fertilisation failure (TROPHY): a multicentre, randomised controlled trial. Lancet Lond Engl 2016; 387:2614–2621.

Fatemi HM, Popovic-Todorovic B. Implantation in assisted reproduction: a look at endometrial receptivity. Reprod Biomed Online 2013; 27:530–538.

Fragouli E, Spath K, Alfarawati S, et al. Altered Levels of Mitochondrial DNA Are Associated with Female Age, Aneuploidy, and Provide an Independent Measure of Embryonic Implantation Potential. PLOS Genet 2015; 11:e10.

Franasiak JM, Forman EJ, Hong KH, et al.The nature of aneuploidy with increasing age of the female partner: a review of 15,169 consecutive trophectoderm biopsies evaluated with comprehensive chromosomal screening. Fertil Steril 2014; 101:656–663.

Franssen MTM, Korevaar JC, Leschot NJ, et al. Selective chromosome analysis in couples with two or more miscarriages: case-control study. BMJ 2005; 331:137–141.

Johnson N, Voorst S van, Sowter MC, Strandell A, Mol BWJ. Surgical treatment for tubal disease in women due to undergo in vitro fertilisation. Cochrane Database Syst Rev 2010;CD002125.

Kasius A, Smit JG, Torrance HL, et al. Endometrial thickness and pregnancy rates after IVF: a systematic review and meta-analysis. Hum Reprod Update 2014; 20:530–541.

Lebovitz O, Orvieto R. Treating patients with "thin" endometrium – an ongoing challenge. Gynecol Endocrinol Off J Int Soc Gynecol Endocrinol 2014; 30:409–414.

Martinelli I, Taioli E, Ragni G, et al. Embryo implantation after assisted reproductive procedures and maternal thrombophilia. Haematologica 2003; 88:789–793.

Mascarenhas M, Kamath MS, Chandy A, Kunjummen AT. Progesterone/Estradiol Ratio as a Predictor in the ART Cycles with Premature Progesterone Elevation on the Day of hCG Trigger. J Reprod Infertil 2015; 16:155–161.

Moffett A, Shreeve N. First do no harm: uterine natural killer (NK) cells in assisted reproduction. Hum Reprod Oxf Engl 2015; 30:1519–1525.

Nastri CO, Gibreel A, Raine-Fenning N, Maheshwari A, Ferriani RA, Bhattacharya S, Martins WP. Endometrial injury in women undergoing assisted reproductive techniques. Cochrane Database Syst Rev 2012; CD009517.

Nejat EJ, Ruiz-Alonso M, Simón C, Meier UT. Timing the window of implantation by nucleolar channel system prevalence matches the accuracy of the endometrial receptivity array. Fertil Steril 2014; 102:1477–1481.

Osman A, Alsomait H, Seshadri S, El-Toukhy T, Khalaf Y. The effect of sperm DNA fragmentation on live birth rate after IVF or ICSI: a systematic review and meta-analysis. Reprod Biomed Online 2015; 30:120–127.

Panagiotopoulou N, Karavolos S, Choudhary M. Endometrial injury prior to assisted reproductive techniques for recurrent implantation failure: a systematic literature review. Eur J Obstet Gynecol Reprod Biol 2015; 193:27–33.

Paulson RJ. Every last baby out of every last egg: the appropriate goal for fertility treatment in women older than 40 years. Fertil Steril 2016; 105:1443–1444.

Potdar N, Gelbaya TA, Konje JC, Nardo LG. Adjunct low-molecular-weight heparin to improve live birth rate after recurrent implantation failure: a systematic review and meta-analysis. Hum Reprod Update 2013; 19:674–684.

Practice Committee of the American Society for Reproductive Medicine; Practice Committee of the Society for Assisted Reproductive Technology. Role of assisted hatching in in vitro fertilization: a guideline. Fertil Steril 2014; 102:348–351.

Qublan HS, Eid SS, Ababneh HA, et al. Acquired and inherited thrombophilia: implication in recurrent IVF and embryo transfer failure. Hum Reprod Oxf Engl 2006; 21:2694–2698.

Raziel A, Friedler S, Schachter M, et al. Increased frequency of female partner chromosomal abnormalities in patients with high-order implantation failure after in vitro fertilization. Fertil Steril 2002; 78:515–519.

RCOG SAC Opinion Paper. The Use of Antithrombotics in the Prevention of Recurrent Pregnancy Loss, 2011.

Rubio C, Bellver J, Rodrigo L, et al. Preimplantation genetic screening using fluorescence in situ hybridization in patients with repetitive implantation failure and advanced maternal age: two randomized trials. Fertil Steril 2013; 99:1400–1407.

Ruiz-Alonso M, Blesa D, Díaz-Gimeno P, et al. The endometrial receptivity array for diagnosis and personalized embryo transfer as a treatment for patients with repeated implantation failure. Fertil Steril 2013; 100:818–824.

Seshadri S, Sunkara SK. Natural killer cells in female infertility and recurrent miscarriage: a systematic review and meta-analysis. Hum Reprod Update 2014; 20:429–438.

Stern C, Pertile M, Norris H, Hale L, Baker HW. Chromosome translocations in couples with in-vitro fertilization implantation failure. Hum Reprod Oxf Engl 1999; 14:2097–2101.

Strandell A, Lindhard A, Waldenström U, et al. Hydrosalpinx and IVF outcome: a prospective, randomized multicentre trial in Scandinavia on salpingectomy prior to IVF. Hum Reprod Oxf Engl 1999; 14:2762–2769.

Tabibzadeh S, Babaknia A. The signals and molecular pathways involved in implantation, a symbiotic interaction between blastocyst and endometrium involving adhesion and tissue invasion. Hum Reprod Oxf Engl 1995; 10:1579–1602.

Teklenburg G, Salker M, Heijnen C, Macklon NS, Brosens JJ. The molecular basis of recurrent pregnancy loss: impaired natural embryo selection. Mol Hum Reprod 2010; 16:886–895.

van der Linden M, Buckingham K, Farquhar C, Kremer JAM, Metwally M. Luteal phase support for assisted reproduction cycles. Cochrane Database Syst Rev 2015; CD009154.

Zhang Y, Trussell JC, Chohan KR. Detecting and minimizing sperm DNA damage. Semin Reprod Med 2013; 31:267–73.

Chapter 12 Surrogacy – a method of family building

Wendy Norton

INTRODUCTION

Third-party reproduction is commonly used by people who are unable to reproduce in the traditional way. Medical and technological advances have revolutionized the field of assisted reproduction, giving rise to growing numbers of people worldwide utilizing surrogacy arrangements as a method of family building. Surrogacy provides an opportunity for individuals or couples to become parents in circumstances where carrying a pregnancy is biologically impossible or medically contraindicated (Shenfield et al. 2005).

Surrogacy is not a new concept: in the book of Genesis in the Bible, Hagar bore Abraham a son as his wife was unable to conceive. Surrogacy has possibly been used for centuries to overcome infertility problems (Brinsden 2003). A 'surrogate' can be defined as a woman who becomes pregnant, carries and delivers a child on behalf of another couple, known as the intended or commissioning parents (Shenfield et al. 2005).

For heterosexual couples, surrogacy may be an option where the female partner has congenital absence of the uterus, e.g. resulting from Müllerian agenesis, or prior hysterectomy due to benign or malignant conditions. Women with significant uterine pathology, e.g. a T-shaped or hypoplastic uterus with a history of infertility or repetitive pregnancy loss, may also be candidates, as are women with untreatable intrauterine scar tissue [Practice Committee of American Society for Reproductive Medicine (ASRM), 2015].

MÜLLERIAN AGENESIS

Müllerian agenesis, also known as Mayer–Rokitansky–Küster–Hauser (MRKH) syndrome is a congenital malformation whereby the Müllerian duct fails to develop. This can lead to absence of a uterus and differing degrees of vaginal hypoplasia. An alternative to surrogacy for women with Müllerian agenesis is uterine transplantation (see Chapter 19).

In addition, surrogacy may also be considered for women for whom a pregnancy could lead to a health risk for either the woman or the child. Examples include severe heart disease, systemic lupus erythematosus, severe renal disease, severe diabetes mellitus, history of breast cancer, cystic fibrosis, Rhesus isoimmunization, a history of severe pre-eclampsia with HELLP syndrome (hemolysis, elevated liver enzymes, and low platelet count) (ASRM 2015; Dar et al. 2015).

In 2009, the UK fertility regulator, the Human Fertilisation and Embryology Authority (HFEA) removed its previous guidance which stated that licensed treatment centers should only offer surrogacy where it was physically impossible or highly undesirable for medical reasons for the commissioning mother to carry a pregnancy (HFEA 2009). The HFEA now allows surrogacy as an option to parenthood for same-sex couples or single people. For same-sex male couples this could involve insemination of either a donor oocyte or an oocyte provided by the surrogate herself. If one of the males provides the sperm, then this allows a biological connection with the child, as well as providing an opportunity to raise a child from birth (Tuazon-McCheyne 2010; ASRM 2015). **Table 12.1** lists the reasons why surrogacy could be considered as a means of creating a family.

This chapter outlines the different types of surrogacy, the steps involved in a surrogacy program, and other key factors to be considered when embarking on a surrogacy arrangement, such as ethical and legal perspectives.

DIFFERENT TYPES OF SURROGACY

There are two types of surrogacy: traditional and gestational. In either case, the intention is that the gestating woman relinquishes the child to the commissioning parents, who want to then assume parental responsibility (Shenfield et al. 2005).

Traditional surrogacy (also known as straight, genetic or partial surrogacy) involves sperm from the intended father and an oocyte from the surrogate. Fertilization is usually achieved by artificial insemination which can be undertaken informally between the parties using home insemination kits, or by intrauterine insemination (IUI) at a fertility clinic. This is a simpler form of surrogacy, as pregnancy can be attempted on a monthly basis and there is a reduced need for medical intervention. The baby is biologically related to the intended father and the surrogate mother, who will have a genetic link by providing the oocyte.

Gestational surrogacy (**Figure 12.1**) (also known as host or full surrogacy) always requires medical intervention as it involves the implantation of an in vitro-derived embryo. There are four options for gametes for creating the embryo, by using:

1. An oocyte and sperm from the intended parents
2. A donated oocyte and sperm from the intended father
3. An oocyte from the intended mother and donated sperm
4. A donated oocyte and donated sperm (use of a donated oocyte and donated sperm for gestational surrogacy is not allowed in the UK, as at least one of the intended parents needs to be biologically related to the child in order to apply for a Parental Order)

Gestational surrogacy has become more prevalent as assisted reproductive technology (ART) has advanced, with the majority of fertility

Table 12.1 Reasons why surrogacy may be considered as an option for parenthood

Conditions in which surrogacy can be considered	
Medical reasons	• Congenital absence of the uterus • Previous hysterectomy (for benign/malignant conditions) • Significant uterine pathology • Medical risk to healthily gestate a pregnancy
Non-medical reasons	• Same-sex male couples • Single men

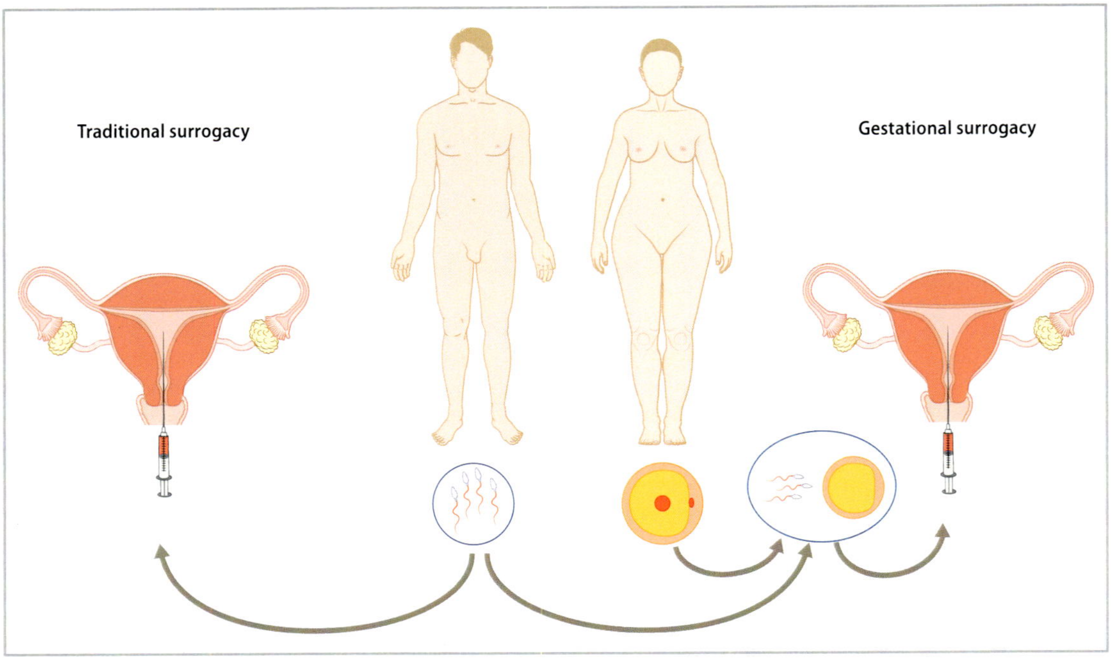

Figure 12.1 Different types of surrogacy. Surrogacy involves two gamete providers (one for the oocyte, one for the sperm) and a uterus. For the latter, there are two types of surrogacy: gestational (where the surrogate provides the uterus but not the oocyte) and traditional (where the surrogate provides both the uterus and the oocyte).

clinics both in the US and the UK only offering this form of surrogacy (FIGO 2008, Norton et al. 2015). This type of surrogacy arrangement involves more time commitment and greater expense, and the success rates will dependent upon the fertility clinic chosen. However, the surrogate will not be genetically related to the child (Zegers-Hochschild et al. 2009).

COMMERCIAL AND ALTRUISTIC SURROGACY

Traditional and gestational surrogacy arrangements are either commercial or altruistic, and this varies widely between jurisdictions, depending on interstate or international surrogacy legislation.

Commercial surrogacy is where the surrogate mother is financially compensated by the commissioning parents, beyond the reimbursement of medical and other reasonable expenses. This is illegal in many countries, including the UK. Altruistic surrogacy is where the surrogate mother chooses to carry the child for reasons other than financial gain, although 'reasonable expenses' can be paid, for example, to cover costs relating to loss of earnings, travelling expenses, maternity clothes (FIGO 2008).

Legal perspectives

Internationally, there is a wide range of legal stipulations regarding surrogacy and third-party reproduction (Armour 2012). This can lead to a very confusing and complicated process. Surrogacy remains illegal in many European countries including France, Germany, Italy, Spain and Switzerland. In contrast, in countries such as Georgia, Ukraine and South Africa, all surrogacy agreements, including commercial surrogacy, are legal and enforceable (see **Figure 12.2**) (Howard 2014). Commercial surrogacy is also acceptable in some US States, where there are increasing numbers of organizations that facilitate contact between couples and surrogates, and assist in the legal side of contracts between parties involved. In the UK, commercial surrogacy is prohibited, following the Surrogacy Arrangements Act (1985). Since Britain's first official surrogate birth in 1985, laws allow for limited payments to cover only what is described as 'reasonable expenses', such as loss of income. It is also a criminal offence to advertise that you are in need of, or willing to enter into a surrogacy arrangement. Surrogacy arrangements are not legally enforceable in the UK, even if a contract has been signed and the expenses of the surrogate have been paid.

Legal parenthood

Different countries have different ways to transfer parental status from the surrogate to the intended parents. For example, some US States authorize pre-birth or post-birth orders for intended parents, thereby establishing a legal relationship between the intended parents and the child upon birth, and removing the need for adoption proceedings (Crockin & Altman 2013).

As the legal status of surrogacy varies across countries and also within different areas of the same country, e.g. between different US States, legal advice is paramount for all parties. To avoid potential conflicts of interest, healthcare professionals assisting in surrogacy cases should encourage all parties involved in these arrangements to seek their own guidance and representation from appropriately qualified legal teams.

In the UK, the woman who gives birth is the legal mother, whilst her husband or civil partner is legally recognized as the second parent of the child. This is irrespective of genetic parenthood or where in the world they live. The only exception to this would be if the surrogate's partner can provide appropriate evidence to demonstrate a factual basis for not consenting (e.g. that they are separated).

In cases where the surrogate is single, or where their partner did not consent to treatment, one of the intended parents can now be formally attributed legal parenthood when the child is born, provided the arrangement took place in an HFEA-licensed clinic and the appropriate consent forms have been signed prior to the commencement of treatment (HFEA, 2016). The surrogate remains the legal mother of the child and has parental responsibility unless, or until, parenthood is transferred to the intended parents, via a Parental Order or adoption after the birth of the child.

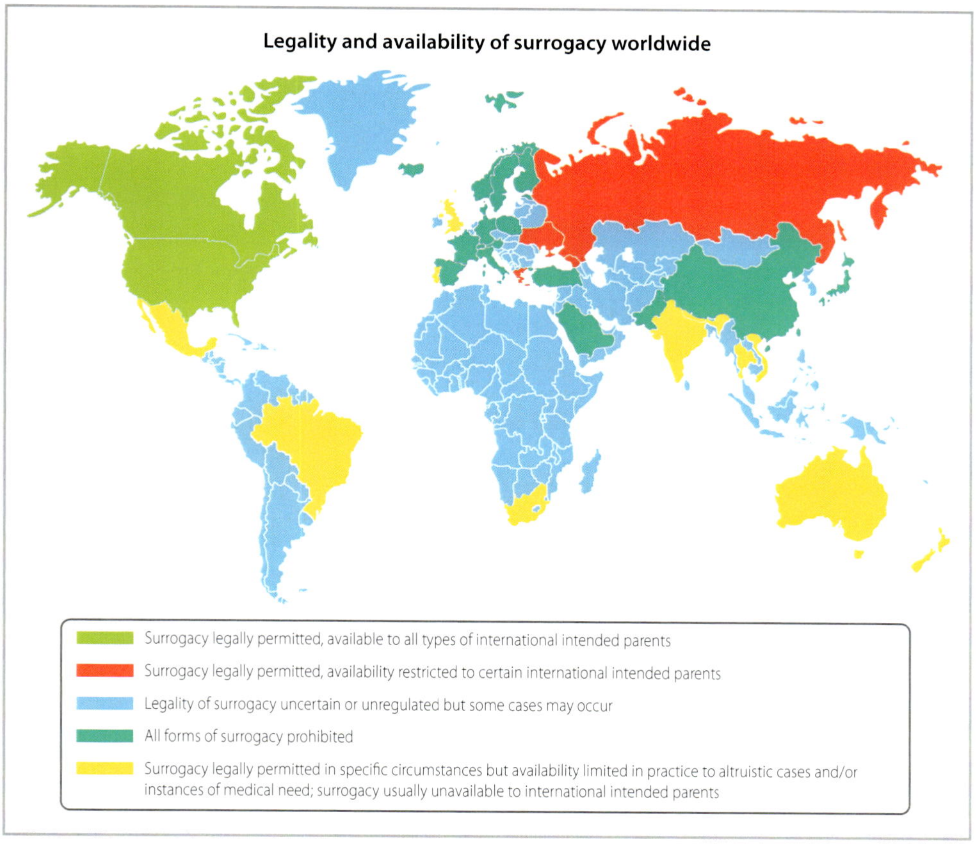

Figure 12.2 The international range of legal stipulations regarding surrogacy . Reproduced with permission from Fertility Road Magazine Spring 2017.

In the UK, the surrogate has the legal right to change her mind and keep the child, even when the baby she gave birth to is not genetically related to her. The birth parents must give full, free and unconditional consent to extinguish their parental rights, and this cannot be given before 6 weeks after the birth. Parental Orders ensure that commissioning parents have legal parentage status, without which the surrogate will retain legal parentage (Baron et al. 2012;Crawshaw et al. 2013). People who are eligible to apply for a Parental Order include couples who are married, in a civil partnership or in an 'enduring family relationship', and where at least one of the commissioning couple is genetically related to the baby, e.g. the sperm provider. This is detailed in the HFE (Parental Orders) Regulations 2010.

INCIDENCE OF SURROGACY

Surrogacy as a method of ART has risen in profile and prevalence. However, there remains limited evidence about the true incidence and nature of surrogacy arrangements. An estimate of the number of surrogacy cases per year can be obtained from assisted conception figures. In 2008, the HFEA reported a 10.2% increase in surrogacy births in the UK, compared to an 8.2% increase of in vitro fertilization (IVF) cycles (HFEA 2008). More recently, the HFEA (2018) reported that the number of patients registered as a surrogate has more than doubled in the past 10 years.

However, not all surrogacy cases take place within a licensed fertility clinic, and there is no current requirement in the UK to collect data on private agreements or arrangements. To assist in capturing this information, statistics relating to the number of couples obtaining a Parental Order are helpful, as they record the number of transfers of legal parentage status from surrogates to commissioning parents. There has been a marked increase in the number of Parental Orders granted, rising from an annual number of 33–50, since their inception in 1995 (Crawshaw et al. 2012) to 189 applications in the UK between 2013 and 2014, concerning 238 children (Children and Family Court Advisory and Support Service [CAFCASS], 2015).

However, it has been suggested that there may be at least 1000 children born annually through overseas surrogacy arrangements whose parents do not subsequently apply for Parental Orders (Blyth et al. 2014). Therefore, there remains no current universal mechanism with which to accurately record or map surrogacy activity.

PLANNING A SURROGACY PROCEDURE

Surrogate criteria

Surrogates can be anonymous, unrelated known individuals, or may be family members. In a largely noncommercial system, surrogates may be family members or friends, whereas in a commercial system the number of unrelated women is higher (Shenfield et al. 2005). Where family members are involved, this may be intragenerational, e.g. between sisters or cousins of similar ages, or intergenerational, e.g. when a mother acts as a surrogate for her daughter (Söderström-Anttila et al. 2002).

Anonymous surrogates are usually found through agencies that specialize in recruiting women to become surrogates, or surrogacy charitable organizations. The UK has a number of charitable, not-for-profit organizations such as COTS (Childlessness Overcome Through Surrogacy), Surrogacy UK and Brilliant Beginnings, which bring together commissioning parents and women willing to act as surrogates. In accordance with the Surrogacy Arrangements Act 1985 and the Human Fertilisation and Embryology Act 1990, it is illegal for an individual or agency to act on a commercial basis to organize or facilitate a surrogacy arrangement for another person. Furthermore, this Act makes it a criminal offence to advertise that you are in need of, or willing to enter into, a surrogacy arrangement.

The criteria to become a surrogate differs across countries. The ASRM (2015) recommends that in order to ensure free and well-considered decision-making, the gestational surrogate should generally fit certain criteria (see **Box**). For those couples opting for traditional surrogacy, a maximum age of <35 years should be considered in line with the decline in fertility after this age (HFEA 2009).

CRITERIA TO BECOME A SURROGATE

- Minimum of 21 years of age
- Maximum upper age of <45 years for gestational surrogacy, as consideration needs to be given to the obstetric complication rate, especially, the incidence of pregnancy-induced hypertension or gestational diabetes
- Ideally have had at least one full term, uncomplicated pregnancy
- Ideally not have had more than a total of five previous deliveries or three deliveries via cesarean section
- Have a stable family environment with adequate support to help her cope with the added stress of pregnancy

Sperm provider

An accurate semen analysis for the commissioning father is essential. This can usually be accessed via a general practitioner, or fertility clinic if gestational surrogacy is the chosen option. It is important that the laboratory performing the analysis is suitably accredited to ensure that the test is accurate and is assessed according to the criteria set by the latest World Health Organization guidelines (WHO 2010). Suboptimal sperm results may indicate the need for intracytoplasmic sperm injection (ICSI) rather than IVF procedures to create embryos, or the use of donor sperm.

In same-sex male couples both men may wish to fertilize donated oocytes to create siblings, so both partners can be biologically related to their children. In the UK, clinics are only able to transfer embryos created by one partner at a time for traceability (HFEA 2009). In such cases, sibling embryos can be cryopreserved for future use. It is also important to consider elective single-embryo transfer (eSET) to reduce the risk of multiple births, which can lead to complications for both the surrogate and the offspring.

Screening

To prevent transmission of infections, e.g. HBV, HCV and HIV, screening is essential for all parties involved in the surrogacy program (see **Box**). In the UK, the intended parents providing gametes for the surrogacy arrangement must be screened in line with requirements for gamete donors (HFEA 2009). This requires the sperm or embryos to be stored in quarantine for a period of time, whilst repeated tests are carried out to minimize the risk of transmitting any infection.

INFECTION SCREENS FOR GAMETE PROVIDERS AND SURROGATES IN THE UK

- HIV 1 and 2: Anti-HIV -1,2
- HBV: HBsAg and Anti-HBc
- HCV: Anti-HCV-Ab
- Gonorrhoea, chlamydia, syphilis
- Cytomegalovirus
- Immunity to rubella and varicella
- Blood group (Rh)

SURROGACY PROCEDURES

Traditional surrogacy

If the commissioning couple opt for traditional surrogacy, these arrangements are often undertaken informally, so couples will make their own insemination arrangement. This may be a more affordable means of conception for some couples and avoid medical intervention.

Timing for this kind of insemination is crucial. Ovulation predictor kits can be used to detect the LH surge, signalling imminent ovulation, and inseminations carried out on the day of the positive surge, and/or the day after. The commissioning father needs to produce a sperm sample which can then be vaginally inseminated by the surrogate using a syringe, or one of the many self-insemination devices that are available to purchase online. Success rates are difficult to gauge as factors such as the surrogate's age and quality of the sperm sample can influence the outcome. If pregnancy has not occurred after six consecutive cycles, additional investigations may be recommended.

Commissioning couples may decide to access IUI programs via a fertility clinic, which may enable them to use fertility drugs to stimulate ovarian activity and undertake ultrasound monitoring to try to optimize their chances of success.

Gestational surrogacy

In the UK, gestational surrogacy must always take place in an HFEA-licensed fertility clinic as it will require an in vitro-derived embryo to be created. It is important that all parties attend for consultation to enable a full medical history to be taken from both the commissioning couple and the surrogate, to detect any underlying conditions that might complicate a pregnancy (ASRM 2015). Physical examinations may need to be carried out, in addition to a review of investigations and screening results. It is important to allow sufficient time for a full discussion of the proposed treatment program, including the associated implications and risks, prior to commencing any treatment cycle (see **Box**).

TO DISCUSS AT CONSULTATION

- Psychological aspects of surrogacy arrangements
- Drug reactions
- Multiple birth
- Ovarian hyperstimulation syndrome
- Miscarriage risk
- Ectopic pregnancy risk
- Birth defects

COUNSELING

The psychological implications and risks involved with surrogacy depend on the type of surrogacy undertaken. Counseling is an essential aspect of any surrogacy arrangement, to ensure all parties are clear about the implications of their decision before proceeding. It is also important for those considering an intra-familial surrogacy arrangement to undergo counseling to assess potential coercion or pressure, and ensure issues relating to the impact of this arrangement on the future child, are discussed in advance. Counseling allows all parties to consider the implications of their involvement that had not been previously understood or acknowledged (Shenfield et al 2005).

Counseling facilitates discussion of a variety of issues and concerns in a supportive environment, such as the practical aspects of the program including the recommendation for eSET, views on multiple pregnancies, and the possibility of miscarriage or termination of pregnancy should a fetal abnormality be detected (awareness of the option for prenatal genetic screening should be discussed).

For the surrogate, it is important to allow time to discuss the psychological issues relating to carrying a baby for another couple, as well as the effect of parting with the child if the pregnancy is successful. The commissioning mother may also worry about her ability to bond with a child carried by another woman, and may have concerns that the surrogate mother may decide to keep the child after delivery (ASRM 2015). Counseling also offers the opportunity to discuss the type of relationship that the commissioning couple and surrogate wish to have and how this will be managed, as well as the possible impact of a surrogacy arrangement on both parties' wider circle of family, including the surrogate's children, and friends.

People considering informal surrogacy arrangements, rather than those undertaken via fertility clinics, may access counseling via the surrogacy agencies or charitable organizations. Alternatively, details of counseling services may be available via general practitioners. Many surrogacy agencies and organisations encourage the drawing up of a surrogacy contract to document the agreed outcomes from these discussions. These 'contracts' are not legally binding in all countries, such as the UK, but may serve to clarify the agreed intentions of all parties and the nature of the relationship. However, the commissioning parents should be well aware that the surrogate has the legal right to make decisions about her pregnancy against their will and against the original agreement (Shenfield et al. 2005).

Embryo creation

All parties should be advised to obtain legal advice prior to signing the relevant consent forms to ensure they have made free and well-informed decisions (HFEA 2009). For gestational surrogacy, the embryo is created via IVF and ICSI using gametes from one or both of the commissioning couple, or donated gametes. The embryo is then transferred into the host surrogate, who will have been receiving hormonal treatment to synchronize her cycle and prepare her endometrium for implantation. It is strongly recommended that only one embryo should be replaced in order to prevent multiple pregnancies (Shenfield et al. 2005). In special circumstances, the replacement of a maximum of two embryos can be considered.

Success rates

It is difficult to determine a success rate for surrogacy, as it depends on many factors, such as the fertility of the surrogate, the age of the oocyte donor, the quality of the sperm and oocytes, and the chosen clinic's IUI or IVF success rates (HFEA 2009). However, evidence has suggested that for gestational surrogacy programs, the clinical pregnancy rate per embryo transfer has been between 19% and 33%, and between 30% and 70% of the couples have become parents as a result of the arrangement (Beski et al. 2000, Brinsden et al. 2000, Corson et al. 1998, Dar et al. 2015, Goldfarb et al. 2000, Meniru & Craft 1997, Parkinson et al. 1998, Raziel et al. 2005, Soderstrom-Anttila et al. 2002, Wood et al. 1999)

CROSS-BORDER SURROGACY

Commissioning parents may enter into arrangements with surrogates in other countries possibly due to lower costs, and more availability of surrogates (Crockin & Altman 2013, Gamble 2009). As well as the factors already discussed, international surrogacy arrangements raise other considerations (see **Box**).

CONSIDERATIONS FOR INTERNATIONAL SURROGACY ARRANGEMENTS

- The chosen country's stance on commercial surrogacy
- Whether surrogacy contracts are enforceable in the chosen country
- Issues relating to the child's nationality
- The child's entry clearance into the country of the commissioning parent, e.g. passport and visa requirements. This needs careful consideration, as the current country of residence may not be the native home, and thus they may not have resident status where they are presently living
- Differences between countries in relation to who is recognised as the child's legal parents. Although foreign birth certificates may name the intended parents, this may not automatically be recognised in the intended parents' home country.

This global variation can leave the commissioning parents and the child vulnerable in a variety of ways. It is therefore essential that advice is sought before going overseas in order to clarify the legal positions.

ETHICAL CONSIDERATIONS

Surrogacy continues to raise debate worldwide in relation to the complex emotional and ethical issues when using third party reproduction. High profile media coverage of the rare occasions when surrogacy has gone wrong has emphasised concerns about the ethics of surrogacy practices. These include the commercialization of human reproduction and the commodification of the child (Horsey 2015), and the possibility of exploitation and coercion of women to act as surrogates (Deonandan et al. 2012, Pande 2011)

There have been concerns regarding the psychological impact for the surrogate in relinquishing the baby she may have formed a bond with prenatally (FIGO 2008), as well as fears that the intended parents will abandon the baby if there is a birth defect. Others have portrayed global surrogacy arrangements as a win–win situation for both the surrogate and the commissioning parents (Carney 2010, Hochschild 2009), proposing that women should be acknowledged as having autonomous control over their own bodies (Purdy 1992). Additionally, some studies report a very positive experience for the majority of surrogates (Jadva et al. 2003, van den Akker 2007, Temen 2010).

Concerns have also been raised about the effect on children's psychological development and family functioning. A longitudinal study of psychological adjustment of children born through reproductive donation, which included 30 surrogacy families, showed that absence of a genetic connection to either the mother or the father was not associated with adjustment difficulties (Golombok et al. 2011). However, surrogacy children did display higher levels of adjustment problems at age 7 years. The authors concluded that while children's scores remained within the normal range, the lack of a gestational connection may place children at increased psychological risk. At age 10 years, most children felt positive about their surrogate mother and surrogate birth (Jadva et al. 2012).

CONCLUSION

Surrogacy arrangements can be complex as the interests of the intended parents, the surrogate, and the future child may differ. All parties require clear, consistent, balanced, and evidence-based information. Healthcare professionals have a duty to inform all those involved about the medical, social, psychological, moral and legal issues involved in surrogacy (Shenfield et al. 2005). If appropriate pathways are followed and legal representation sought by all parties involved, then surrogacy can offer a viable route to family building for many people. As the legal position differs worldwide it is essential that healthcare professionals keep themselves abreast of current evidence and legal perspectives in this rapidly evolving area.

REFERENCES

Armour KL. An overview of surrogacy around the world: trends, questions and ethical issues. Nurs Womens Health 2012; 16:231–236.

Baron J, Blyth E, Haigh A. Counselling and Surrogacy in Licensed Clinics in the UK, 2nd edn. New York: BICA Publications, 2012.

Beski S, Gorgy A, Venkat G, Craft IL, Edmonds K. Gestational surrogacy: a feasible option for patients with Rokitansky syndrome. Hum Reprod 2000; 15:2326–2328.

Blyth E, Crawshaw M, van den Akker O. What are the best interests of the child in international surrogacy? BioNews Commentary 2014.

Brinsden PR, Appleton TC, Murray E, et al. Treatment by in vitro fertilisation with surrogacy: experience of one British centre. BMJ 2000; 320:924–928.

Brinsden PR. Gestational Surrogacy. Hum Reprod Update 2003; 9:483–491.

Carney S. Cash on delivery: Gestational dormitories. Routine C-sections. Quintuple embryo implants. Brave new world? Nope surrogacy tourism. Mother Jones 2010:69–73.

Children and Family Court Advisory and Support Service (CAFCASS). Study of Parental Order Applications made in 2013/14. London: CAFCASS, 2015 (online only).

Committee of the Society for Assisted Reproductive technology. Recommendations for practices utilizing gestational carriers: a committee opinion. Fertil Steril 2015; 103:e1–e8.

Corson SL, Kelly M, Braverman AM, English ME. Gestational carrier pregnancy. Fertil Steril 1998; 69:670–674.

Crawshaw M, Blyth E, van den Akker OBA. The changing profile of surrogacy in the UK: Implications for national and international policy and Practice. Journal of Family Welfare & Social Law 2012; 34:265–275.

Crawshaw M, Purewal S, van den Akker O. Working at the margins: The views and experiences of court social workers on Parental Orders' work in surrogacy arrangements. Brit J Soc Work 2013; 43:1225–1243.

Crockin S, Altman A. Statutory and case law governing the practice of 3rd party reproduction. In: Sauer M (Eds), Principles of Oocyte and Embryo Donation. Springer-Verlag 2013.

Crockin SL. Growing families in a shrinking world: legal and ethical challenges in cross-border surrogacy. Reprod Biomed Online 2013; 27:733–741.

Dar S, LazerT, Swanson S. Assisted reproduction involving gestational surrogacy: an analysis of the medical, psychosocial and legal issues: experience from a large surrogacy program. Hum Reprod 2015; 30:345–352.

Deonandan R, Green S, van Beinum A. Ethical concerns for maternal surrogacy and reproductive tourism. J Med Ethics 2012; 38:742–745.

FIGO Committee for Ethical Aspects of Human Reproduction and Women's Health. FIGO Committee Report: Surrogacy. Int J Gynaecol Obstet 2008; 102:312–313.

Gamble N. Crossing the line: the legal and ethical problems of foreign surrogacy. Reprod Biomed Online 2009; 19:151–152.

Goldfarb JM, Austin C, Peskin B. Fifteen years' experience with an in-vitro fertilization surrogate gestational pregnancy programme. Hum Reprod 2000; 15:1075–1078.

Golombok S, Readings J, Blake L, et al. Families created through surrogacy: mother-child relationships and children's psychological adjustment at age 7. Dev Psychol 2011; 47:1579–1588.

Her Majesty's Stationery Office. Human Fertilisation and Embryology Act 1990. London: HMSO, 1990.

Her Majesty's Stationery Office (HMSO). Human Fertilisation and Embryology (Parental Orders) Regulations. London: HMSO, 2010.

Her Majesty's Stationery Office. Surrogacy Arrangements Act 1985. London: HMSO, 1985.

Hochschild A. Childbirth at the global crossroads. The Amercan Prospect 2009.

Horsey K. Surrogacy in the UK; Myth busting and reform; report of the Surrogacy UK Working Group on Surrogacy Law Reform (Surrogacy UK). Matlock: Surrogacy Working Group, 2015.

Howard S. Taming the international commercial surrogacy industry. BMJ 2014; 349:6334.

Human Fertilisation and Embryology Authority (HFEA). Annual Report. London: HFEA, 2008.

Human Fertilisation and Embryology Authority. Code of practice, 8th edn. Revised October 2015. London: HFEA, 2009.

Human Fertilisation and Embryology Authority. Surrogacy and Legal Parenthood. London: HFEA, 2013.

Human Fertilisation and Embryology Authority. The Human Fertilisation and Embryology (Parental Orders) Regulations 2010. London: HFEA, 2010.

Jadva V, Blake L, Casey P, Golombok S. Surrogacy families 10 years on: relationship with the surrogate, decisions over disclosure and childrens' understanding of their surrogacy origins. Hum Reprod 2012; 27:3008–3014.

Human Fertilisation and Embryology Authority (HFEA). Fertility treatment 2014-2016 trends and figures. London: HFEA, 2018 (online only).

Jadva V, Murray C, Lycett E, MacCallum F, Golombok S. Surrogacy: the experiences of surrogate mothers. Hum Reprod 2003; 18:2196–2204.

Meniru GI, Craft IL. Experience with gestational surrogacy as a treatment for sterility resulting from hysterectomy. Hum Reprod 1997; 12:51–54.

Norton W, Crawshaw M, Hudson N, Culley N, Law C. A Survey of UK fertility clinics' approach to surrogacy arrangements. Reproductive BioMedicine Online 2015; 31:327–338.

Pande A. Transnational commercial surrogacy in India: gifts for global sisters? Reprod Biomed Online 2001; 23:618–625.

Parkinson J, Tran C, Tan T, et al. Perinatal outcome after in-vitro fertilization-surrogacy. Hum Reprod 1998; 14:671–676.

Practice Committee of the American society for Reproductive Medicine and Practice

Purdy L. Another look at contract pregnancy. In: Holmes HB (Ed), Issues in Reproductive Technology. New York: New York University Press, 1992.

Raziel A, Schachter M, Strassburger D, et al. Eight years' experience with an IVF surrogate gestational pregnancy programme. Reprod Biomed Online 2005; 11:254–258.

Shenfield F, Pennings G, Cohen J, et al. ESHRE Task Force on Ethics and Law 10: surrogacy. Hum Reprod 2005; 20:2705–2707.

Soderstrom-Anttila V, Blomqvist T, Foudila T, et al. Experience of in vitro fertilization surrogacy in Finland. Acta Obstet Gynecol Scand 2002; 81:747–752.

Temen E. Birthing a Mother: The Surrogate Body and Pregnant Self. University of California: London Press, 2010.

Tuazon-McCheyne J. Two dads: gay male parenting and its politicisation – a co-operative inquiry action research study. Aust N Z J Fam Ther 2010; 31:311–323.

van den Akker OB. Psychological aspects of surrogate motherhood. Hum Reprod Update 2007; 13:53–62.

Wood EG, Batzer FR, Corson SL. Ovarian response to gonadotrophins, optimal method for oocyte retrieval and pregnancy outcome in patients with vaginal agenesis. Hum Reprod 1999; 14:1178–1181.

World Health Organisation. WHO Laboratory Manuel for the Examination & Processing Of Human Semen, 5th edn. Cambridge: Cambridge University Press, 2010.

Zegers-Hochschild F, Adamson GD, de Mouzon J, et al. The International committee for Monitoring Assisted Reproductive Technology (ICMART) and the World Health Organization (WHO) Revised glossary on ART Terminology, 2009. Hum Reprod 2009; 24:2683–2687.

Chapter 13 Support and counseling

Susan Seenan, Kate Brian

INTRODUCTION

There have been many research studies in recent years looking at the psychosocial impact of infertility and treatment. It is well-established that not being able to conceive causes women considerable distress and anxiety, and that the provision of good support at the clinic and through counseling services is important.

In 1997, a survey of 980 mainly female patients carried out for the UK's National Infertility Awareness Campaign (now known as Fertility Fairness) looked at the emotional impact of infertility and found that patients experienced a range of negative responses (Kerr et al. 1999). These included tearfulness (97%), depression/isolation (94%), anger (84%), inadequacy (72%), guilt/shame (62%) and loss of libido/sex drive (80%). One in five of those who responded to the survey said they had experienced suicidal feelings, which illustrates how significant the emotional response to fertility problems and treatment can be.

Support group meetings offer patients the opportunity to discuss their feelings of depression, sadness and isolation. This can become more important as people experiencing infertility begin to feel increasingly alone as friends and colleagues conceive and become absorbed in family life.

Feelings of shame and failure are common, and many women report that their fertility problems make them feel inferior. Pregnancy announcements from others can be difficult and the jealousy and anger that women experience can lead to concerns that their entire personality has changed as a result of their infertility. Dealing with family and friends can be challenging as it may seem that others are unable to appreciate how they feel and often make suggestions which can be at best unhelpful. Some women say that they have lost friends as a result of their fertility treatment.

Research confirms that coping at work can also be difficult, particularly as there is no statutory right to take time off for treatment. As a result, patients often feel uncomfortable about disclosure and many have concerns about confidentiality and negative attitudes from colleagues (Payne et al. 2015).

In the UK, a National Infertility Awareness Campaign study questioned patients about relationships with their partners, and found that around a third reported that this had been strained by their fertility experiences, while a similar number said that going through this together had improved their relationship (Kerr et al. 1999). When positive support is available from partners and family, this can help patients to cope with the stresses caused by fertility problems and treatment. However, other forms of assistance such as counseling and support groups, as well as a supportive attitude from medical staff at the fertility clinic, also play a vital role.

COUNSELING

In the UK, the importance of the provision of counseling for people undergoing fertility treatment is recognized in law by the Human Fertilization and Embryology Act 1990 which states that people should be given "a suitable opportunity to receive proper counseling" if they are having IVF, using donor gametes or embryos and/or want to donate or store gametes or embryos.

Furthermore, the UK has the Human Fertilization and Embryology Authority (HFEA), an independent regulator for IVF treatment which came into effect in 1991. The HFEA is an 'arm's-length body' of the UK government's Department of Health. An arm's-length body is an organisation that delivers a public service, is not a ministerial government department, and which operates to a greater or lesser extent at a distance from governmental ministers. The HFEA works independently on behalf of the UK government. All HFEA-licensed fertility clinics must give patients the opportunity to receive counseling (Licence Condition T60, see Box). Similar instructions about counseling apply where there is an intended second parent (Licence Condition T61, see Box).

HFEA LICENCE CONDITIONS FOR COUNSELING

HFEA issues 'licence conditions' in their Code of Practice. There are three licence conditions relating to counseling:

T60

A woman must not be provided with treatment services using embryos or donated gametes unless she and any man or woman who is to be treated together with her have been given a suitable opportunity to receive proper counseling about the implications of her being provided with treatment services of that kind, and have been provided with such relevant information as is proper.

T61

A woman must not be provided with treatment services where there is an intended second parent unless, either before or after both have consented to the man or woman being the intended second parent, she and the intended second parent have been given a suitable opportunity to receive proper counseling about the implications of the woman being provided with treatment services and have been provided with such relevant information as is proper.

T62

The reference in licence conditions T60 and T61 above to the intended second parent is a reference to:

(a) any man with respect to whom the agreed fatherhood conditions in Section 37 of the Human Fertilisation and Embryology Act 2008 ('the 2008 Act') are for the time being satisfied in relation to treatment provided to the woman mentioned in licence conditions T60 and T61; and

(b) any woman with respect to whom the agreed female parenthood conditions in Section 44 of the 2008 Act are for the time being satisfied in relation to treatment provided to the woman mentioned in licence conditions T60 and T61.

Fertility clinics meet this requirement in a variety of ways. Some patients are offered counseling regularly throughout their treatment, whilst others may only be given information about the existence of the counseling service once when they first visit the clinic. Some clinics employ counselors who work from the clinic; whilst other clinics give patients the contact details for a counselor who is based elsewhere. Funding for counseling depends on the clinic: some clinics incorporate a number of counseling sessions into the cost of treatment, while other clinics ask patients to pay for their own counseling as independent events.

We know that the take-up of counseling is relatively low and that many patients may rely on their own networks of friends and family for support during treatment rather than seeking professional help (Boivin et al. 1999).

There may be several reasons why patients do not use fertility counseling services. An online survey in 2014 of more than 200 patients by the 'British Infertility Counseling Association' and patient charity Fertility Network UK found that a majority (61%) felt that the potential benefits of counseling had not been made clear to them (Payne and van den Akker 2016). A minority (20%) reported that they had not been made aware that counseling was on offer at all, although some of these patients had not been having IVF/ICSI or donor treatment but were instead either waiting to start treatment (6%), having intrauterine insemination (IUI) (5%) or ovulation induction (3%) which may explain this. Counseling is normally not offered to these groups of patients.

Of those who knew that counseling was on offer but had chosen not to see a counselor, many patients felt that they did not have enough information about how counseling might help (45%), while others said they did not need counseling (32%), could not afford counseling (12%) or were worried about how it might affect their treatment if the clinic felt they were not coping (8%).

The survey results make it clear that the way in which counseling is presented is important. Patients should not be worried that accepting support might be seen in a negative light by clinic staff. It would also be helpful for patients if the offer of counseling could be made in more than one way (e.g. not just in literature or on the clinic website, but also when talking to patients during consultations so that the benefits can be discussed) and at more than one stage during treatment process.

FERTILIITY COUNSELING PROCESS

Factors explored during fertility counseling include:

- Current situation, pathway to current situation and hopes for the future
- Validation of loss and appropriate grieving around unmet desire for a child, conceived without assistance
- Acknowledgement of the appropriateness of trauma, validating thoughts and feelings and acknowledging impact of treatment re-traumatising past experiences
- Validation of unconscious/conscious fertility-related conflicts and why cognitive behavioral therapy (CBT) techniques can be unhelpful. Extreme thoughts, both negative and positive, can take place
- Social, legal and ethical implications of treatment for individual(s), the partner, within relationship, for wider networks, including the latest research into interpersonal neurobiology and importance of pregnancy for 'hard wiring' and fetal – maternal/paternal attachment and attunement, especially when using donor conception for any child conceived
- It is important to understand the need for transparency and to tell a child early on in their development if donor gametes are used, via use of attachment theory
- Impact of not conceiving without assistance on self and relationship
- Current coping strategies and ensure awareness of appropriate additional strategies, including mindfulness and other ongoing support which is available
- Implications around choosing not to continue and validate autonomy in choosing to proceed with treatment
- Implications of genetic testing if appropriate
- Social, legal and ethical implications around relationship in individual appointments and group sessions if using known donor conception and/or surrogacy
- Acknowledgement of the impact if assisted conception does not end with a positive pregnancy test
- Ensure appropriate ending with access to ongoing support, explaining potential for continued trauma around secondary infertility in the future, support not just available if treatment unsuccessful

SUPPORT GROUPS

SUPPORT GROUPS

Many countries have national support groups to help people with concerns about fertility. In Europe, an umbrella organization has been formed called Fertility Europe to represent patient associations in more than 20 European countries. The aims of Fertility Europe are to:

- build a strong European network among European patients and professionals in order to achieve the exchange of best practice
- promote education in the field of protection of reproductive health and a pro-active approach to family planning
- improve the situation concerning the rights of those affected by difficulties in conceiving in many areas.

Fertility Europe puts up a 'Wall of Hope' at the annual meeting of the European Society of Human Reproduction and Embryology where goodwill messages are posted for those trying to conceive. See **Table 13.1** for individual country members of Fertility Europe.

In the UK, a campaign group called Fertility Fairness (previously the National Infertility Awareness Campaign), was set up over 20 years ago. Their aim is to fight for the right for people to have full and equal access to investigations and treatments for infertility via the state funding by the UK's National Health Service (NHS). This includes the right to access up to three full cycles of IVF treatment free on the NHS, as recommended by the UK's National Institute for Health and Care Excellence (NICE).

Support groups can be peer-led and run by volunteers which may meet in cafes, community centers or even people's homes. Some group meetings take place at fertility clinics, and may be run by an individual member of staff or by a team of volunteers (who are either going through the treatment or have completed their treatment) with staff assistance.

There has been an increase in the numbers of groups run by people who have businesses in the field, such as fertility coaches or complementary therapists. These can work well but can also raise challenges if the group is seen as a way of attracting clients for the business. There are also many individuals offering private fertility support services, including complementary therapists, fertility yoga teachers, coaches, hypnotherapists and former fertility patients.

In the UK, there are currently 37 fertility support groups in England, 14 groups in Scotland, four in Northern Ireland, three in Wales and two in the Channel Islands. The aim of these groups is not to offer any form of counseling or therapeutic support, but rather to provide a forum in which people experiencing fertility problems can get together and share experiences. The groups tend to be fairly small, and people often like to dip in and out of them during their fertility tests and treatment. Although there are some members who attend every meeting, it is more common for people to come to meetings as and when they feel they need it. There may be times during the treatment journey when a support group is very welcome, and other times when members do not feel ready to talk or share their feelings.

Although people may prefer a local support group to be closer to their home, this does not necessarily translate into attendance at a group; sometimes patients report that just knowing the group is there if they need it can in itself be beneficial, even if they do not attend meetings.

In London, there are presently nine support groups. The group in central London has been contacted by around 80 patients who have expressed an interest in attending meetings, and yet meetings are rarely attended by more than 20 people, despite being free to attend with no requirement to book ahead. The important message, however, is that groups are accessible to all, as and when they need support.

Even though clinics promote awareness of support groups, the majority of people who attend meetings tend to find out about them via social media platforms, rather than from the staff at the clinic they are attending.

Specialist support groups

There is also a need for specialist support groups. For example, patients with secondary infertility do not always feel comfortable turning up at groups which are mainly attended by those experiencing primary infertility. It can be difficult for others in the group when someone who is already a parent wants to express their distress at being unable to conceive again. Thus, a specialist support group for people with secondary infertility is useful.

Similarly, there is often a need to run specialist groups for people from different cultures, especially in countries that have people from many different ethnicities.

Online support

Online support for patients has been growing in popularity, and one of the most popular online forums in the UK, Fertility Friends, currently reports more than 92,000 members. The popular women's websites Mumsnet and Netmums both have active fertility and conception sections too. These websites offer an opportunity to read about other people's experiences of fertility problems and treatment, to share emotional responses and to ask other patients questions.

Participants can choose their own name when posting onto the forum and therefore remain anonymous. Some people find this easier, and it may allow them to be more open about any challenging issues they are facing. The websites also provide a place where support is available at any time as there is nearly always someone out there to respond – so there is an immediacy which more traditional methods of support are unable to provide. This can be particularly helpful in addressing the isolation and loneliness which many patients experience. Closed group Facebook pages can offer another form of support and online support meetings mean participants can talk to a specialist from home.

Online support can be particularly beneficial when patients are going through a treatment cycle. A system of 'cycle buddies' enables them to connect with others who are at the same stage of treatment. Some may also post their own treatment diaries online as they go through a treatment cycle, which can give them an outlet for their feelings while also providing an opportunity for others to read about their experiences.

Although there are some very clear advantages to using online support networks, there are some negative points too. Patients often use these networks to ask one another questions about the latest treatments, drugs or technologies, and there is no shortage of other patients keen to give their own opinion on issues such as drug dosage, IVF protocols and the pros and cons of reproductive immunology or any adjunct treatment.

Patients may even interpret results from one another's tests and scans. It is apparent that the responses from other patients are often accepted as factual, informed and accurate, when in fact this may be far from the case. The large numbers of patients asking one another medical questions online does raise questions about why they are discussing these medical issues with one another rather than asking the professionals who are caring for them at their clinic.

Support for male partners

Research has suggested that women experience more stress as a result of fertility problems than men and that they are more impacted by fertility problems than their male partners (Greil et al. 2010). However, there is often more of a focus on women's experiences of fertility problems in psychosocial research and more work is needed on men's perceptions of fertility problems and treatment and their needs for support (Culley et al. 2013).

While support groups are open to both men and women, the majority of those who come along to the meetings are women attending alone. Some men attend meetings with their partners but they are in a minority. It is unusual for a man to attend a support group meeting without his partner. The sections dedicated to men on fertility websites are markedly less busy than the main areas where most users are women, and the dedicated men's fertility support website www.mensfe.net has fewer people posting than the sites used by women.

Women are also more likely to visit a fertility counselor, and complementary therapists see more women for fertility problems too. In the UK, an example of such a group is the Association of Reproductive Reflexologists. Support groups and online networks may not be the best way to help male fertility patients, and new initiatives and research in this area would be helpful.

Support in the clinic

Research supports the view that patients would like medical staff at clinics to have a more supportive attitude and to be aware of their emotional welfare (Schmidt et al. 2003).

The European Society of Human Reproduction and Embryology (ESHRE) has produced guidance for clinic staff about how best to offer care and support to patients in a fertility clinic which provides a helpful list of key points for staff to take into consideration. The guidance suggests that clinic staff should be aware of the importance patients place on an understanding and empathetic attitude, on continuity of care and not being rushed, on counseling being available and on good patient information (Gameiro et al. 2015).

The provision of good, patient-friendly and jargon-free information is important, and patients would like to have clear explanations when they are given the results of tests or information about the treatment that is on offer.

Patients are not always aware of the impact of reproductive aging on their fertility and on their chances of IVF success. When treatment is unsuccessful, many do not appear to have been informed of the role age may play in this.

The wide range of treatment add-ons currently available is often confusing for patients, especially as clinicians are not always agreed about the benefits. It can be hard for patients to know who they should listen to or trust when they are being given conflicting opinions about the relative merits of various treatments. Patients want reliable and accurate information about the benefits of any treatment they are being offered and about the costs they can expect to incur, and they do not always receive this when it comes to the additional treatments which are being offered at some fertility clinics.

FUNDING AND FINANCIAL ISSUES

In 2013, the NICE guideline (NG156) was updated and certain sections of the guidance were amended (NICE 2013). The new guideline continued to recommend three full cycles of IVF for eligible women of

39 years and under, and also recommended one full cycle for a small group of women aged 40–42 years. In order to qualify for the one cycle, women in this age group must have been trying to conceive for at least 2 years without having any fertility treatment and must be diagnosed as having 'a good ovarian reserve'. The updated guideline clarified the definition of a full cycle of IVF to make it clear that this included the fresh cycle and also the cryopreservation and subsequent transfer of all suitable embryos.

The recommendation that the NHS should provide three full cycles of IVF for women of 39 years and under has still not been implemented in many areas. The campaign group Fertility Fairness and patient charity Fertility Network UK have worked to raise awareness of the 'postcode lottery' for IVF treatment and the problems it causes for fertility patients. Fertility Fairness carries out an annual audit of provision to see what is being funded in each area and to check the criteria used for access to treatment.

In England, fertility treatment is now commissioned locally by clinical commissioning groups (CCGs), and the most recent audit found that just 28% of CCGs were funding three cycles of treatment. The majority, 57%, were offering one cycle of treatment and 24% were offering two. What is more, 44% of CCGs were not using the definition of a 'full' cycle as laid out by NICE but were instead choosing to follow their own more limited definition. Scotland, Wales and Northern Ireland have each adopted their own national criteria, but they differ from one another in what they provide. Only NHS Scotland currently implements full NICE guidance. NHS Wales funds, two fresh cycles and all related frozen embryo transfer (FET) cycles, including the first year of cryo-storage. NHS Northern Ireland currently funds one fresh cycle and one FET cycle.

For patients, this lack of clarity about what is available causes confusion, anxiety and heartache. Many are aware of NICE guidance and are then confused to find that they are unable to access the treatment, they thought, they were eligible for because of where they live. Others find their access to treatment is restricted by the eligibility criteria set locally by their CCG.

These criteria vary from one area to another but may include restrictions relating to patient factors such as their BMI, whether they smoke or whether a couple has existing children from previous relationships. Many patients are reduced to borrowing to fund treatment, and some have reported selling their belongings, crowd-funding or opting for egg sharing agreements in order to access IVF. The stress of infertility is exacerbated by financial concerns for many patients at a time when the most recent figures from the HFEA show that a minority of IVF treatment cycles (41.3%) were funded by the NHS.

Lack of funding in the UK has led some patients to consider traveling overseas for fertility treatment where IVF can sometimes be cheaper. The cost of fertility treatment is known to be one potential driver for patients who opt for cross-border treatment along with availability of donor gametes, success rates and short waiting times (Culley et al. 2011). Despite the potential challenges of traveling abroad for treatment around language and logistics, patient satisfaction is often relatively high. An unpublished survey of patient views about cross-border fertility treatment carried out by Fertility Network UK in 2008 found that the majority of patients who had been treated abroad had been happy with their treatment.

However, one concern is multiple pregnancies, as the HFEA's 'One at a Time' policy in the UK has successfully brought down the multiple birth rate from one in four to one in six after fertility treatment. Overseas clinics may not always follow the same strategies to reduce their multiple pregnancy rate, and patients may not be made aware of the risks that they could face.

REDUCING MULTIPLE BIRTHS – THE 'ONE AT A TIME' CAMPAIGN

In an attempt to reduce the multiple birth rate following fertility treatment in the UK, the HFEA launched a campaign called 'One at a time' in 2007. The campaign is part of a national collaboration between the HFEA and patient groups, fertility professionals, neonatal experts and commissioners. Together, the group aims to share best practice and develop professional guidance, and publish information for patients and professionals about multiple births and single embryo transfer. For IVF treatment where several embryos are produced, the group advocates transferring one embryo per cycle to the uterus, rather than transferring two or three embryos in a single attempt.

See Table 14.1 for the risks associated with multiple births.

SUPPORT AFTER UNSUCCESSFUL TREATMENT

Making a decision to end treatment is not easy for a fertility patient. There are many reasons why they may decide to stop. Sometimes it may be a matter of not being able to afford to pay to continue but the psychological burden of going through treatment is often the most important factor (Gameiro et al. 2012).

Once the decision to stop fertility treatment has been made, patients sometimes report feeling that perhaps they were being given false hope at the clinic about their chances of success while they were being treated, and that this had made them reluctant to give up (Peddie et al. 2005). It is important to recognize that patients often feel isolated and abandoned by the clinic when they leave after unsuccessful treatment. The need to offer support and counseling at this point should not be overlooked (**Figure 13.1**). The experience of unsuccessful treatment and living without children can continue to resonate throughout former fertility patients' lives and for some women feelings of social isolation can become even stronger as they grow older (Wirtberg et al. 2007).

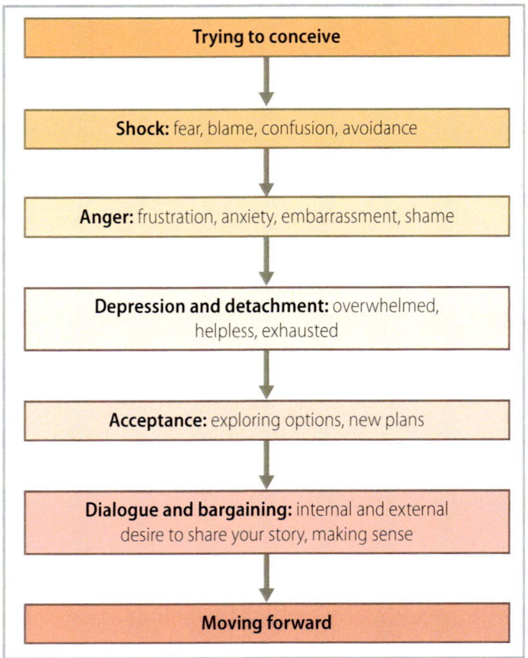

Figure 13.1 A flow diagram to help validate the emotional reaction of those exploring fertility.

Table 13.1 Support groups throughout Europe. Most groups have a Facebook page (information obtained from Fertility Europe)

Country	Organisation	Website
Belgium	De Verdwaalde Ooievaar Netwerk Fertiliteit (The Lost Stork – Fertility Network)	www.deverdwaaldeooievaar.be
Bulgaria	Iskambebe (I want a baby foundation)	www.iskambebe.bg
	Sdruzhenie Zachatie (Association Conception)	www.zachatie.org
Croatia	Association RODA (Parents in Action)	www.roda.hr
Czech republic	Adam	www.adamcr.cz
Finland	Lapsettomien yhdistys Simpukka ry (Infertility Association Simpukka)	www.simpukka.info
France	Maia	www.maia-asso.org
Greece	Magna Mater	www.magnamater.gr
	Kiveli	www.kiveli.gr
Iceland	Tilvera	www.tilvera.is
Ireland	NISIG – National Infertility Support & Information Group	www.nisig.com
Israel	CHEN – Patient Fertility Association	www.amotatchen.org
Italy	Amica Cicogna (Friend Stork)	www.amicacicogna.it
Malta	Malta Infertility Network	www.fertilitysupport.com.mt
Montenegro	Nas San (Our Dream)	
The Netherlands	Freya – Vereniging voor vruchtbaarheidsproblemen (Freya – Fertility problems association)	www.freya.nl
Norway	Ønskebarn (WishChild)	www.onskebarn.no
Poland	Nasz Bocian (Our Stork)	www.nasz-bocian.pl
Portugal	Associação Portuguesa de Fertilidade (Portuguese Fertility Association)	www.apfertilidade.org
Romania	Asociatia SOS Infertilitatea (SOS Infertility Association)	www.infertilitate.com
Serbia	Sansa za roditeljstvo (Wish for parenthood)	www.sansazaroditeljstvo.org.rs
Sweden	Barnlängtan (Child longing)	www.barnlangtan.com
United Kingdom	Fertility Network UK	www.fertilitynetworkuk.org
Turkey	Çider (I Want a Child Support Association)	www.cocukistiyorum.com

The ESHRE guideline for staff working in clinics suggests that they should give patients time to discuss the implications of stopping their treatment, and that those who have decided to give up and have not been successful should be referred for counseling or psychology support (Gameiro et al. 2015).

CONCLUSION

It is clear that the provision of good support at every stage of fertility tests, and treatment is a key part of good quality care for women and their partners. Offering counseling services and ensuring that patients are aware of the potential benefits, making sure that they know about support groups and that they have good, accessible information will make all the difference to women's experience of fertility treatment, regardless of the outcome.

ACKNOWLEDGEMENTS

We are grateful to Tracey Sainsbury, Fertility Counsellor, member of Fertility Network UK Advisory Panel, for advice regarding the figure and table used in this chapter.

REFERENCES

Boivin J, Scanlan L, Walker S. Why are infertile patients not using psychosocial counselling? Hum Reprod 1999; 14:1384–1391.

Culley L, Hudson N, Lohan M. Where are all the men? The marginalization of men in social scientific research on infertility. Reprod Biomed Online 2013; 27:225–235.

Culley L, Hudson N, Rapport F, et al. Crossing borders for fertility treatment: motivations, destinations and outcomes of UK fertility travelers. Hum Reprod 2011; 26:2373–2381.

Gameiro S, Boivin J, Peronace L, Verhaak C. Why do patients discontinue fertility treatment? A systematic review of reasons and predictors of discontinuation in fertility treatment. Hum Reprod Update 2012; 18:652–669.

Gameiro S, Boivin J, Dancet E, et al. ESHRE guideline: routine psychosocial care in infertility and medically assisted reproduction-a guide for fertility staff. Hum Reprod 2015; 30:2476–2485.

Greil A, Slauson-Blevins K, McQuillan J. The experience of infertility: A review of recent literature. Social Health Illn 2010; 32:140–162.

Kerr J, Brown C, Balen A. The experiences of couples who have had infertility treatment in the United Kingdom: results of a survey performed in 1997. Hum Reprod 1999; 14:934–938.

National Institute for Health and Care Excellence (NICE). Fertility: for people with fertility problems. CG no. 156. London: NICE, 2013.

Payne N, van den Akker O. Fertility Network UK Survey on the Impact of Fertility Problems. Final Report 2016. London: Fertility Network UK, 2016.
Payne N, van den Akker O, Lewis S, Constantinou C. Experiences of combining work and fertility treatment. J Fertility Counselling 2015; 22:13–16.
Peddie V, van Teijlingen E, Bhattacharya S. A qualitative study of women's decision-making at the end of IVF treatment. Human Reproduction 2005; 20:1944–1951.
Schmidt L, Holstein B, Boivin J, et al. Patients' attitudes to medical and psychosocial aspects of care in fertility clinics: findings from the Copenhagen Multi-centre Psychosocial Infertility (COMPI) Research Programme. Hum Reprod 2003; 18:628–637.
Wirtberg I, Möller A, Hogström L, Tronstad SE, Lalos A. Life 20 years after unsuccessful infertility treatment. Hum Reprod 2007; 22:598–604.

Chapter 14 Management of early pregnancy

Karen Sohan

DIAGNOSIS OF PREGNANCY

The aim of fertility treatment is to achieve a successful pregnancy and a healthy newborn. With any form of fertility treatment there is a waiting period before success of the procedure can be determined. During this time, the woman is encouraged to use the hormonal supports (commonly known as luteal support) and other medications that positively influence implantation. Psychologically, waiting can be exhausting as there is anxiety that the technique might be unsuccessful. Written and verbal information provided by the clinic about what to expect during this period can be helpful and is recommended.

Any woman who is planning a pregnancy should be advised about the importance of taking folate which has been shown to reduce the chance of neural tube defects (Murphy et al. 2000; see Chapter 4). The minimum recommended prophylactic dose is 400 μg. This should ideally be commenced preconceptually for maximum effect, but can be started as soon as the pregnancy is diagnosed in the first trimester. By the 11th week, the baby's spine is formed and folic acid is not expected to have an impact.

About 2 weeks (typically 10–14 days) following embryo transfer (ET), the woman is advised to do a blood test for determination of beta-human chorionic gonadotropin (β-hCG) levels, the first detectable hormone of pregnancy. A β-hCG level >10 mIU/mL indicates a positive test. Blood β-hCG levels are recommended for the early detection of pregnancy as blood tests are more sensitive than urine pregnancy tests. At this stage, a pregnancy is referred to as 'biochemical,' since imaging with ultrasound scanning will not detect the presence of a pregnancy.

If the test is negative, the woman is instructed to stop all medication. The withdrawal of hormonal support usually results in vaginal bleeding within days. This can be emotionally distressing as the woman realizes that the assisted reproductive technologies (ART) procedure has been unsuccessful. It is extremely important to address the emotional issues associated with a failed ART attempt. The woman and her partner should be invited to meet with medical staff at the earliest convenient time to discuss events. Telephone consultations, while helpful, should not be the only form of counseling offered.

When the test is positive, the β-hCG should be repeated after 48 hours. In about two-thirds of viable intrauterine pregnancies, the level will increase by a factor of two or more (Seeber 2012). The range of β-hCG that is considered normal for a given gestational age is wide, so even if the levels are not following the expected pattern, further β-hCG tests and transvaginal ultrasound may be requested. Further investigations over time provide useful information in making the diagnosis and are considered good clinical practice. At about 21 days post-ET, a transvaginal ultrasound scan can be performed (see Box).

INFORMATION PROVIDED BY AN ULTRASOUND SCAN IN EARLY PREGNANCY

- Viability (whether the pregnancy is alive or not)
- Location (to check that the pregnancy is located in the uterine cavity and not elsewhere, e.g. an ectopic pregnancy in the fallopian tube)
- Number of pregnancies (singleton or multiples)
- Normality of the fetus(es)

The first embryonic structure that is visible with transvaginal scanning is the gestational sac. This appears as a hypoechoic area surrounded by an echogenic rim within the uterine cavity, usually at or near the fundus (**Figure 14.1**) (Timor-Tritsch et al. 1988). The serum β-hCG level above which a gestational sac should be seen (known as the discriminatory zone for β-hCG) is 1500–2000 mIU/mL (Barnhart et al. 1994). This is followed by the appearance of the yolk sac (a round structure with a sonolucent center) within the gestational sac, typically when the mean gestational sac diameter is 5–6 mm (**Figure 14.2**). By 28 days post-ET, the embryonic pole is visible as a linear echogenic structure adjacent to the yolk sac (**Figure 14.3**).

If the uterus contains a fluid-filled area but no other embryonic structures are identifiable within it, the woman is counseled that there is a pregnancy of unknown location. A fluid-filled sac without any embryonic structures can occur in both intrauterine and ectopic pregnancies and therefore the woman should be appropriately counseled (NICE Clinical Guideline 154, 2012).

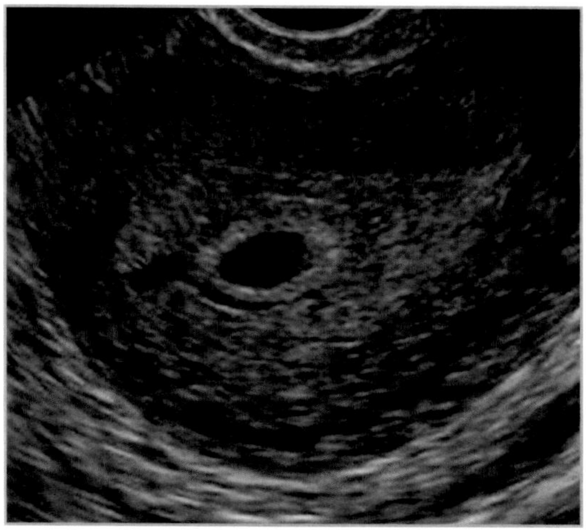

Figure 14.1 The initial scan following a positive pregnancy test. The first embryonic structure that is visible with transvaginal scan is the gestational sac. This appears as a hypoechoic area surrounded by an echogenic rim within the uterine cavity, usually at/or near the fundus. The fluid-filled intrauterine sac is usually detectable when the sac has a diameter of 2–3 mm.

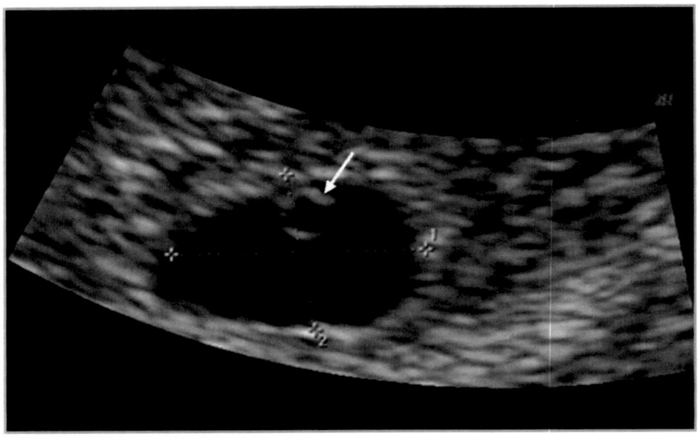

Figure 14.2 An ultrasound scan showing a gestational sac. The gestational scan contains a yolk sac, a round structure with a sonolucent center within the gestational sac, typically when the mean gestational sac diameter is 5–6 mm.

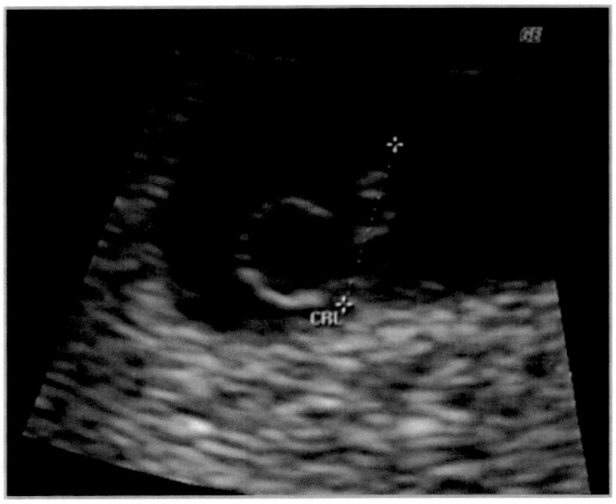

Figure 14.3 An ultrasound scan performed at 28 days after embryo transfer. The embryonic pole is visible as a linear echogenic structure adjacent to the yolk sac.

When the yolk sac or fetal node is seen in the gestational sac then the location of the pregnancy is confirmed as intrauterine.

If the yolk sac is visible or there is a fetal node without a pulsation suggestive of a heartbeat, then the pregnancy is classified as an intrauterine pregnancy of unknown viability and a repeat ultrasound is arranged.

A viable intrauterine pregnancy is confirmed only when a fetal node with a heartbeat is observed in the intrauterine cavity.

ECTOPIC AND HETEROTOPIC PREGNANCY

It is estimated that the risk of ectopic pregnancy is about 1.4% following ART (Santos-Ribeiro et al. 2016). Heterotopic pregnancy is rare and refers to the presence of both an intrauterine and ectopic pregnancy.

It is important to exclude an ectopic pregnancy as this has the potential for morbidity, and in severe cases mortality in women. As the placental tissue expands in an intrauterine pregnancy, the uterus enlarges to accommodate the developing pregnancy as it is designed to do so. In an ectopic site, such as the fallopian tube, the tube is unable to expand as required. As the pregnancy develops, it leads to rupture and internal hemorrhage, which may be life-threatening if not detected at an early stage. The medical team caring for women who have undergone ART are particularly vigilant to exclude an ectopic pregnancy.

It is important to advise women about suspicious symptoms for which they must seek emergency treatment. The common symptoms are lower abdominal pain, especially unilateral, irregular vaginal bleeding, shoulder tip pain, dizziness and syncope (fainting).

The combination of serial β-hCG and transvaginal ultrasound is important when an ectopic pregnancy is suspected and the patient is hemodynamically stable. If the β-hCG has not doubled after 48 hours, and measures >1000 mIU/mL and the transvaginal ultrasound shows an empty uterus or a fluid-filled sac with no embryonic structures, an ectopic pregnancy should be suspected. Sometimes the location of the pregnancy is not evident and multiple blood tests and ultrasound are required to make the diagnosis. If an ectopic pregnancy is diagnosed or there is a high index of suspicion, management may be surgical or medical (Capmas et al. 2014, Mol et al. 2008).

Laparoscopy or keyhole surgery is the treatment of choice if:

- An ectopic pregnancy is suspected and the patient is in significant pain
- Transvaginal ultrasound shows an adnexal mass of ≥35 mm
- Transvaginal ultrasound shows a live ectopic pregnancy, i.e. a fetal node with a clear heartbeat
- The β-hCG level is >5000 mIU/mL

The final procedure is either salpingotomy (removal of the damaged part of the tube containing the ectopic) or salpingectomy (removal of the entire tube), depending on the extent of damage to the fallopian tube. In the rare instances where the patient is hemodynamically unstable, laparotomy (open surgery) may be required in the interest of time.

Methotrexate, a drug that targets placental tissue, may be utilized if the patient is well and:

- β-hCG levels are <1500 mIU/mL
- Transvaginal ultrasound shows an unruptured ectopic with an adnexal mass of <35 mm

If the β-hCG levels are between 1500 and 5000 mIU/mL with an unruptured ectopic and adnexal mass of <35 mm, either laparoscopy or methotrexate can be utilized.

Women receiving methotrexate treatment will require serial β-hCG tests to monitor the success of treatment as the β-hCG levels return to nonpregnancy values with time. Methotrexate users must be advised that if their symptoms worsen, they must attend the emergency department.

MISCARRIAGE

The risk of miscarriage (nonviable pregnancy) with pregnancies from ART can be as high as 40% (Barlow et al. 1988).

In some instances, following the initial positive β-hCG, the woman may begin to experience lower abdominal cramps and vaginal bleeding. When this occurs very early in pregnancy, embryonic structures are not detectable on transvaginal scan. A repeat β-hCG (minimum of 48 hours following bleeding) may show a nonpregnant value. A decrease in β-hCG levels to nonpregnant values may also occur in asymptomatic women. In these cases, the pregnancy is described as biochemical since the only evidence that a pregnancy was achieved was the elevation of the β-hCG level.

Since women who have had fertility treatment have serial ultrasounds, the diagnosis of miscarriage is based on the ultrasound findings in many women without symptoms (NICE Clinical Guideline 154, 2012). If the mean sac diameter (MSD) is measured as ≥25 mm and there is no yolk sac or embryonic structures, an anembryonic pregnancy (blighted ovum) is diagnosed (**Figure 14.4**). If the MSD is measured as <25 mm on the first ultrasound scan, then a repeat ultrasound scan should be arranged a minimum of 7 days after the first scan.

If the fetal node is present and the crown-rump length (CRL) is measured as ≥7 mm and there is no heartbeat, the diagnosis of early fetal demise is made. If the CRL is measured as <7 mm and there is no heartbeat, a repeat ultrasound scan should be arranged a minimum of 7 days after the first scan.

If a woman has been diagnosed with an intrauterine pregnancy and she begins to bleed or experiences lower abdominal pain, an ultrasound scan should be arranged to exclude a miscarriage. If the ultrasound shows an empty uterus, thickened endometrium only or a fetal node without a heartbeat, then a diagnosis of miscarriage is made. The management will depend on the woman's clinical condition and the diagnosis.

In some instances, it is not possible to confirm viability with a single scan and repeat scans are arranged. If the ultrasound findings are inconclusive, a repeat ultrasound should be arranged, in a minimum of 7 days. Even when the clinician is certain that the pregnancy is not viable at the first visit, it is good clinical practice to offer a repeat scan. Sometimes, this needs to be performed for the emotional well-being of the patient.

Once the diagnosis of miscarriage is confirmed the woman should be counseled and options about management discussed. These would include conservative, medical and surgical management (Trinder et al. 2006).

In the case of ART pregnancies, the woman usually starts to bleed within a week of stopping all medications and therefore it is reasonable to use conservative management as the first-line of treatment. The woman is advised to repeat the blood β-hCG or perform a urine pregnancy test 2 weeks after bleeding to ensure that the miscarriage is complete. If either is positive, then the woman should return to the clinician for assessment. If bleeding or abdominal pain persists, or the woman fails to start bleeding within 2 weeks, a repeat ultrasound should be arranged.

In some instances, the woman may not wish to wait, in which case medical management with misoprostol should be administered. When the diagnosis is an early embryonic demise, a single dose of misoprostol 800 μg, vaginally or orally, should be prescribed (Chen et al. 2008). The woman should be counseled about possible side-effects of the medication, such as vomiting, diarrhea and abdominal cramps. A blood β-hCG or a urine pregnancy test should be performed 2 weeks after bleeding occurs. If bleeding does not occur within 24 hours then the clinician should review to determine further care.

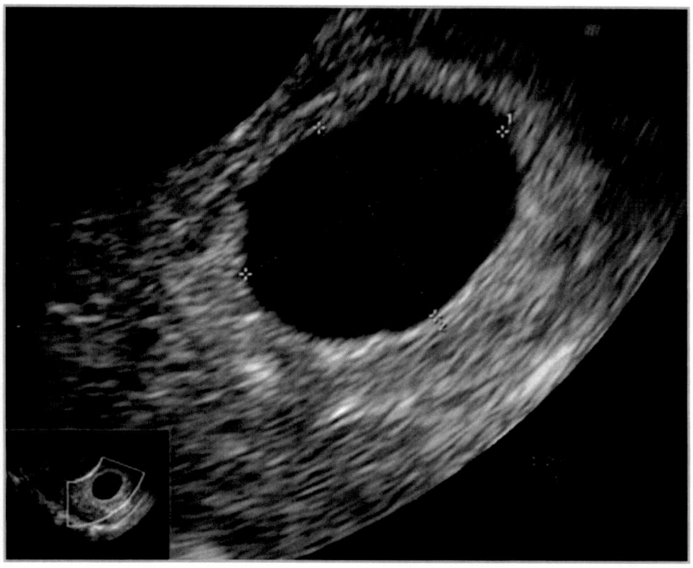

Figure 14.4 An ultrasound scan showing early embryonic demise: empty gestational sac >25 mm in diameter.

If surgical management is the treatment of choice, this can be performed either on an outpatient basis using local anesthesia via manual vacuum aspiration, or as a hospital procedure in theater under general anesthesia.

The importance of the psychological support for a woman who has lost her most wished pregnancy cannot be underestimated (Lok et al. 2007), especially following fertility treatment. Women experience a wide range of emotions which may vary from sadness to guilt. In addition, a pregnancy loss can have a profound impact on the partner as well. There are usually more questions than answers, as in many instances it is not possible for the clinician to give a reason for the miscarriage. Care should be taken to arrange appropriate counseling, which may be time-consuming and may involve referral to other professionals as needed (see Chapter 13). Certainly, consideration should be given to inform the woman's general practitioner and the local miscarriage support group, as these can both provide the much-needed help at this most difficult time.

MULTIPLE PREGNANCY

ART has historically been associated with multiple pregnancies following the transfer of more than one embryo after IVF. Multiple pregnancies and births are the greatest health risks of fertility treatment (**Table 14.1**).

At least 50% of twins and 90% of triplets are born prematurely before 37 weeks of gestation. As such, there are strict guidelines produced by many professional bodies about how many embryos should be transferred. Since 2004, the embryo transfer policy in the UK states that a maximum of two embryos may be transferred in the woman who is less than 40 years of age, with no exceptions, and a maximum of three may be transferred in the woman 40 and over. However, in 2009, the HFEA introduced a policy to further minimize the risk of multiple pregnancies, following an expert group report and public consultation. The HFEA's overall aim was to reduce the UK IVF multiple birth rate to 10%. According to the HFEA Multiple Births Report 2015, there has been a dramatic decrease in multiple pregnancy rates from 27% in 2004 to 16% in the first half of 2014. It should be noted though that the desired multiple pregnancy rate of 10% stipulated by the HFEA has still to be achieved.

When a multiple pregnancy has been confirmed, it is important to determine the chorionicity, which usually can only be accurately performed in the first trimester (Carroll et al. 2004). It cannot be assumed that because two embryos were transferred, the presence of a twin pregnancy indicates that the two embryos implanted. This is because a single embryo can split into two prior to implantation, leading to identical twins. The management of twin pregnancy is influenced by the chorionicity, i.e. whether the fetuses have a single placenta (monochorionic) or separate placentae (dichorionic).

Monochorionic pregnancies have a higher risk to both the mother and babies, and have to be monitored more closely for complications peculiar to the sharing of one blood supply (Christensen 2015). The risk of first trimester miscarriage, congenital abnormalities, intrauterine growth restriction, and extreme preterm birth are higher with monochorionic twin pregnancies. Chorionicity is determined by ultrasound in the first trimester by locating the membrane insertion into the placenta. If this looks like a 'T' then this is deemed a monochorionic twin pregnancy and if it appears as a lambda sign then it is dichorionic.

Table 14.1 The risks associated with multiple births. Iatrogenic multiple pregnancies pose health risks to both the offspring and the mother

Condition	Risk
Preterm labor and birth	Risk of extremely preterm birth (gestational weeks 20–27) is 0.8% (singleton), 2.6% (twins), 7.4% (triplets) Risk of very preterm birth (28–32 weeks) is 2.5% (singleton), 11.0% (twins) 37.4% (triplets) Risk of preterm (33–36 weeks) is 8.7% (singleton), 39.3% (twins), 43.9% (triplets)
Pre-eclampsia	A multiple birth is twice as likely to raise blood pressure in pregnancy, increasing the risk of placental abruption (early detachment of the placenta)
Anemia	A multiple birth is twice as likely to cause anemia
Miscarriage	Vanishing twin syndrome (and bleeding) is more likely in multiple pregnancies
Postpartum hemorrhage	Increased risk to the mother of bleeding after delivery with multiple pregnancy
Cesarean delivery	Increased risk of a cesarean section

Since the risk of preterm delivery is increased with multiple pregnancies, some clinicians may choose to monitor cervical length at the end of the first trimester to determine if a cervical cerclage is indicated (Melamed et al. 2016).

TESTS FOR CHROMOSOMAL ABNORMALITY

Many women undergoing fertility treatment are >35 years and therefore the risk of chromosomal abnormality in the fetus should be discussed. While this should ideally be performed preconceptually, it is necessary to discuss it again once an intrauterine pregnancy is diagnosed. The woman and her partner should be provided with accurate up-to-date information, and they should make the decision as to what they would like to be done without influence from the attending physician.

The risk of chromosomal abnormalities increases with maternal age (Snijders et al. 1999). The commonest chromosomal condition is Down syndrome or trisomy 21. Each individual is made up of 23 pairs of chromosomes (one from each parent so that an individual has 46 chromosomes). In the majority of cases of Down syndrome, there is an extra copy of chromosome 21 so the individual has 47 chromosomes. Several screening tests are available which can identify the woman as high or low-risk for trisomy 21. These include ultrasound, maternal serum markers via noninvasive prenatal diagnosis (NIPT; see Chapter 16) and a combination of these. At present, a combined test involving measurement of the nuchal translucency (fluid at the back of the fetal neck) by ultrasound and serum protein markers from a sample of the maternal blood is recommended by the National Health Service (NHS) in the UK. This is performed in the first trimester (before 12 weeks). It has a Down syndrome detection rate of nearly 90% for a 3% positive rate (Wright et al. 2010).

For NIPT, a single blood sample is required in the majority of cases. Cell-free DNA is analyzed to screen for trisomy 21 and with improved techniques detection rates, sensitivity and specificity close to 100% have been reported. Since this test involves a single blood sample from the mother, it is anticipated that in time it will replace the combined testing as its sensitivity is higher and is not user dependent (e.g. accurate nuchal translucency measurements are dependent on the technician performing the ultrasound) (Hyett 2016).

If the woman is deemed to be high risk from the screening test, then she can be offered a diagnostic test via chorionic villus sampling (CVS) or amniocentesis. However, any needle test has a risk of miscarriage, with the risk of miscarriage from a CVS being 2% compared to 1% with amniocentesis. The apparent higher risk with CVS is because the procedure is performed at earlier gestation and will include some pregnancies which would have spontaneously miscarried.

CONCLUSION

This chapter has provided an overview of the management of early pregnancy. The methods used to diagnose pregnancy and also detect ectopic and heterotopic pregnancies have been discussed.

With ART, there are heightened risks relating to miscarriage, multiple pregnancies and the normality of the offspring. However, provided patients are fully informed and risks are mitigated, then the pregnancies can be carefully monitored, to result in the birth of much desired healthy babies.

REFERENCES

Barnhart K, Mennuti MT, Benjamin I, et al. Prompt diagnosis of ectopic pregnancy in an emergency department setting. Obstet Gynecol 1994; 84:1010–1015.

Barlow P, Lejeune B, Puissant F, et al. Early pregnancy loss and obstetrical risk after in-vitro fertilization and embryo replacement. Hum Reprod 1988; 3:671–675.

Capmas P, Bouyer J, Fernandez H. Treatment of ectopic pregnancies in 2014: new answers to some old questions. Fertil Steril 2014; 101:615–620.

Carroll SG, Soothill PW, Abdel-Fattah SA, et al. Prediction of chorionicity in twin pregnancies at 10-14 weeks of gestation. BJOG 2002; 109:182–186.

Chen BA, Creinin MD. Medical management of early pregnancy failure: efficacy. Semin Reprod Med 2008; 26:411–422.

Hyett J. Combined first trimester or cffDNA screening. BJOG 2016; 123:98.

Lok IH, Neugebauer R. Psychological morbidity following miscarriage. Best Pract Res Clin Obstet Gynaecol 2007; 21:229–247.

Melamed N, Pittini A, Hiersch L, et al. Serial cervical length determination in twin pregnancies reveals 4 distinct patterns with prognostic significance for preterm birth. Am J Obstet Gynecol 2016; 215:476.e11.

Mol F, Mol BW, Ankum WM, van der Veen F, Hajenius PJ. Current evidence on surgery, systemic methotrexate and expectant management in the treatment of tubal ectopic pregnancy: a systematic review and meta-analysis. Hum Reprod Update 2008; 14:309–319.

Murphy M, Whiteman D, Stone D, et al. Dietary folate and the prevalence of neural tube defects in the British Isles: the past two decades. BJOG 2000; 107:885–889.

National Institute for Health and Care Excellence. Ectopic pregnancy and miscarriage: diagnosis and initial management in early pregnancy of ectopic pregnancy and miscarriage. NICE Clinical Guideline 154. London: NICE, 2012.

Santos-Ribeiro S, Tournaye H, Polyzos NP. Trends in ectopic pregnancy rates following assisted reproductive technologies in the UK: a 12-year nationwide analysis including 160 000 pregnancies. Hum Reprod 2016; 31:393–402.

Seeber BE. What serial hCG can tell you, and cannot tell you, about an early pregnancy. Fertil Steril 2012; 98:1074–1077.

Snijders RJ, Sundberg K, Holzgreve W, Henry G, Nicolaides KH. Maternal age- and gestation-specific risk for trisomy 21. Ultrasound Obstet Gynecol 1999; 13:167–170.

Timor-Tritsch IE, Farine D, Rosen MG. A close look at early embryonic development with the high-frequency transvaginal transducer. Am J Obstet Gynecol 1988; 159:676–681.

Trinder J, Brocklehurst P, Porter R, et al. Management of miscarriage: expectant, medical, or surgical? Results of randomised controlled trial (miscarriage treatment (MIST) trial). BMJ 2006; 332:1235–1240.

Wright D, Spencer K, Kagan KK, et al. First-trimester combined screening for trisomy 21 at 7–14 weeks' gestation. Ultrasound Obstet Gynecol 2010; 36:404–411.

Chapter 15 Management of genetic disorders

Semra Kahraman, Caroline Pirkevi

CHROMOSOMAL ABNORMALITIES

Chromosomal structure and origin of abnormalities

Chromosomal abnormalities are very common. It is estimated that 40% of spontaneously aborted 1st trimester pregnancies are due to them. Less than 1% of fetuses carrying such abnormalities survive to term and they are subsequently affected by the chromosome imbalance.

Chromosomes are present in the nucleus of each cell and are made up of DNA, the genetic material, tightly coiled several times around proteins called histones. Chromosomes are not visible under the microscope during the resting phase of the cell. However, during cell division, as DNA becomes more tightly packed, chromosomes become visible under microscope.

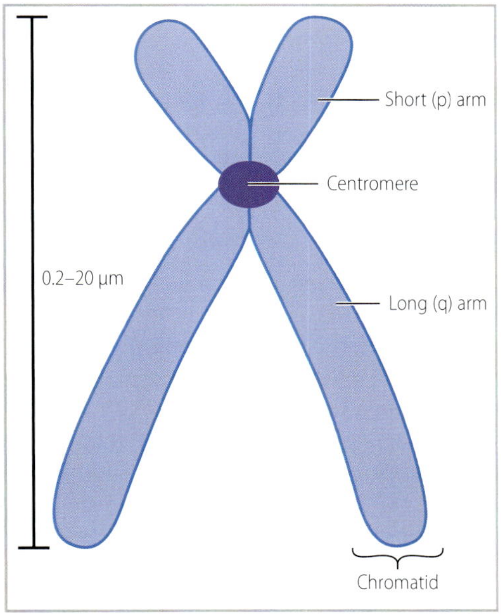

Figure 15.1 A prophase chromosome after replication showing the short and long arms with centromere positioning to produce two chromatids.

Each cell contains 46 chromosomes: 22 pairs of autosomes and one pair of sex chromosomes (X and Y), i.e. one set of 23 from each parent. Gametes, with their one set of 23 chromosomes, are termed haploid or 'n'; the cells of the offspring, with two sets of 23, are diploid or '2n'. The members of a chromosome pair are called homologous chromosomes, one homolog from each parent; by definition they are non-homologous with the other chromosomes in the set.

Each chromosome has a constriction point called the centromere (**Figure 15.1**). After DNA replication has taken place (see **Figure 15.6**) the chromosome has two identical chromatids, and the centromere plays an important role in the separation of these into daughter cells during cell division (mitosis and meiosis) (**Figure 15.2**). For division, a 'spindle' of microtubules is assembled from protein subunits. Microtubules attach to the centromere and pull the chomosome's daughter chromatids towards opposite ends of the cell before it divides. This separation ensures that each daughter cell has a full set of chromosomes.

Chromosomes can be described by the position of their centromere (**Figure 15.3**):

- Metacentric, with the centromere near the centre of the chromosome.
- Submetacentric, with an off-centre centromere, such that one 'arm' of the chromosome is longer than the other.
- Acrocentric, with the centromere very near to one end of the chromosome.

The shorter arm is designated by the letter 'p' (for petite) and the longer arm is designated by the letter 'q' (as 'q' follows 'p' alphabetically). The 'acrocentric' chromosome has the centromere very near one end (**Figure 15.3a**). Centromere position and size are the easiest ways to tell chromosomes apart. In addition the 'banding pattern', i.e. the size and location of bands produced by Giemsa staining, is unique for each chromosome (**Figure 15.3b**). The number and appearance of a cell's chromosomes are termed its karyotype.

A region of a chromosome or a gene's location on a chromosome (its locus) can be described by a combination of the chromosome

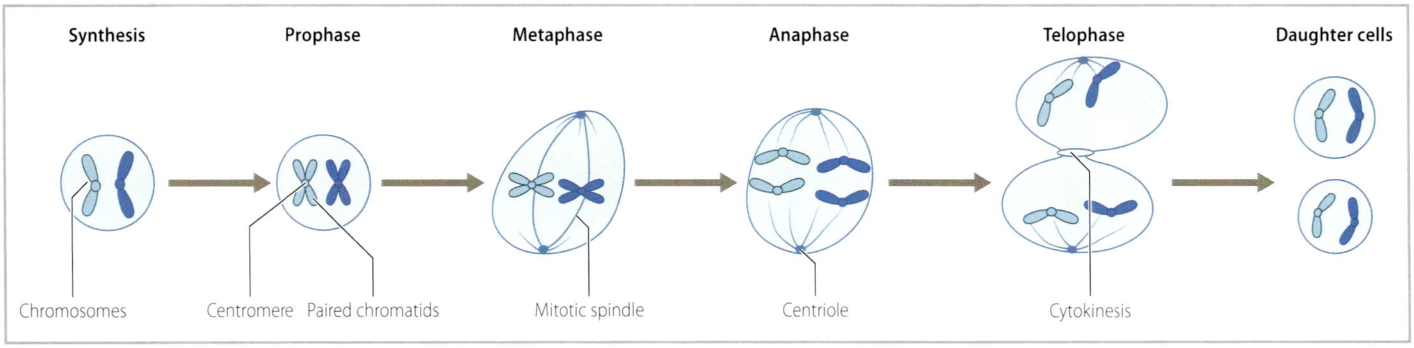

Figure 15.2 During cell division, microtubules attach to centromeres and pull the chromosomes to opposite ends of the cell.

number (e.g. chromosome 15), the chromosome arm (p or q) and its position with respect to banding and sub-banding (e.g. 11 or 13), for example 15q11 or 15q13 (see **Figure 15.7**).

Chromosome abnormalities are produced by misrepair of broken chromosomes, improper recombination or mal-segregation of chromosomes during meiosis I or II. Chromosomal abnormalities can also arise postmeiotically, in the preimplantation embryo, as it enters multiple cell divisions during early embryo development.

It is well documented that chromosomal abnormalities originate during female meiosis and especially in meiosis I (Kuliev 2012). Furthermore, a strong correlation between maternal age and chromosomal abnormalities in oocytes and embryos is well established. As age increases, the number of oocytes with a normal set of chromosomes (2n) decreases. Under the age of 35 years, the proportion of embryos with a normal number of chromosomes (euploid) is approximately 50%. However, this proportion decreases to 14% by the age of 42–43 years, and is only 6% at age 44 years (Kahraman et al. 2016). In contrast, no method has yet been made available for testing the outcome of male meiosis as the present methods used to analyze the sperm genome involves sperm destruction, making them useless for fertilization (Kuliev 2012). For that reason, analysis of oocytes, cleavage-stage embryos or blastocysts is especially valuable for preimplantation genetic testing (PGT).

The main numerical structural chromosome abnormalities and abnormalities arising from unequal contributions from the two parents [uniparental disomy (UPD)] are discussed below.

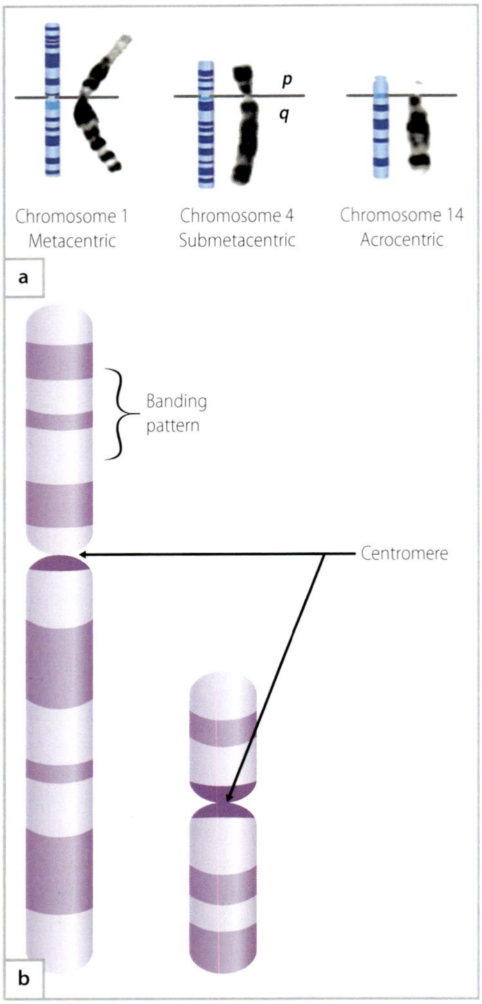

Figure 15.3 (a) Identification of different chromosomes can be based on the position of the centromere in relation to the height of the chromosome. (b) Identification of chromosome based on size; band pattern and centromere positioning.

Numerical chromosomal abnormalities

In diploid cells, the normal number of chromosomes is 46 – two sets of 23. This is termed euploid and abbreviated as 2n, where n is 23. Numerical chromosomal abnormalities involve gain or loss of complete chromosomes and fall into three categories:

- Polyploid: having more than two sets of 23 chromosomes (e.g. 3n or 4n)
- Haploid: having only one set of 23 chromosomes (1n)
- Aneuploid: having a loss or gain of one or more specific chromosomes.

Polyploidy

The most common cause of polyploidy is two sperm fertilizing a single oocyte (dispermy). Polyploidy can also be caused by a gamete being diploid (either the sperm or the oocyte) but fertilization with diploid sperm is highly unlikely. Examples of triploidy are 69,XXX; 69,XXY; and 69,XYY (the X and Y sex chromosomes are included in the total number and their pattern is designated by adding the letters). They account for 1% of conceptions and very seldom survive to term (Toufaily et al. 2016). The triploid condition is not compatible with life and the affected fetus often does not survive past the first trimester (Toufaily et al. 2016).

Tetraploidy is rarer and is always lethal. To date, only 10 live births with the condition have been reported (Wada et al. 2016). Tetraploidy (e.g. 92,XXYY) is mostly due to a post-meiotic error, namely a cytoplasmic failure to complete all stages of the first zygotic division (**Figure 15.4**). In this case, DNA originating from two haploid gametes

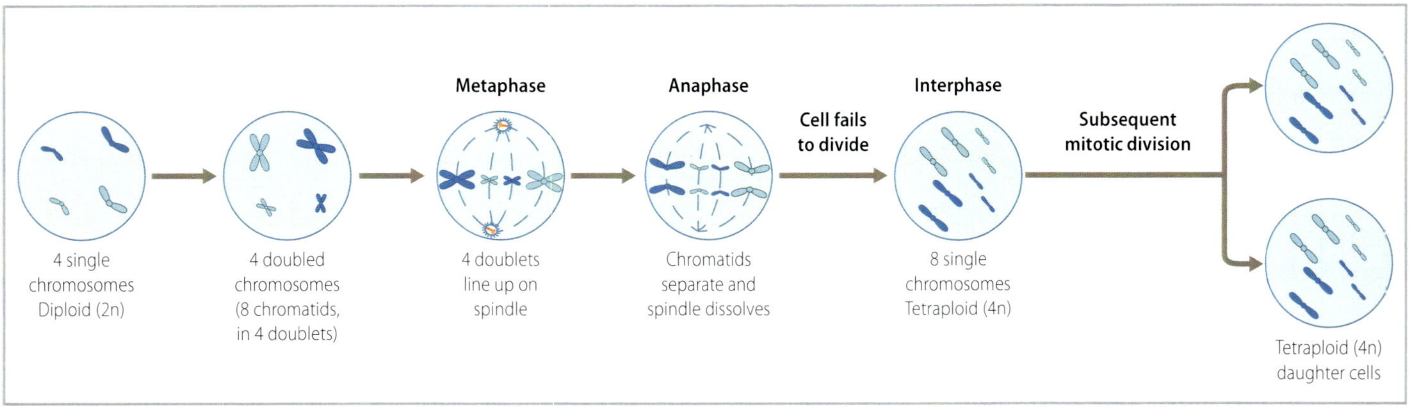

Figure 15.4 Mitotic polyploidy. The formation of a tetraploid cell from a diploid mother cell.

replicates to give a content of 4n, but the cell then fails to complete its first mitotic division. As a result all subsequent cells are 4n.

Aneuploidy

An aneuploid cell has one or more individual chromosomes additional to, or missing from, the euploid set. This is termed trisomy and monosomy, respectively (see **Table 15.1** for examples of trisomy). Aneuploid cells arise through two main mechanisms:

- nondisjunction
- anaphase lag.

Nondisjunction happens when paired chromosomes fail to separate in anaphase of meiosis I or when sister chromatids fail to disjoin at meiosis II or at mitosis. Nondisjunction happens when paired chromosomes fail to separate in anaphase of meiosis I (**Figure 15.5**) or when sister chromatids fail to disjoin at meiosis II or at mitosis.

Anaphase lag happens because of improper attachment of the chromosomes to the microtubular spindle during anaphase. As a result, one sister chromatid is simultaneously attached to microtubules emanating from both poles. The lagging chromosome or chromatid fails to incorporate into one of the daughter cells prior to cell division.

Mosaicism

Mosaicism is the result of nondisjunction or chromosome lag occurring in one of the mitotic divisions of the early embryo. A proportion of normal cells and a proportion of aneuploid cells then coexist in the same embryo. Mosaicism within preimplantation embryos is discussed on pages 117–118.

Structural chromosomal abnormalities

Structural chromosomal abnormalities result from misrepair of chromosome breaks. These may occur either as a result of damage to chromatin, e.g. by radiation or chemicals, or from malfunction of the recombination system. If the break occurs in the G2 phase of the cell cycle (**Figure 15.6**), when chromosomes consist of two chromatids, it is referred to as a chromatid break and affects only one of the two sister chromatids. However, if the break occurs in the G1 phase and is not repaired by specialized enzymes before entering the S phase, it will further cause a chromosome break, affecting both chromatids.

Structural abnormalities can arise if a cell cycle checkpoint is passed despite failure to meet the conditions for passing it, for

Table 15.1 Common trisomies and sex chromosome variations

Syndrome	Karyotype	Prevalence	Phenotype	Congenital malformations/ complications associated with syndrome	Average life expectancy
Down syndrome	95% of patients have 3 separate chromosome 21s (Trisomy 21); 3–4% of patients have an unbalanced Robertsonian translocation	1/700 births	Upslanting eyes and epicanthal folds, brushfield spots, dysplastic ear, excess nuchal skin, single transverse palmar crease and clinodactyly of 5th finger, sandal gap of toes 1–2, protruding tongue, diastasis recti	Cardiac, gastrointestinal, thyroid, orthopedic, hearing, vision, hematologic	55–60 years; major cause of early mortality is congenital heart disease; risk of infections and pneumonia; increased risk of Alzheimer's disease
Edwards syndrome	Trisomy 18	1 in 5000 to 1 in 7000 births, withan excess of affected females	Microcephaly, short palpebral fissures, short upturned nose, micrognathia, clenched hands, overlapping fingers, camptodactyly, talipes valgus	Cardiac anomalies, coarctation, pulmonic stenosis, hydronephrosis, Wilms' tumor, polycystic kidneys, ectopic kidney, thyroid and adrenal hypoplasia, Meckel's diverticulum, hernias, omphalocele	Mean life expectancy 4 days; 1–5% live >1 year
Patau syndrome	75% of patients have a separate extra chromosome 13 (trisomy 13); 20% de novo translocations; 5% inherited translocations; 5% cases mosaic	1 in 12,000 births	Microcephaly, microphthalmia, cleft lip and palate, polydactyly, rocker-bottom feet, postaxial polydactyly, aplasia cutis congenital or scalp defects	Cardiac defects, renal anomalies	Mean life expectancy 130 days; 86% die during the first year
Turner syndrome	50% of patients are 45,X; the remainder are variants with other X chromosome abnormalities (isochromosome, ring, mosaicism)	1 in 5000 female births	Increased nuchal fold thickness, webbed neck, nipples widely spaced, carrying an increased angle/ cubitus valgus, short 4th metacarpals, lymphedema, cystic hygroma	Cardiac and renal abnormalities, short stature, delayed puberty, infertility, hearing impairment, learning disabilities	Shorter mean life expectancy, mostly due to heart problems and diabetes
Klinefelter syndrome	47,XXY	1 in 1000 male births	Tall stature, gynecomastia, hypogonadism	Infertility, learning disabilities, problems with socialization, many never diagnosed	Mean life expectancy may be reduced by 2 years, but cases are multifactorial, e.g. severe mental illness can impact on life expectancy, as can risk of acquiring type 2 diabetes, breast cancer and/or autoimmune diseases

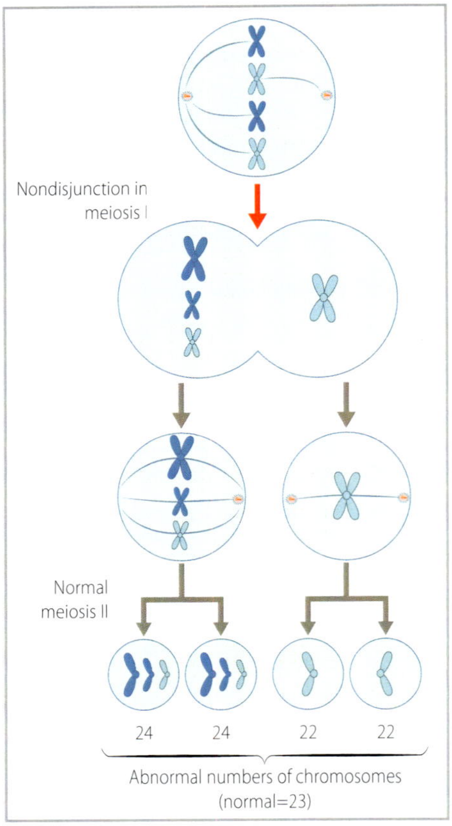

Figure 15.5 Anaphase I-nondisjunction in meiosis I.

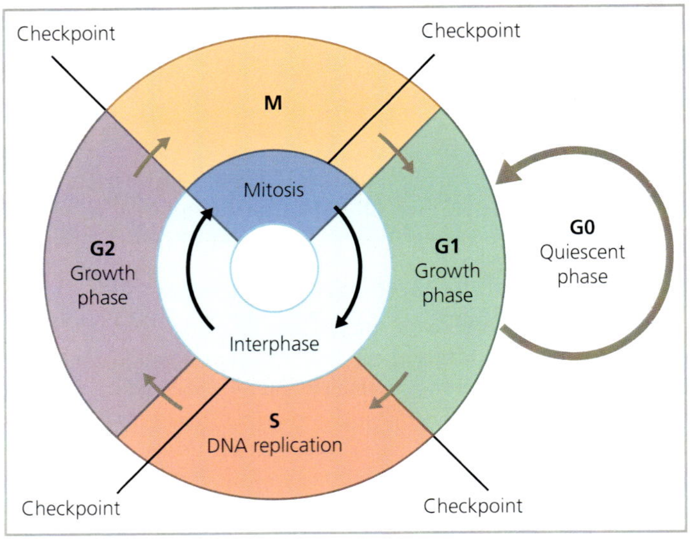

Figure 15.6 The cell cycle. For much of the cell cycle, the cell is in interphase (G0, G1, S and G2 phases), with mitosis (M) comprising only a minority of the cycle time. DNA replication takes place mid-interphase. At each checkpoint, specific conditions must be favorable for the cycle to progress beyond it, e.g. DNA integrity at the end of G1, chromosome duplication at the end of G2 and spindle attachment in late M.

Table 15.2 Structural chromosomal abnormalities: balanced versus unbalanced translocations

	Gain or loss of chromosomal information	Extra/less DNA in resulting cell	Examples
Balanced	No	No	Balanced rearrangements included inverted or translocated chromosomal regions. Since the full complement of DNA material is still present, balanced chromosomal rearrangements may go undetected since it may not result in disease. A disease can arise as a result of a balanced rearrangement if the breaks in the chromosomes occur in a gene, resulting in an absent or nonfunctional protein, or if the fusion of chromosomal segments results in a hybrid of two genes producing a new protein product whose function is damaging to the cell
Unbalanced	Yes	Yes	Unbalanced rearrangements include deletions, duplications, or insertions of a chromosome segment. Ring chromosomes can result when a chromosome undergoes two breaks and the broken ends fuse into a circular chromosome. An isochromosome can form when an arm of the chromosome is missing and the remaining arm duplicated

example, if broken chromosomes have been repaired but the wrong ends have been joined together. Resulting chromosomes may be acentric (without a centromere) or dicentric (with two centromeres). This means they will not be stable during mitosis, causing malsegregation or elimination of the genetic material. However, a structurally abnormal chromosome with a single centromere can still maintain stability, whilst propagating through mitotic divisions.

Meiotic recombination between mispaired chromosomes, i.e. between non-homologous chromosomes, is a common cause of translocations.

Structural chromosomal abnormalities are termed balanced when there is no net gain or loss of chromosomal material, and unbalanced when there is net gain or loss. Generally, balanced abnormalities, inversions and balanced translocations have no effect on the phenotype (**Table 15.2**).

Unbalanced abnormalities can arise directly, through deletion, or rarely duplication, or indirectly by malsegregation of chromosomes during meiosis in a carrier of a balanced abnormality.

Reciprocal translocation

A reciprocal translocation is an exchange of segments between nonhomologous chromosomes. If the pair of translocated chromosomes are inherited together there will be no change in the information content, apart from the breakpoint, which, if it occurs within a gene, may result in that gene being damaged. Thus most reciprocal translocations are balanced chromosomal abnormalities. However, if the pair of translocated chromosomes are not inherited together in a gamete, then some segments of chromosomes may be missing in the resulting zygote and some may be present in triplicate. Such zygotes are not likely to be viable, because usually both members of a pair of reciprocally translocated chromosomes must be inherited together.

Robertsonian translocation

A Robertsonian translocation is caused by breaks at or near the centromeres of two acrocentric chromosomes, namely chromosomes 13,

14, 15, 21 and 22. The breaks are in the proximal short arms and the distal parts of the two short arms are lost. The result is a single chromosome comprising two long arms, one from each of the acrocentric chromosomes. Loss of the short arms is without any phenotypic effect because these contain only arrays of ribosomal RNA genes. Therefore, Robertsonian translocations are regarded as balanced, despite having longer 'q' arms and shorter 'p' arms.

Inversion

Inversions occur when a single chromosome undergoes breakage and rearrangement within itself. Pericentric inversions include the centromere, with a break point in each arm. Paracentric inversions do not include the centromere, both breaks occurring in one arm of the chromosome.

Insertion

Insertions are due to unequal crossover during meiosis and signify that a large DNA sequence has been introduced into a chromosome.

Uniparental disomy

Normal chromosomal complements may be pathogenic if they have the wrong parental origin. 46,XX conceptuses in which both genomes originate from the same parent (uniparental diploidy) never develop correctly in humans.

For some individual chromosome pairs, having both homologs derived from the same parent (UPD) also causes abnormality due to imprinting. Imprinting is an epigenetic process that involves DNA methylation and histone methylation without altering the genetic sequence. A small number of genes are imprinted with their parental origin and are expressed differently according to the origin. For example, 46,XX or 46,XY individuals who inherit both copies of chromosome 15 from their father develop Angelman's syndrome; if both copies of chromosome 15 are maternally inherited, Prader–Willi syndrome results (**Figure 15.7**).

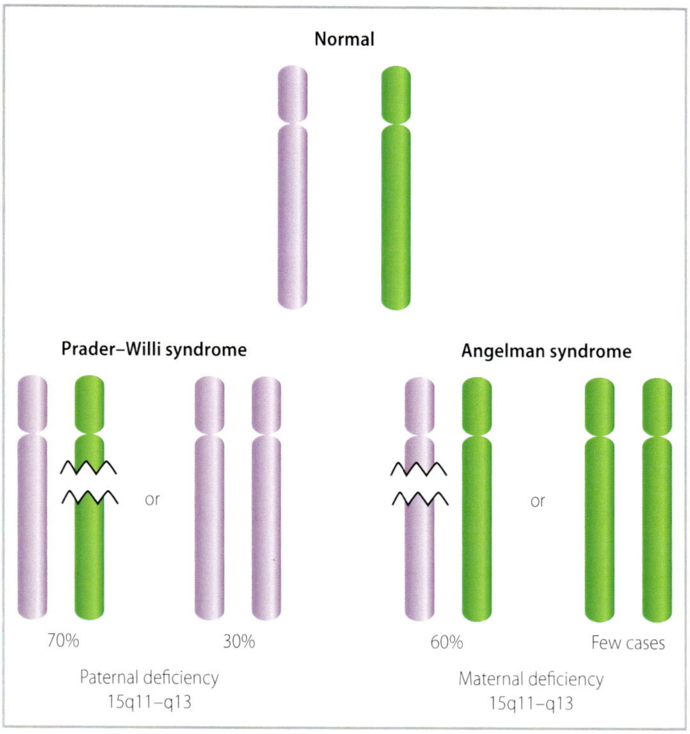

Figure 15.7 How paternal and maternal deficiency in the region q11 to q13 on chromosome 15 results in Prader–Willi syndrome or Angelman syndrome.

COMMON GENETIC DISORDERS

Besides numerical and structural chromosomal abnormalities causing genetic syndromes, there are single-gene (monogenic) disorders. These include frameshift, nonsense and deletion mutations which prevent any active protein being made. Trinucleotide repeat expansion mutations are also responsible for monogenic diseases.

These disorders follow simple patterns of inheritance predictable from the Mendelian laws of of genetics. One classification is according to whether the affected gene is located on the X chromosome or one of the 22 autosomes and whether the trait is recessive or dominant. They are said to be X-linked, autosomal recessive or autosomal dominant, respectively. Two of these inheritance patterns are shown in Chapter 10 (autosomal recessive in Figure 10.1a and X-linked in Figure 10.2).

Over 5000 disorders are listed in the Online Mendelian Inheritance in Man database, representing a significant fraction of the total number of human genes, estimated between 30,000 and 35,000.

Monogenic autosomal recessive disorders

Autosomal recessive disorders require the inheritance of two defective alleles. When both parents are carriers, i.e. heterozygous at the locus concerned, each child born has a 25% risk of being affected, 50% chance of being a carrier and 25% chance of being normal (see Figure 10.1a). Some diseases caused by single-gene defects are present in certain populations at a much higher frequency than would be expected from spontaneous mutation alone. One reason for an elevated frequency is that the heterozygote benefits from some protective advantages. This is the case in some African populations, amongst whom carriers of sickle cell anemia or thalassemia are more resistant to the malaria that is endemic in African countries. Examples of the major monogenic recessive disorders are listed and discussed below.

α- and β-thalassemias

Thalassemias are autosomal recessive inherited blood disorders. People with thalassemia are susceptible to health problems which include severe anemia, poor growth and skeletal abnormalities during infancy, and spleen and gallstones problems in adulthood.

The α- and β-thalassemias are the most common inherited single-gene disorders in the world, with the highest prevalence in areas where malaria was or still is endemic.

The red blood cell protein hemoglobin is a tetramer consisting of two α-globin and and two β-globin polypeptide chains, each complexed with a molecule of iron-containing haem. The α- and β-thalassemias are manifestations of a decrease in or absence of fully functioning α- and β-globin, respectively. There are two α-globin genes, occupying 30 kb of chromosome 16 and producing two types of α-globin, and one β-globin gene which is 70 kb in size and located on chromosome 11, with a total of 6 globin alleles contributing to a person's hemoglobin. The severity of a type of thalassemia depends on the number of defective alleles. Thus, for α-thalassemia, the disease phenotype ranges from asymptomatic, mild or moderate anemia to hydrops fetalis. β-thalassemia results also in variable phenotypes ranging from clinically asymptomatic individuals to severe anemia.

The total annual incidence of symptomatic individuals in β-thalassemia is estimated at 1 in 100,000 throughout the world and 1 in 10,000 people in the European Union.

Cystic fibrosis

Cystic fibrosis is an autosomal recessive disorder common among Northern Europeans. It affects approximately 1 in 2000 people and has an estimated carrier frequency of 1 in 25 (Massie and Delatycki, 2013).

The primary defect is decreased chloride ion export and increased sodium ion absorbance leading to insufficient hydration of epithelial surfaces. In the lungs, this results in a sticky mucus that cannot be cleared by the action of the epithelial cilia resulting in chronic bacterial infection and inflammation.

Mutations take place on the cystic fibrosis transmembrane conductance regulator (CFTR) gene. This gene is extremely large, occupying approximately 230 kb of chromosome 7 and consisting of 27 exons. Over 550 different mutations of the CFTR gene have been described but two-thirds of cystic fibrosis mutant alleles carry the delta F508 mutation.

Monogenic autosomal dominant disorders

When the defective allele is dominant, the disorder affects people who have two copies of the defective gene *and* people who have one defective copy and one normal copy (i.e. are heterozygous for the gene). Thus, at least half the children of an affected person will have the disorder: for a gene 'a' with a normal allele *a* and a defective allele *A*, the unaffected parent must be *aa*, and if the affected parent is *Aa* then half the children will be *aa* and half *Aa*; in contrast, if the affected parent is *AA*, all children will be *Aa* and have the disorder.

Myotonic dystrophy

Myotonic dystrophy is the most common neuromuscular disorder showing adult onset and affecting 1 in 8500 individuals. It also shows a range of symptoms from cataracts and frontal baldness in mildly affected individuals to multisystem failure in severely affected individuals with symptoms including muscular dystrophy, myotonia, endocrine dysfunction, mental retardation, cardiac abnormalities, and testicular atrophy in males.

The disorder is caused by expansion of the CTG codon, which is then repeated. This codon repeat is located in the DMPK gene. The repeat is polymorphic in normal populations with repeat numbers in the range of 5–35. This expands in affected individuals to 50 to >3000. Repeat length, disease severity and age of onset are approximately correlated.

X-linked disorders

The pattern of inheritance of X-linked disorders is shown in Figure 10.2. The best known is hemophilia. Another is Duchenne muscular dystrophy.

Duchenne muscular dystrophy

Duchenne muscular dystrophy (DMD) is characterized by progressive failure of muscle growth and wasting, leading to weakness, paralysis and respiratory difficulties. In addition, the heart, smooth muscle and central and peripheral nervous systems may be affected. It is a sex-linked disease affecting 1 in 3300 boys.

DMD is caused by mutations in the dystrophin-encoding *DMD* gene. The dystrophin protein links the actin cytoskeleton to the muscle sarcolemma.

The DMD gene is the largest genetic locus known in the human genome and is composed of 79 exons, scattered across 2.4 Mb.

PREIMPLANTATION GENETIC TESTING

Preimplantation genetic testing is a field including cytogenetic and molecular techniques for the testing of biopsy samples taken from embryos generated by in vitro fertilization (IVF) techniques.

PGT for structural rearrangements or monogenic disorders

PGT for structural rearrangements (PGT-SR) or monogenic disorders (PGT-M), formerly known as preimplantation genetic diagnosis (PGD), allows for the diagnosis and subsequent transfer of chromosomally normal (euploid) and disease-free embryos to the uterus. PGT-SR and PGT-M offer couples with an increased risk of transmitting genetic disorders the chance to give birth to healthy children preventing thereby complications such as maternal or fetal health problems, psychological and financial burden caused by the termination of a pregnancy.

PGT-M was first performed in 1990 by Alan Handyside and his colleagues using polymerase chain reaction (PCR). The aim was to prevent transmission of a sex-linked disorder (Handyside et al. 1990). The technique is now applied to many different conditions for a variety of indications, including monogenic disorders, preimplantation human leukocyte antigen (HLA) typing for hematopoietic stem cell transplantation, numerical and structural chromosomal abnormalities and selection of euploid embryos for elective single embryo transfer (eSET).

The biopsy technique and timing, the choice of genetic diagnosis techniques for mutational and chromosomal abnormalities and the appropriate genetic counseling play important roles in establishing a successful PGT program.

PGT for aneuploidy

PGT for aneuploidy (PGT-A), formerly known as preimplantation genetic screening (PGS), is used for the purpose of selecting preimplantation embryos with the correct chromosomal number (euploid) for transfer to patients. This avoids transfer of embryos with abnormal chromosome number (aneuploidies), and therefore should increase the take-home baby rates following IVF treatment.

Aneuploidy is the major cause of the first trimester miscarriages, and thus has a significant contribution to IVF failures (Munné et al. 2004). Therefore, PGT-A could be considered for IVF with the following clinical indications:

- Advanced female age
- Previous history of chromosomally abnormal fetus
- Repeated pregnancy losses
- Translocation carriers
- Inversion carriers

PGT-A is used for people experiencing recurrent first trimester miscarriages in order to selectively remove chromosomally abnormal embryos from transfer. Also, women of advanced maternal age are at a higher risk of producing chromosomally abnormal oocytes, and thus their offspring may have an increased chance of chromosomal abnormalities. Lastly, carriers of balanced translocations (e.g. Robertsonian or reciprocal translocations or inversions) may have fertility problems due to unbalanced chromosome segregation. As a result, such couples may suffer from multiple pregnancy losses.

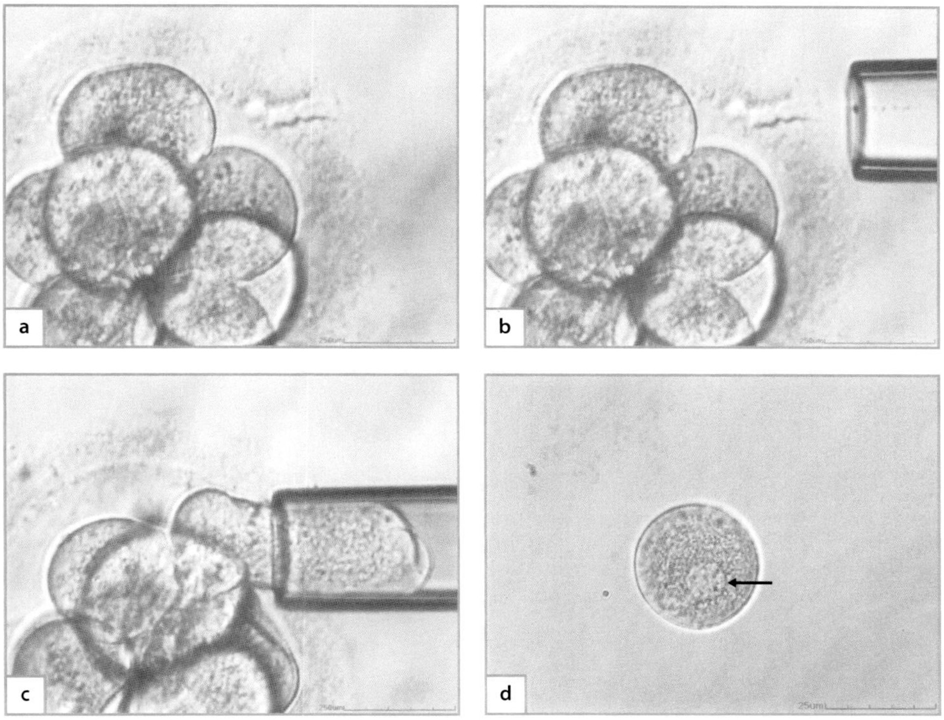

Figure 15.8 A blastomere biopsy pipette is placed through the zona pellucida opening; the nucleus-containing and targeted blastomere is gently aspirated into the pipette and slowly released into the medium. In (d), the black arrow on the last frame shows the nucleus within a single blastomere.

Biopsy stages in IVF

There are currently three sources of genetic material available for PGT: polar bodies from oocytes, blastomeres from cleavage-stage embryos and cells from blastocyst stage embryos.

Polar body biopsy

Polar body biopsy can be applied either before fertilization (to remove the first polar body) or after fertilization (to remove both the first and second polar body simultaneously). Polar bodies give only maternal information and therefore cannot be used to diagnose paternal mutations, HLA typing, chromosomal abnormalities caused by paternal meiosis, mitotic errors or gender (Christopikou et al. 2013, Geraedts et al. 2011). As a result of these limitations, polar body biopsy is mostly restricted to diagnose aneuploidies in advanced maternal age, in maternally inherited disorders, such as X-linked anomalies, and in maternal translocations. It should also be noted that in some countries, polar body diagnosis is the only option available due to legal restrictions.

Cleavage-stage biopsy

Blastomere biopsy is accomplished at the cleavage stage, typically on day 3 of in vitro development. This technique was used for PGT for many years, but there is increasing evidence that biopsy at this time may have a negative impact on embryo viability and implantation potential (Cimadomo et al. 2016).

In this method, one or two blastomeres are retrieved from embryos with more than six cells (**Figure 15.8**). With cleavage-stage biopsy, both maternal and paternal meiotic errors can be detected. In addition, blastomere biopsy gives enough time for genetic analysis to be performed before the embryo reaches the blastocyst stage. This can then allow for a fresh transfer provided there is timely shipment of biopsied samples to the genetics laboratory and reporting of results.

Blastocyst biopsy

Blastocyst-stage embryo biopsy is the removal of a small part of the TE (usually 5–6 cells) from a hatching blastocyst (**Figure 15.9**). The major advantage of this method is the amount of genetic material available for testing. Having more than one cell to work with reduces the risk of diagnostic errors caused mostly by technical problems, such as hybridization or amplification failures and absence of a nucleus. The allele drop-out rate (see page 118) is also lower, thereby increasing the reliability and accuracy of the diagnosis (Forman et al. 2011). The routine policy is to perform the TE biopsy on day 5–6 and then immediately vitrify the biopsied blastocyst. Subsequently, if euploid embryos are diagnosed, a single blastocyst transfer is performed in a 'frozen embryo transfer' cycle.

A blastocyst should contain over 100 cells, so the removal of 5–6 TE cells is very unlikely to have a detrimental effect on blastocyst development or fetal development, since this originates from the inner cell mass (ICM) which is left fully intact and unharmed. This need to be considered when comparing to cleavage-stage biopsy, where cell have yet to develop into TE or ICM cells (Scott et al. 2013).

The PGT for single-gene disorders has become an effective alternative to prenatal diagnosis. Moreover, PGT is an excellent option for families having an affected child who is in need of bone marrow transplantation. Preimplantation HLA typing can facilitate birth of an HLA-matched donor infant (Kahraman et al. 2011, Verlinsky et al. 2001) and hematopoietic progenitor cells from this donor could then be transplanted to the affected child with successful cure results (Kahraman et al. 2014).

Mosaicism in trophectoderm biopsies

Embryonic mosaicism is defined as the presence of karyotypically different cell lines within the preimplantation embryo and is the result of non-disjunction or chromosome lag occurring in one of the mitotic divisions of the early embryo (Capalbo et al. 2016). A proportion of normal cells and a proportion of aneuploid cells then coexist in the same embryo (see page 113).

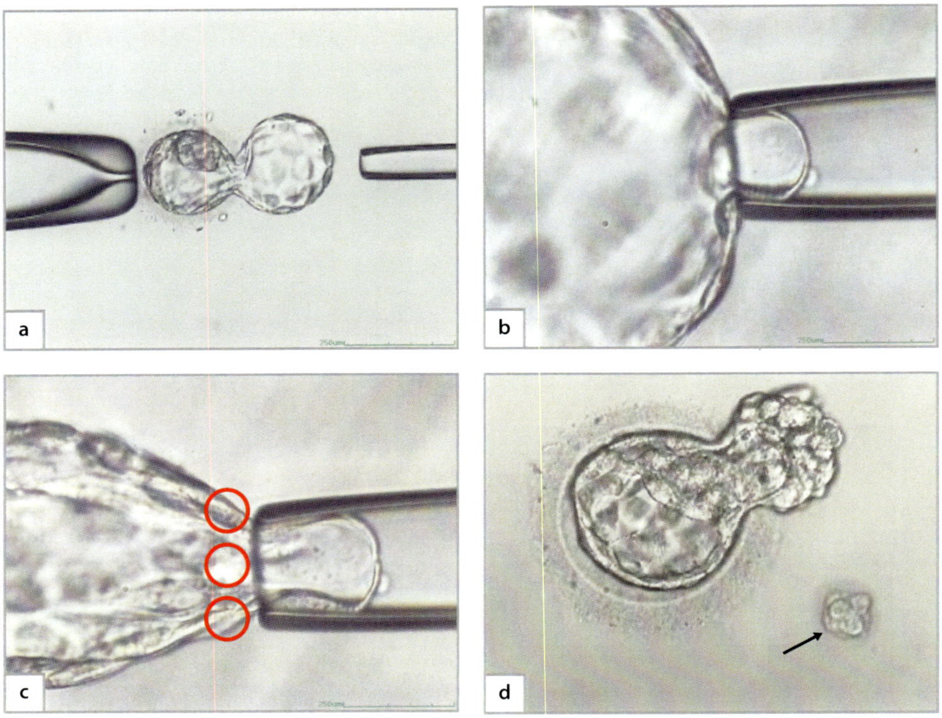

Figure 15.9 Stages of blastocyst biopsy. (a) Day 5 expanded blastocyst with trophectoderm (TE) cells protruding through an opening in the zona pellucida (ZP) made on day 3 or 4 with a micro-laser. (b) Aspiration of the protruding TE cells through the ZP. (c) Laser shots are applied to break down the tight junctions between TE cells (red circles indicate the site of laser beams). (d) Aspirated TE cells (range 4–6 cells). The arrow points to the biopsied TE cells.

The rate of mosaicism within preimplantation embryos not only varies based on the stage of the embryo, but also with the chromosomal detection technique used. The rate of mosaicism among blastocysts with the use of array comparative genomic hybridisation (aCGH) is estimated to be 4.8–32% and may vary based on the aCGH protocols used (Sachdev et al. 2017). The ability of aCGH to detect mosaicism is dependent on the percentage of aneuploid cells within the trophectoderm (TE) biopsy specimen and aCGH is able to pick up mosaicism when >50% of cells are abnormal (Mamas et al. 2012). On the other hand, next-generation sequencing (NGS) has a greater ability to detect mosaicism in blastocysts' samples. The use of mixed model aneuploidy cell lines showed that NGS is able to detect mosaicism when as few as 17% of the cells are aneuploid (Goodrich et al. 2016).

Euploid embryos should always be preferentially transferred over mosaic embryos and in the absence of euploid embryos, certain types of mosaic embryos should be preferentially transferred over others. Transfer of embryos with mosaic trisomies 2, 7, 13, 14, 15, 16, 18, and 21 may pose the most risk of having a child affected with a trisomy syndrome; however, the transfer of embryos with mosaic monosomies or other mosaic trisomies are not devoid of risk.

Recently, Gratti and colleagues (2018) have proposed an evidence-based scoring system for transfer of mosaic embryos using the observed risk of a mosaic trisomy affecting the fetus, being involved in UPD or resulting in a miscarriage. This risk was determined by considering the outcome of over 72,000 pregnancies assessed by chorionic villus sampling and 3800 losses assessed via products of conception analysis. The investigators then calculated a composite score for mosaicism involving specific chromosomes based on a mathematical combination of the risks of an affected fetus, UPD or miscarriage, with zero representing no risk (highest priority for transfer) and five representing the highest risk (transfer best avoided). Using this system, they have given a score of 5 for mosaic trisomies 13, 14, 16, 18, and 21, and 45 X; an intermediate score between 4 and 5 for chromosome trisomies 8, 20, 47,XXX and 47,XXY; a score of 3 for mosaic trisomies 6, 9, and 15; a score of 2 for mosaic trisomies of chromosomes 2, 7, 11, 17, and 22; a score of 1 for mosaic trisomies 47,XYY, 4 and 5; and a score of zero for trisomic mosaics of chromosomes 1, 3, 10, 12, and 19 (Munné 2018).

Therefore, until more data are available, patients should be encouraged to undergo another cycle to obtain euploid embryos, when possible, rather than transferring a mosaic embryo.

ANALYTICAL METHODS FOR DETECTING CHROMOSOMAL ABNORMALITIES

Multiplex polymerase chain reaction

A common PGT method for single gene disorders involves the usage of single cell multiplex PCR for amplification of short tandem repeat (STR) polymorphic markers located in close proximity to the mutation site. Those polymorphic STR markers are repeats of DNA which are mostly heterozygous and highly variable in size among individuals. STR length values linked to the mutated allele can be determined via fragment analysis using paternal and maternal genomic DNA prior to PGT and genotype of the generated embryos can be diagnosed by linkage analysis during PGT (**Figure 15.10**). In addition to direct mutation techniques via restriction length polymorphism (RFLP) or minisequencing, the use of multiple STR markers linked to the mutation site assists in overcoming diagnostic problems arising from ADO, which is a one of the major causes of misdiagnosis during PGT (Harper et al. 2012). In ADO if a gene is heterozygous, i.e. there are two different alleles rather than duplicates of a single allele, unequal sampling of the alleles can result in failure to detect one of them; the allele is lost, hence the name allele drop-out.

Also, amplification of the single cell genome by whole genome amplification allows the combination of PGT for single gene disorders with aneuploidy testing.

Fluorescence in situ hybridization

In 1993, Munné and his colleagues developed a diagnostic method combining the principles of fluorescent in situ hybridization (FISH) and the fixation of a single blastomere biopsied from a cleavage-stage

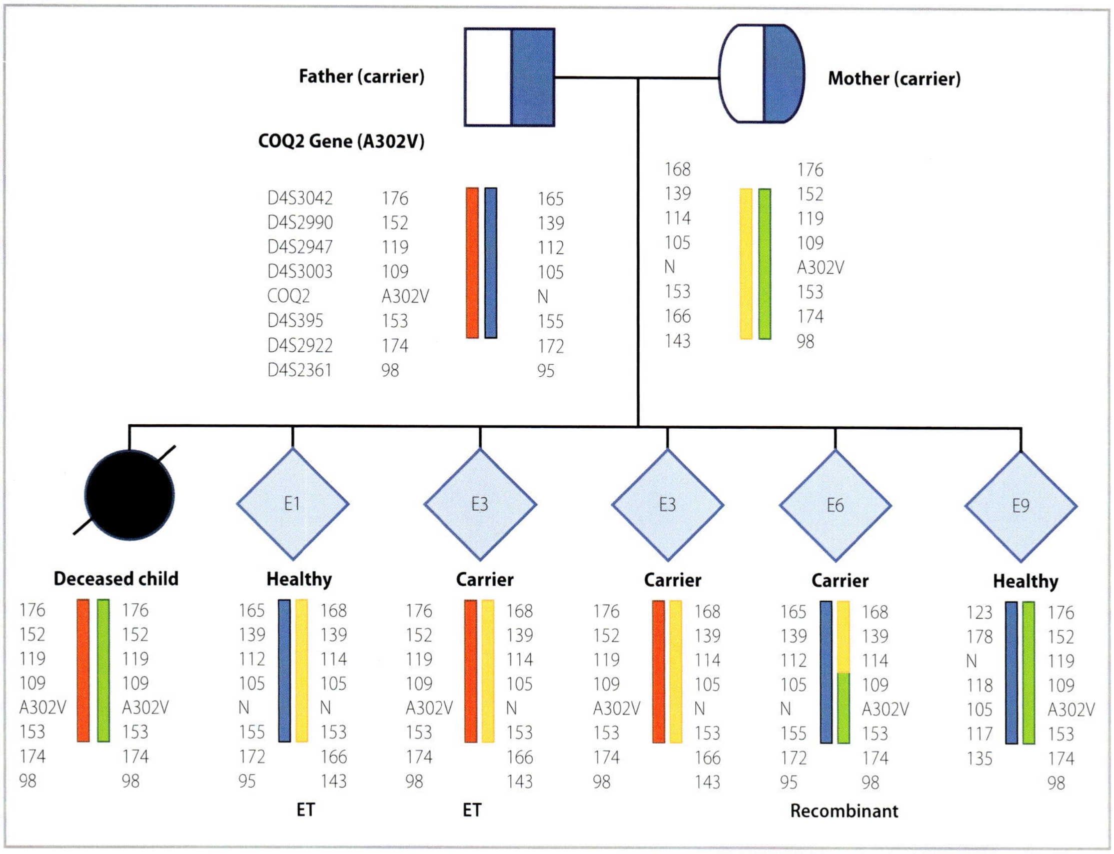

Figure 15.10 Case sample of linked short tandem repeat (STR) marker analysis for coenzyme Q deficiency (COQ2 gene). Preliminary work was done on the DNA of parents and the DNA of deceased child using specifically designed STR markers to identify informative markers to be used in the preimplantation genetic diagnosis case. Seven informative STR markers (4 upstream and 3 downstream of the gene) were used for detection of mutation A302V in COQ2 gene. Two embryos (1 healthy and 1 carrier) were transferred resulting in the birth of a healthy singleton. Embryos 6 and 9 were cryopreserved for possible future use. ET, Embryo transfer.

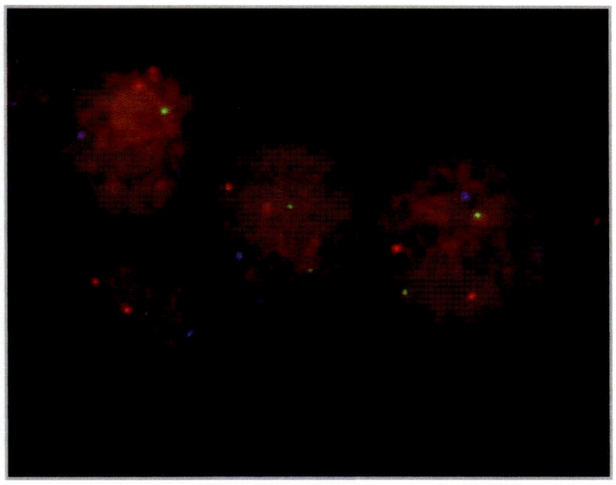

Figure 15.11 A fluorescent in situ hybridization (FISH) technique image of trophectoderm (TE) cells belonging to a chromosomally normal embryo (chromosome 13 was labeled with spectrum red, chromosome 18 with spectrum blue, chromosome 21 with spectrum green, Abbott, Vysis) (with courtesy from Istanbul Memorial Hospital, 2011).

human embryo in an attempt to provide an alternative to the PCR technique for the gender determination of the embryos (Munné et al. 1993b). Subsequently, a short FISH procedure using fluorochrome and digoxigenin labelled DNA probes specific to chromosomes mostly involved in miscarriages (13, 18, 21, X and Y) was developed in order to screen for aneuploidy (**Figure 15.11**) (Munné et al. 1993a).

FISH is also used for the diagnosis of unbalanced products and embryos belonging to balanced rearrangement carriers. For translocation and inversion carriers, a preclinical work up study is performed beforehand to confirm the rearrangement breakpoint regions and to test for the efficiency of the probes that will be used in PGT. In this preclinical study, at least ten metaphase cells and 100 interphase cells should be analyzed with the same probe combination to assess signal specificities and any possibility of polymorphism in the probe-specific regions that may cause difficulties in signal interpretation during the PGT study. With FISH, only a maximum of 9–12 chromosomes can be screened, and thus FISH can still not detect 20–40% of all aneuploid embryos (Munné et al 2010).

As the quality of FISH results is highly dependent on the quality of the nucleus, several factors need consideration. This includes:

- The skills of the embryologist who performs the biopsy and prepares the biopsied cells prior to assay
- The skills of the geneticist who performs the fixation and assay
- A failing in any of the above can lead to inconclusive results

Any of the above may very well lead to inconclusive results.

Array comparative genomic hybridization

Array comparative genomic hybridization (aCGH) is a technique whereby hybridization is performed on chips [usually bacterial artificial chromosomes (BACs)] or arrays, and the analysis is then performed with specialized software (Le Caignec et al. 2006). The whole procedure is completed within 12 hours.

Briefly this technique includes the following steps:

- Extraction of genomic DNA
- Whole genome amplification
- Fluorescent labeling of samples and references
- Mixing of differentially labeled probes
- Hybridization on arrays
- Washing, scanning and analysis by the computer program

The software does the analysis by first calculating the ratio of intensity coming from red and green fluorescent dyes for each position and second, by comparing it with the male and female reference DNAs. Briefly, the decision of chromosomal status is being made by processing the standard deviation (SD) after smoothing and normalizing the data. When SD for a specific chromosome is higher than +0.3, the software calls it as a 'gain' (usually a trisomy) and if this ratio is below -0.3 it calls a 'loss' (usually a monosomy) (**Figure 15.12**).

aCGH is also capable of detecting segmental aneuploidies as small as 2Mb and imbalances formed by abnormal segregations due to rearrangements (**Figure 15.13**) (Alfarawati et al. 2011, Fiorentino et al. 2011, Viaggi et al. 2012).

aCGH can diagnose unbalanced products formed from any Robertsonian translocations and from the vast majority of reciprocal translocations carriers. However, the diagnosis of reciprocal translocations smaller than 2 Mb length has not yet been validated by either aCGH nor by any other array systems. This is a remaining indication for FISH-based PGT in translocation carriers. aCGH has the ability to screen not only translocated chromosomes but also the ones which are not involved in the rearrangements.

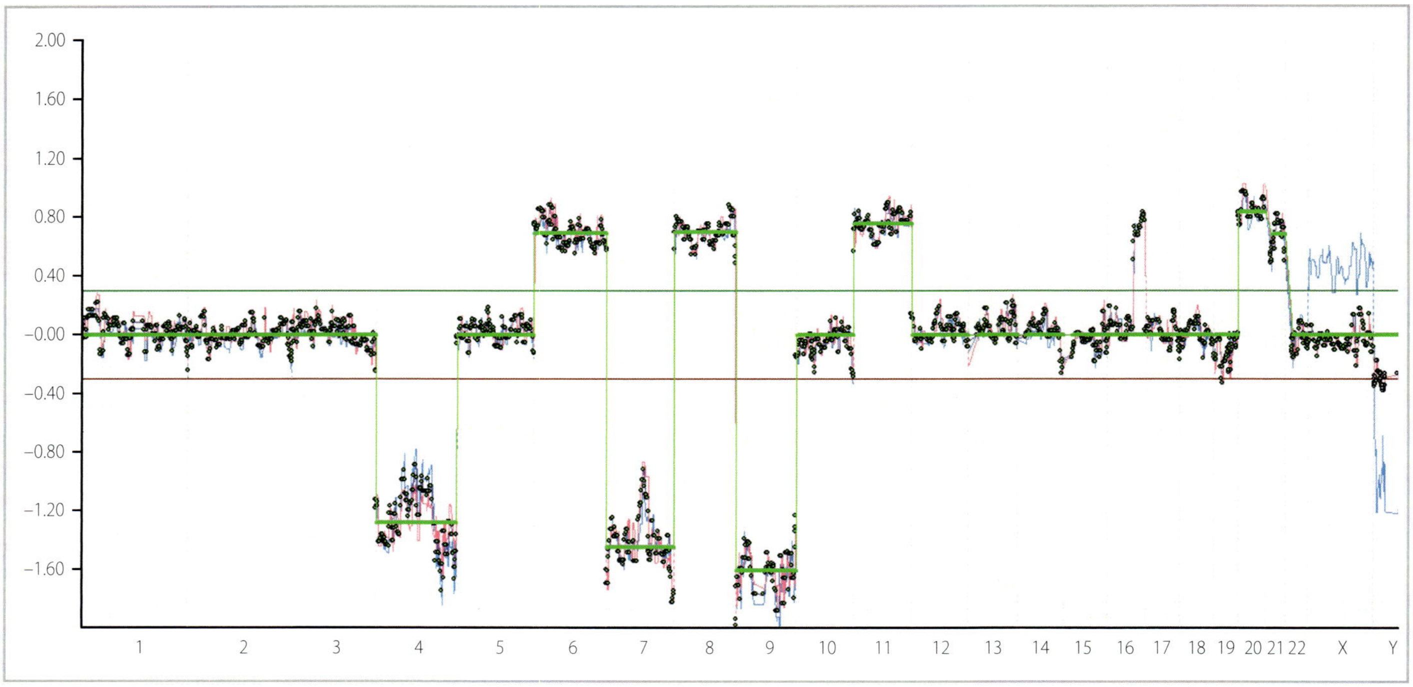

Figure 15.12 A typical comparative genomic hybridization trace of an embryo with complex abnormality.

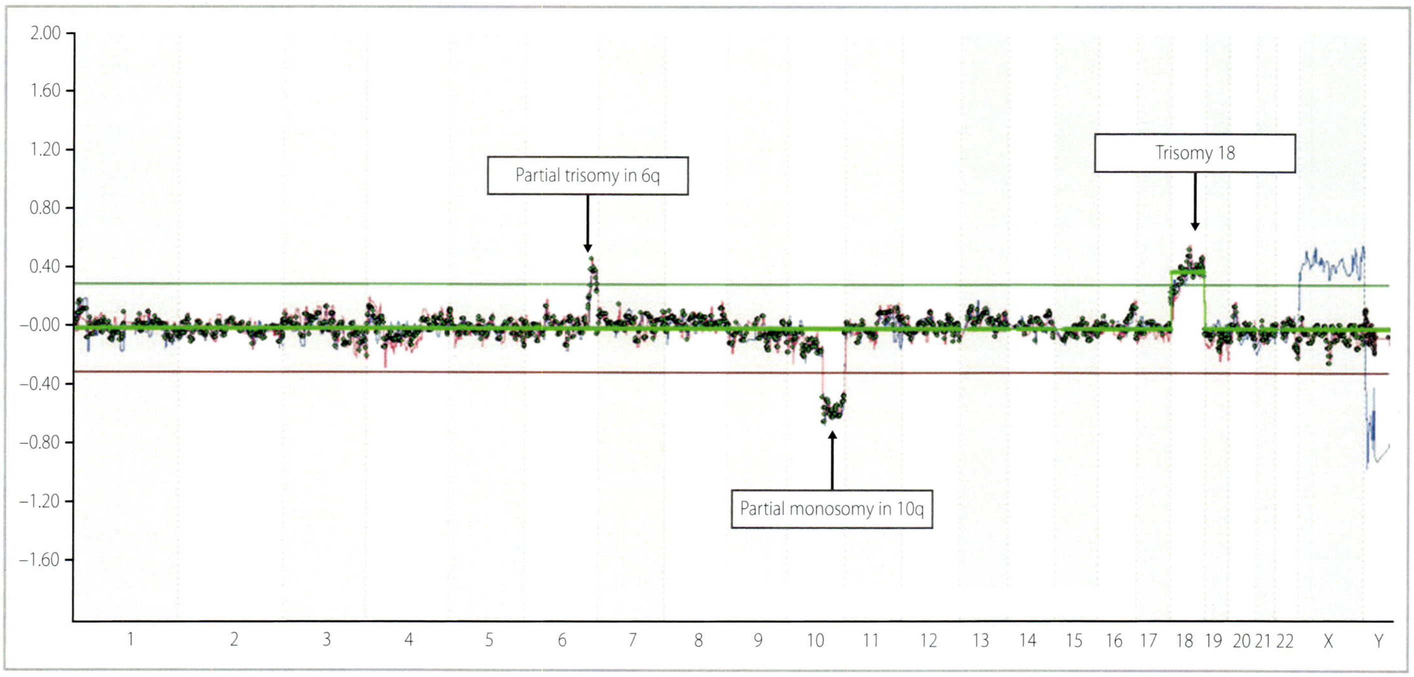

Figure 15.13 An unbalanced embryo generated by a balanced translocation carrier with 46,XY,t(6;10)(q25.1;q22.1) karyotype. Note that besides the unbalanced chromosomal state, a trisomy 18 is present.

The high rates of aneuploidies observed in non-translocated chromosomes have shown the importance of aneuploidy screening by aCGH in both young and advanced maternal age groups (Beyazyurek 2012). However, aCGH cannot detect:

- polyploidies, such as triploidy and tetraploidy
- balanced chromosomal rearrangements such as translocations and inversions
- uniparental disomies

Since the total amount of DNA in the biopsy sample is the same in reference DNAs.

The possibility of interchromosomal effect (ICE) as a cause for the increased incidence of aneuploidies in embryos belonging to Robertsonian translocation carriers has been proposed by a retrospective study using FISH (Gianaroli et al. 2002). More recently, Alfarawati and colleagues reported ICE in Robertsonian translocation carriers but not in reciprocal translocation carriers. Using aCGH, the authors claimed that ICE is more pronounced in cleavage-stage embryos, but not in blastocysts and might be attributed to mitotic instability (Alfarawati et al. 2012).

PGT-A with aCGH can be used to help select a single euploid embryo for eSET, and thereby decrease the multiple pregnancy rate following IVF treatment. In order to determine whether performing comprehensive chromosomal screening on blastocysts can reduce the risk of multiple gestation, Yang and colleagues assessed clinical outcomes after single blastocyst transfer by comparing morphological evaluation alone and combined with aCGH in good prognosis patients. According to their randomized controlled trial, blastocyst transfer after aCGH testing significantly increased ongoing pregnancy rates (Yang et al. 2012).

Next generation sequencing

Nowadays, NGS is the gold standard for high resolution genome-wide DNA copy number variations analysis. With the use of NGS, it is now possible to identify mosaicism and mitochondrial DNA levels in the embryo biopsy. With NGS, DNA polymerase catalyzes the incorporation of fluorescently-labeled deoxyribonucleotide triphosphates (dNTPs) into a DNA template strand during sequential cycles of DNA synthesis and during each cycle, incorporated nucleotides are called by fluorophore excitation. The essential modification performed in NGS technology is that, instead of sequencing a single DNA fragment, NGS extends this process across millions of fragments in a massively parallel fashion. NGS has been performed on TE cells and on blastomeres for detection of aneuploidies and unbalanced chromosomal rearrangements with successful results (Fiorentino et al. 2014, Yan et al. 2015, Yin et al. 2013).

Furthermore, results to date indicate that the NGS technique is comparable to aCGH for the diagnosis of aneuploidy, with >99% concordance, suggesting that these methods have equivalent accuracy (Kung et al. 2015).

CONCLUSION

Although noninvasive techniques, such as time-lapse analysis and noninvasive assessments of embryos and oocytes, are being developed in order to generate an alternative to PGT, invasive techniques still remain the most reliable methods in order to eliminate affected and chromosomally abnormal embryos. In the last couple of decades, preventive medicine has gained more attention worldwide. Together with the implementation of more powerful, comprehensive and cost-effective techniques such as karyomapping and NGS have strengthened the place of PGT in ART and increased the demand for PGT.

Altered levels of mitochondrial DNA have been found to be associated with female age and thus provide an independent measure of embryonic implantation potential (Fragouli et al. 2015). The quantity of mtDNA appears to be significantly higher in embryos from older women but also in aneuploid embryos, independent of age. The retrospective analysis of mtDNA quantities after the transfer of euploid embryos showed that blastocysts that successfully implanted tended to contain lower mtDNA quantities than those failing to implant. Authors suggest that mtDNA content represents a novel biomarker with potential value for IVF treatment, revealing chromosomally normal blastocysts incapable of producing a viable pregnancy (Fragouli et al. 2015)(see Chapter 18).

For the time being, the choice of PGT technique depends mostly on the indication (where the purpose is either mutation testing or chromosomal analysis), the cost, availability and the applicability of the technique. As conditions and indications for PGT testing are extending enormously, the techniques have been urged to evolve toward a universal method for the simultaneous diagnosis of diverse genetic conditions such as monogenic disorders, HLA typing, rearrangements, aneuploidy screening and the selection of the best embryo that has the highest implantation capacity which will be possible in the near future.

REFERENCES

Alfarawati S, Fragouli E, Colls P, Wells D. Embryos of robertsonian translocation carriers exhibit a mitotic interchromosomal effect that enhances genetic instability during early development. PLoS Genet 2012; 8:e1003025.

Alfarawati S, Fragouli E, Colls P, Wells D. First births after preimplantation genetic diagnosis of structural chromosome abnormalities using comparative genomic hybridization and microarray analysis. Hum Reprod 2011; 26:1560–1574.

Beyazyurek C, Yapan C, Ekmekci GC, et al. Aneuploidy screening reveals high incidence of abnormalities of chromosomes which are not involved in the rearrangements. Reprod Biomed Online 2012; 24:S40.

Capalbo A, Ubaldi FM, Rienzi L, Scott R, Treff N. Detecting mosaicism in trophectoderm biopsies: current challenges and future possibilities. Hum Reprod 2017; 32:492-498.

Cimadomo D, Capalbo A, Ubaldi FM, et al. The Impact of Biopsy on Human Embryo Developmental Potential during Preimplantation Genetic Diagnosis. Biomed Res Int 2016; 2016:7193075.

Christopikou D, Tsorva E, Economou K, et al. Polar body analysis by array comparative genomic hybridization accurately predicts aneuploidies of maternal meiotic origin in cleavage stage embryos of women of advanced maternal age. Hum Reprod 2013; 28:1426–1434.

Fiorentino F, Biricik A, Bono S, et al. Development and validation of a next-generation sequencing-based protocol for 24-chromosome aneuploidy screening of embryos. Fertil Steril 2014; 101:1375–1382.

Fiorentino F, Spizzichino L, Bono S, et al. PGD for reciprocal and Robertsonian translocations using array comparative genomic hybridization. Hum Reprod 2011; 26:1925–1935.

Forman EJ, Ferry KM, Gueye NA, et al. Trophectoderm biopsy for single-gene disorder preimplantation genetic diagnosis (PGD) is significantly more reliable than day 3 blastomere biopsy. Fertil Steril 2011; 96:S222.

Fragouli E, Spath K, Alfarawati S, et al. Altered levels of mitochondrial DNA are associated with female age, aneuploidy, and provide an independent measure of embryonic implantation potential. PLoS Genet 2015; 11:e1005241.

Geraedts J, Montag M, Magli MC, et al. Polar body array CGH for prediction of the status of the corresponding oocyte. Part I: clinical results. Hum Reprod 2011; 26:3173–3180.

Gianaroli L, Magli MC, Ferraretti AP, et al. Possible interchromosomal effect in embryos generated by gametes from translocation carriers. Hum Reprod 2002; 17:3201–3207.

Goodrich D, Tao X, Bohrer C, et al. A randomized and blinded comparison of qPCR and NGS-based detection of aneuploidy in a cell line mixture model of blastocyst biopsy mosaicism. J Assist Reprod Genet 2016; 33:1473-1480.

Gratti FR, Gallazzi G, Branca L, et al. An evidence-based scoring system for prioritizing mosaic aneuploid embryos following preimplantation genetic screening. Reprod. Biomed (Online) 2018;36:442-449.

Handyside AH, Kontogianni EH, Hardy K, Winston RM. Pregnancies from biopsied human preimplantation embryos sexed by Y specific DNA amplification. Nature 1990; 344:768–770.

Harper JC, Wilton L, Traeger-Synodinos J, et al. The ESHRE PGD Consortium: 10 years of data collection. Hum Reprod. Update 2012; 18:234–247.

Kahraman S, Beyazyurek C, Ekmekci CG. Seven years of experience of preimplantation HLA typing: a clinical overview of 327 cycles. Reprod Biomed Online2011; 3:363–371.

Kahraman S, Beyazyurek C, Yesilipek MA, et al. Successful haematopoietic stem cell transplantation in 44 children from healthy siblings conceived after preimplantation HLA matching. Reprod Biomed Online 2014; 29:340–351.

Kahraman S, Cil AP, Ogur C, et al. Probability of finding at least one euploid embryo and euploidy rate with FISH and array CGH based on age and the number of retrieved oocytes. J Reprod Biotechnol Fertil 2016:1–9.

Kung A, Munné S, Bankowski B, Coates A, Wells D. Validation of next-generation sequencing for comprehensive chromosome screening of embryos. Reprod Biomed Online 2015; 31:760–769.

Le Caignec C, Spits C, Sermon K, et al. Single-cell chromosomal imbalances detection by array CGH. Nucleic Acids Res 2006; 34:e68.

Massie J, Delatycki MB. Cystic fibrosis carrier screening. Paediatr Respir Rev 2013; 14:270–275.

Mamas T, Gordon A, Brown A, Harper J, Sengupta S. Detection of aneuploidy by array comparative genomic hybridization using cell lines to mimic a mosaic trophectoderm biopsy. Fertil Steril 2012; 97:943-947.

Munné S. Origins of mosaicism and criteria for the transfer of mosaic embryos. Reprod Biomed Online 2018; 36:369-370.

Munné S, Bahçe M, Sandalinas M, et al. Differences in chromosome susceptibility to aneuploidy and survival to first trimester. Reprod Biomed Online 2004; 8:81–90.

Munné S, Fragouli E, Colls P, et al. Improved detection of aneuploid blastocysts using a new 12-chromosome FISH test. Reprod Biomed Online 2010; 20:92–97.

Munné S, Lee A, Rosenwaks Z, Grifo J, Cohen J. Diagnosis of major chromosome aneuploidies in human preimplantation embryos. Hum Reprod 1993a; 8:2185–2191.

Munné S, Weier HU, Stein J, Grifo J, Cohen J. A fast and efficient method for simultaneous X and Y in situ hybridization of human blastomeres. J Assist Reprod Genet 1993b; 10:82–90.

Sachdev NM, Maxwell SM, Besser AG, Grifo JA. Diagnosis and clinical management of embryonic mosaicism. Fertil Steril 2017 ;107:6-11.

Scott RT Jr, Upham KM, Forman EJ, Zhao T, Treff NR. Cleavage-stage biopsy significantly impairs human embryonic implantation potential while blastocyst biopsy does not: a randomized and paired clinical trial. Fertil Steril 2013; 100:624–630.

Toufaily MH, Roberts DJ, Westgate MN, Holmes LB. Triploidy: Variation of Phenotype. Am J Clin Pathol 2016; 145:86–95.

Verlinsky Y, Rechitsky S, Schoolcraft W, Strom C, Kuliev A. Preimplantation diagnosis for Fanconi anemia combined with HLA matching. JAMA 2001; 285:3130–3133.

Viaggi CD, Cavani S, Pierluigi M, et al. Characterization of a complex rearrangement involving chromosomes 1, 4 and 8 by FISH and array-CGH. J Appl Genet 2012; 53:285–288.

Wada Y, Kakiuchi S, Mizuguchi K, et al. A female newborn having mosaicism with near-tetraploidy and trisomy 18. Am J Med Genet 2016; 170:1262–127.

Yan L, Huang L, Xu L, et al. Live births after simultaneous avoidance of monogenic diseases and chromosome abnormality by next-generation sequencing with linkage analyses. Proc Natl Acad Sci USA. 2015 29; 112:15964–15969.

Yang Z, Liu J, Collins GS, et al. Selection of single blastocysts for fresh transfer via standard morphology assessment alone and with array CGH for good prognosis IVF patients: results from a randomized pilot study. Mol Cytogenet 2012; 5:24.

Yin X, Tan K, Vajta G, et al. Massively parallel sequencing for chromosomal abnormality testing in trophectoderm cells of human blastocysts. Biol Reprod 2013; 88:69.

FURTHER READING

Tur-Kaspa I. Clinical management of in vitro fertilization with preimplantation genetic diagnosis. Semin Reprod Med 2012; 30:309–322.

Fragouli E, Alfarawati S, Spath K, et al. The origin and impact of embryonic aneuploidy. Hum Genet 2013; 132:1001–1013.

Gardner DK, Meseguer M, Rubio C, Treff NR. Diagnosis of human preimplantation embryo viability. Hum Reprod Update 2015; 21:727–747.

Kuliev A. Practical preimplantation genetic diagnosis (2nd edn) Berlin: Springer, 2013.

Chapter 16 Noninvasive prenatal testing

Kathryn Sanders, Tony Gordon

INTRODUCTION

Noninvasive prenatal testing (NIPT) has revolutionized prenatal screening for fetal live birth trisomies (e.g. trisomy 21, Down syndrome, trisomy 18, Edward syndrome; and trisomy 13, Patau syndrome), since it was first introduced clinically in 2012 in the USA. The number of copies of each chromosome in the fetal DNA are counted by sequencing the fetal DNA that is present in the maternal blood plasma. This technology produces an accurate, reliable, sensitive and specific determination of fetal trisomies and, as such, has been rapidly taken up as the preferred method of prenatal screening.

Live birth of children with an extra copy of a chromosome 21 (Down syndrome), chromosome 18 (Edwards syndrome), or chromosome 13 (Patau syndrome) has long been correlated with advanced maternal age. Among these syndromes, Down syndrome has the highest prevalence of live birth, rising from 0.84 per 1000 births for women between 25–29 years old, to 15.22 for women between 40–44 years old, in England and Wales (Wu & Morris 2013).

Conventional methods of prenatal screening for such fetal trisomies, prior to the introduction of NIPT, involve the screening of biochemical markers in the blood of pregnant women, in conjunction with ultrasound scanning. If a high risk of fetal trisomy pregnancy is detected via an invasive prenatal test, then either chorionic villus sampling (CVS) from 11–14 weeks' gestation, or amniocentesis following 15 weeks' gestation, is advised. Biochemical screening has a significant false positive rate (4.2%) and there are elevated risks of complications and/or possible pregnancy loss associated with such invasive prenatal testing. In contrast, NIPT has a comparatively low false positive rate (0.5%) (Bianchi et al. 2014) and has seen rapid uptake in order to reduce the unnecessary use of invasive diagnostic testing.

It has been known since the 1940s that fetal cells are present in the blood of pregnant women as these cells 'leak' from the placenta into the maternal blood stream. Walknowska et al. (1969) first suggested that these cells could be collected for prenatal diagnosis. Subsequently, it became the goal of scientists working in the field of prenatal testing, to isolate these rare fetal cells and produce a noninvasive screening test. However, fetal cells are present in less than 1 in 1 million of the cells in the blood of pregnant women. Furthermore, fetal cells from previous pregnancies can also persist in the maternal blood stream for years. Therefore, producing an effective screening test for these rare cells has been a huge challenge.

It was not until Lo et al. in 1997 first identified that fetal DNA was present in the blood plasma of pregnant women that an alternative method of NIPT became a possibility. NIPT became truly feasible by the early 2010s due to the exponential increase of capacity of DNA sequencers. These sequencers allowed the accurate quantification of fetal trisomies in cell-free DNA (cfDNA) from maternal plasma. The first commercial test became available in 2012 and since that time more than 1 million cfDNA NIPT samples have been processed, leading to a whole new area of prenatal medicine.

STANDARD PRENATAL SCREENING METHODS AND INVASIVE DIAGNOSTIC TESTS

Prenatal screening for fetal trisomy is routinely offered to most pregnant women as a combination of ultrasound scanning to measure nuchal translucency (NT) thickness and several biochemical markers. Various combinations of first and second trimester biochemical markers can be combined with ultrasound scanning to produce the various combined/integrated/quadruple tests (**Tables 16.1**).

The integrated test is considered to have the best performance characteristics of the ultrasound and biochemical test. Although, even with the best combination of ultrasound and biochemical markers, the sensitivity is lower and the false positive rates are significantly higher, than that seen with NIPT, leading to much lower positive predictive values (PPV) for these tests (PPV being the likelihood of being given a positive screen result and that actually being confirmed as a positive test). The integrated and quadruple tests, whilst not being as effective as NIPT for screening for live birth trisomies, do benefit from having reasonable detection rates (85% for integrated test) and false positive rates (1% for integrated test) for open neural tube defects. The results of the integrated and quadruple tests are generally expressed as a risk factor, e.g. 1 in 100 risk of Down syndrome live birth, whereas, many of the different NIPT tests offered provide detected/not detected results.

Table 16.1 Various combinations of first and second trimester biochemical markers can be combined with ultrasound scanning to produce the various combined, integrated and quadruple tests

Test	Types of prenatal screening for fetal trisomy
Combined test	• Blood taken at 10–13 weeks pregnancy • Ultrasound scan for nuchal translucency • Blood screen for pregnancy associated plasma protein-A (PAPP-A) • Blood screen for free ß-human chorionic gonadotropin (free ß-hCG) • Sensitivity (detection rate) of 82–87% and a false-positive rate around 5%
Integrated test	• First stage at 11 weeks pregnancy of ultrasound scan for nuchal translucency/gestational age and blood screen for pregnancy associated plasma protein-A (PAPP-A) • Second stage ideally at 15–16 weeks pregnancy. Blood screen for alpha-fetoprotein (AFP), total hCG, unconjugated estriol (uE3) and inhibin-A (inhibin) • Integration of results from first and second stage to single screening result • Sensitivity (detection rate) of 88–95% with a 2–5% false-positive rate for Down syndrome
Quadruple test	• Blood sample taken at 15–16 weeks' pregnancy • Blood screen for AFP, total hCG, uE3 and inhibin-A (inhibin)

Integrated and quadruple tests are intended for screening and are not fully diagnostic tests, since they determine the potential for the presences of live birth trisomies. This is in contrast to CVS and amniocentesis, which are considered diagnostic tests, since they can accurately confirm the absence/presence of live birth trisomies.

Chorionic villus sampling

CVS is performed from the 11th to the 14th weeks of pregnancy (**Figure 16.1**). A small sample of placental tissue containing chorionic villus cells is removed by ultrasound-guided aspiration. CVS can be carried out either by a transcervical or transabdominal method (with the latter most commonly performed). The sample cells are then either cultured directly by a cytogenetics laboratory to provide a karyotype, or the DNA is extracted from the sample for a microarray test. Both methods detect the presence of a fetal trisomy, as well as other cytogenetic abnormalities (usually as indicated from an ultrasound scan). However, as CVS is an indirect test of the placenta rather than the actual fetus, confined placental mosaicism (CPM) can occur, because the cytogenetics of the placenta may be different to the cytogenetics of the fetus.

Amniocentesis

Amniocentesis is performed between the 15th and 20th weeks of pregnancy. The process involves the use of a needle to remove a sample of the amniotic fluid from the amniotic sac. As with CVS, the amniotic fluid is either cultured to provide a cytogenetic karyotype, or DNA extracted from the amniotic fluid and a microarray test performed. Amniocentesis is the most diagnostic prenatal test for live birth trisomies that can be performed, since the process tests cells that are essentially direct from the fetus.

The timing of testing

Early testing is preferred as this is when termination is safest and can reduce the amount of distress encountered. There are similar risks of miscarriage associated with both CVS and amniocentesis of 0.5–1%, although the exact risk can also depend on the skill of the practitioner.

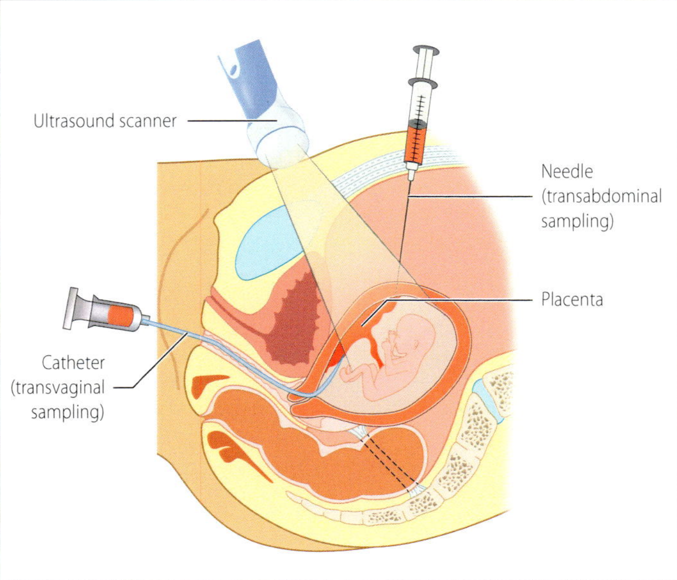

Figure 16.1 Chorionic villus sampling.

CVS is the method of choice for the first trimester, as amniocentesis prior to 15 weeks is not generally offered. This is because amniocentesis can lead to a higher risk of club foot and miscarriage in the first trimester (Alfirevic et al. 2003). The associated risk of miscarriage from both invasive procedures is a major consideration, especially if it has been conducted due to a false positive screen. The minimization of prenatal screening false positives, and therefore minimization of invasive procedures, has been a major advantage of NIPT and one of the main reasons for its rapid uptake. NIPT can also be carried out from 10 weeks of pregnancy, offering a means of screening pregnancies at a more advantageous early stage.

NONINVASIVE SCREENING

Biology

Cell-free fetal DNA (cffDNA) is formed due to a natural process of cell death (apoptosis) in the placenta. This is part of the constant turnover of trophoblast within the placenta to maintain its healthy function. Apoptosis leads to the release of small fragments of DNA, around 150 base pairs into the maternal blood stream. CffDNA appears in greater amounts as the pregnancy progresses, with male sequences cfDNA being detectable after 6–7 weeks and averaging at around 11–13% of total cfDNA.

NIPT is not offered until 10 weeks of gestation, since this is when the fraction of fetal DNA is greater than 2–4% of total cffDNA and averages around 11–13% of the total cfDNA. The fetal fraction is important in NIPT, as a higher fetal fraction can lead to more accurate results. When a maternal blood sample is taken for NIPT, it is centrifuged to separate the plasma from the blood cells. The cffDNA remains in the plasma, together with a larger proportion of maternal cfDNA. It has been demonstrated that cffDNA is most commonly present in smaller fragments than that of maternal cfDNA, averaging <0.3 kb and >1 kb, respectively. Therefore, by enrichment of the smaller fragments (<0.3 kb) of cfDNA, it is possible to direct the testing toward the DNA that is representative of the fetus, as opposed to the mother (Li et al. 2004).

There are two further areas of cffDNA biology that need to be considered in relation to screening tests.

Firstly, the biological source of cffDNA must be considered. It is widely accepted that the majority of cffDNA originates from the trophoblast of the placenta (Masuzaki et al. 2004). As a result, NIPT is not a fully diagnostic test, but rather a screening test. This is because NIPT is not directly testing the fetal genome, but the placenta as a proxy for the fetus, much like that carried out in CVS testing. Due to the similarity of the source of DNA for NIPT and CVS testing, a positive NIPT test result should not be confirmed by CVS testing but by amniocentesis.

Secondly, cffDNA is present in an excess of maternal cfDNA, and despite enhancement of smaller DNA fragments, many tests (although not all) cannot differentiate and quantify between fetal and maternal DNA. This is a problem if there is an underlying maternal chromosomal abnormality, as this may lead to a false positive NIPT result. In rare cases, the pregnant women may be mosaic for trisomy 21 (Down syndrome) and since the maternal genome is present in often 10–20 times greater concentration in the cfDNA than the fetal DNA, even a low level maternal mosaic trisomy 21 can lead to a false-positive NIPT. The most frequently seen maternal chromosome abnormalities, when sex chromosomes are included in screening, is low level mosaic Turner syndrome (where a single chromosome X is missing, alternatively known as 45,X). Again, for some NIPT tests where the cffDNA cannot be distinguished from maternal DNA, this can lead to a false positive screen for Turner syndrome.

Factors such as maternal basal metabolic index (BMI) and whether the conception was a result of IVF can cause the fetal fraction to be too low to produce a result. With high BMI, there appears to be a 'dilution effect', where there is more maternal cfDNA circulating, causing the fetal fraction to reduce, possibly due to an increased turnover of adipocytes. For the latter, it has been suggested that there may be problems with impairment of placentation in IVF pregnancies, which can result in a lower amount of cffDNA in the maternal blood plasma (Bevilacqua et al. 2015).

The NIPT false positives associated with confined placental mosaicism can be a sign of placental dysfunction. These false positive results can be an indicator of other problems that can occur later during pregnancy. Follow-up testing with amniocentesis, which rules out chromosomal abnormalities in the fetus, could be an indication that the chromosomal abnormality is in fact present but only in the placenta. This could potentially interfere with the normal functioning of the placenta. Placental dysfunction can lead to a higher rate of miscarriage, intrauterine growth restriction and hypertension.

It has also been shown that high levels of fetal fraction can also be linked to pre-eclampsia. Increased levels of apoptosis, and thus increased levels of cfDNA in the maternal circulation, can be due to oxidative stress on the placenta. It has been suggested that those patients that have false positive results and high levels of fetal fraction should be closely monitored during their pregnancy (Taglauer et al. 2014).

Technology

The first successful application of NIPT was possible due to the introduction of massively parallel genomic sequencers that enabled millions of sequence reads to be made in parallel from each cfDNA sample. This has made it possible to sequence multiple samples at the same time and reduce the turn-around time. This has further reduced the cost of testing and made this form of prenatal screening more commercially viable.

There are currently three different methods to carry out NIPT:

- Quantitative massively parallel shotgun sequencing (MPSS)
- Quantitative targeted massively paralleled sequencing (MPS)
- Qualitative single nucleotide polymorphism (SNP) based targeted sequencing.

Here, we briefly discuss the differences in these methods and how this can affect the performance of the tests.

Massively parallel shotgun sequencing

The MPSS reads from all chromosomes rather than from specific chromosomes (i.e. 13, 18, 21, X and Y). Maternal and fetal DNA are sequenced at the same time, but it is not possible to distinguish between the maternal and fetal DNA. An algorithm is used to count the number of chromosomes, and a ratio is produced to see if one chromosome is over- or under-represented. The accuracy of this test is related to fetal fraction, in that the higher the fetal fraction, the easier it is to distinguish when one chromosome has a higher representation than the others. The algorithm uses a reference database of previously analyzed population to determine thresholds for trisomy. When the number of reads per sample is lowered, this allows for more samples to be analyzed in the same run, although a lower number of reads can result in an increase in no results returned. There can be variation in the efficiency of amplification in individual chromosomes; this can alter the ratio of reads, which can result in false positives.

Sex chromosome detection is not as sensitive in this method as with other chromosomes. When testing for chromosomes 13, 18, 21, X and Y, this accounts for only about 14% of the reads from sequencing, therefore, the rest of the genome which has been sequenced would be wasted. However, this means that there is potential to expand screening to all other chromosomes (Kotsopoulou et al. 2015).

Targeted massively paralleled sequencing

Targeted MPS is similar to MPSS but only amplifies those chromosomes of interest, i.e. 13, 18, 21, X and Y. The chromosomes are then counted in the same manner. A benefit to targeted MPS is that more samples can be sequenced simultaneously and at higher reads (**Figure 16.2**).

Qualitative single nucleotide polymorphism

Qualitative SNP-based targeted sequencing using a genotype analysis as opposed to a counting analysis. This method targets SNPs on specific chromosomes. This method gives information regarding chromosome copy number but can also give further information and allow for more complex analysis such as, inheritance patterns. The maternal and fetal DNA contributions are identified.

Some forms of this testing are not suitable for patients that have received oocyte donation, as the maternal information is not available. One test that is commercially available, simultaneously, tests for DNA which is exclusively from the mother; this information is used to remove her DNA from the cfDNA that is detected in the plasma (Kotsopoulou et al. 2015). SNP-based targeted sequencing offers very low false positives and the ability to detect triploidy.

Clinical applications

The NIPT is most commonly available to women who are at a higher risk of having a pregnancy with a live birth trisomy. High risk pregnancies are those associated with advanced maternal age (35 years or older at delivery), positive screening test results (as previously mentioned), history of pregnancies with a trisomy, previous miscarriage, multiple gestation and parental balanced Robertsonian translocation.

It has been suggested that NIPT should be available for all pregnancies; however, the benefits of this are questionable. For example, women who are considered low risk can still have pregnancies which result in a live birth trisomy. In the United States, it is estimated that 1 in 1300 pregnancies will be affected by trisomy 21 for a woman of 25 years old (Newberger 2000), and this increases to 1 in 400 at 35 years of age. However, 80% of all children born with Down syndrome are born to mothers under 35 years (Bunt and Bunt 2014). Yet, there is concern that the number of true positive results from NIPT will be outweighed by an increased number of false positive results leading to unnecessary invasive procedures and possible miscarriages as a result.

It is highly recommended that women seeking NIPT are adequately counseled before the testing. There is concern that with the rapid uptake of NIPT, clinics are not able to keep up with providing appropriate counseling. It should be emphasized that NIPT is a screening test and not diagnostic. Despite this, it is still a highly sensitive and specific screening test, by comparison to conventional screening methods mentioned previously.

A study in 2016 by Mackie et al. reviewed the results from 117 studies to determine the accuracy of NIPT. The results for fetal trisomies were, for sensitivity and specificity, respectively:

- Trisomy 21: 99.4% and 99.9%
- Trisomy 18: 97.7% and 99.9%
- Trisomy 13: 90.6% and 100%

Factors that can lead to a false positive result include those mentioned previously, and CPM, where the aneuploidy is confined to the placenta and the fetus is unaffected.

It is recommended that counseling is offered for other problems that can arise due to a false positive and aneuploidy confined to the placenta, e.g. placental dysfunction, suggesting that further monitoring later in the pregnancy could be beneficial.

Maternal chromosomal abnormalities could be identified from screening and can lead to a false positive result for the fetus. This should be explained to women before NIPT to determine if they would like these findings disclosed. It has also been shown that false positives for multiple aneuploidies can come about when there is undetected cancer in the mother.

Another factor which can cause false positive results is if there has been co-twin demise. If it is known that one twin has 'vanished,' it is important to counsel patients that a positive result could be due to a chromosomal abnormality in the demised twin. Although the twin is no longer detectable, the placenta could still be intact and able to contribute to the cffDNA in the maternal circulation.

In these instances, it can be recommended to wait a couple of weeks and repeat the NIPT to see if the result is still positive prior to carrying out an invasive procedure.

False negative results are much rarer than false positives. It is estimated that potentially 0.2% of cases in high risk patients could be missed and 0.02% in the low risk patients (Van Opstal et al. 2016), whilst this is rarer than false positives. The two main factors which can lead to a false negative result are, confined placental mosaicism and low-level trisomy mosaicism. As with CPM seen in false positives, the trophoblasts from the placenta could be chromosomally normal, presenting a normal karyotype with NIPT. Whilst, in fact, the fetus has a trisomy, therefore this would be missed by NIPT. Low-level trisomy mosaicism is where not all cells in the fetus and the placenta possess the trisomy. Where the trisomy is very low, for example <30% of the cells are effected, the fetal fraction which represents the trisomy will be further reduced. Therefore, the normal cells will have a greater representation, indicating a negative NIPT result and the low-level trisomy would be missed. However, low-level trisomy mosaicism is known to present a problem for prenatal clinicians, as it is not clear what percentage level will result in an affected live birth. For example, Tang et al. 2017 have reported on cases of low-level trisomy 3 mosaicism, where investigation through amniocentesis has presented mosaicism between 8 and 10% but resulted in a normal live birth. Normal outcomes have also been seen at 16 and 22% mosaic, but congenital anomalies at 36%. It is important that patients are counseled that there is a chance for false negative results. It is also recommended that follow up screening for structural abnormalities should be offered to all patients, to aid in detection of those low-level mosaic trisomies that may be missed by NIPT.

It is advantageous to be able to apply NIPT to twin pregnancies as the risk of aneuploidies in these pregnancies is higher than with singletons. The risk of miscarriage associated with invasive techniques for testing are also higher in twin pregnancies. Twin pregnancies present challenges when it comes to NIPT. It is important to understand that, in the case of twins, the amount of cffDNA does not double. It appears that cffDNA increases by approximately a third when comparing twins to a singleton and the contribution of cffDNA from each twin can vary. With dizygotic twins (those from two different oocytes) there is a greater challenge than with monozygotic (those from the same oocyte), as it is not possible to identify which fetus is affected when a trisomy is detected. If one twin has a trisomy, that twin could be under-represented in terms of cffDNA and a false negative result could occur. This is particularly true of trisomy 18 and trisomy 13 as these are often related to a low fetal fraction. Despite this, testing is possible with NIPT, accepting that the accuracy is not as high as that seen in singleton pregnancies and there is a higher testing failure rate seen (Bevilacqua et al. 2015). It is not possible to be conclusive with the sex of the twins, however in the case of Y chromosome being detected it indicates that at least one of the fetus is likely to be male.

The most common NIPT offered is for trisomy 21, trisomy 18, trisomy 13 and sex chromosome aneuploidy. However, testing for microdeletions, cri-du-chat and Prader–Willi/Angelman syndrome is beginning to emerge. These tests may not be as sensitive as that seen in conventional NIPT, due to the biological nature of these microdeletions and the early stage of testing. Most importantly, NIPT does not screen for all birth defects and it is important that women have additional screening for all other chromosomal abnormalities and neural tubal defects. One downside to the increased uptake of NIPT is that there has been an increase in the number of infants born with the conditions which are not screened for using cffDNA. This is thought to be linked to the decrease in the amount of invasive procedures carried out (Beaudet 2016).

Overall, there are less pregnancies being exposed to invasive procedures because of the uptake of NIPT. For women who receive a positive NIPT, it is vital to ensure that they are fully informed regarding the importance of follow up diagnostics for confirmation. While NIPT can be offered early in the pregnancy, the wait for a subsequent invasive diagnostic test may seem unacceptable to some women. For example, one study found that 6.2% of cases had terminated directly after a positive NIPT result (Dar et al. 2014).

It has been suggested that offering early amniocentesis might be worth considering for patients who are unwilling to wait and would otherwise opt for termination of pregnancy following a positive NIPT result (Zelig et al. 2016).

THE FUTURE OF NONINVASIVE PRENATAL SCREENING

NIPT is a relatively recent advance to the world of prenatal screening, and as such we would expect to see new developments and improvements in the future. With improvements in technology, expanding the scope and reducing the cost of NIPT seems increasingly possible.

It would be ideal to expand the limits of testing for NIPT, so that it would be possible to screen for a wide range of fetal abnormalities in one test. The first area of expansion of NIPT, is to screen for all chromosomal trisomies, or rare autosomal trisomies (RATs). It has been suggested that trisomies on other chromosomes can influence the algorithm, resulting in false positive results for those chromosomes that are reported and test failures (Bianchi et al. 2017). Therefore, while it might be beneficial to offer as much information regarding all chromosomes, avoidance of false positive results needs to be considered.

An area of much recent focus is that of microdeletion screening. NIPT for microdeletions involves more time and cost to detect subchromosomal abnormalities. For example, 71.8% of these abnormalities can be detected at 3.5M reads, yet this increases to 94.5% with 10M reads (Liu et al. 2016). It is hoped that in the future, with improved technology and cost-effectiveness, microdeletion screening will become a more viable option.

Another future possibility is for NIPT to screen for single gene disorders, such as cystic fibrosis, sickle cell anemia and Huntingdon's disease. One suggestion has been to involve analysis of both parents to identify the affected alleles which may be inherited from the male and female. However, the challenge remains of the fetal DNA existing within an abundance of maternal DNA. To identify whether the fetus has inherited the affected alleles, the cfDNA will need to be analyzed for relative mutation balance or imbalance. For example, a mother who is a carrier of a single gene disorder, possessing one affected allele and one unaffected allele will have 50:50 (affected, unaffected, respectively) represented in her cfDNA. Where there is a fetal fraction of 10% the mutant allele load will increase (55:45) when affected, decrease (45:55) when unaffected or remain the same (50:50) when a carrier, depending on fetal inheritance of the affected alleles. Another method is analysis of haploblocks, to build a picture of the direction of allele inheritance. As these methods involve the sequencing of, at least the parents and the fetus there is increased cost involved. It is therefore, thought that targeted sequencing for the genes affected may be more cost effective; however, methods to avoid allele drop-out would be necessary to increase accuracy.

There are still some unanswered biological questions relating to fetal cfDNA. For example, whilst, it is widely accepted that the majority of cffDNA originates from trophoblast cells from the placenta, the amount contributed from the source is not known, or, if it is the only source. Details of the mechanism of cffDNA production and the nature of cfDNA clearance, both maternal and fetal, from maternal plasma during pregnancy, is not fully understood. Further knowledge in these areas would greatly benefit NIPT to aid in future developments and increased accuracy.

Advances in technology could see a return to analysis of whole fetal cells. If whole genome amplification (WGA) and analysis was successfully applied to isolated whole fetal cells, it would make it possible to screen for all abnormalities, including copy number variation, microdeletions and point mutations. WGA and analysis of whole fetal cells, would then make prenatal testing truly diagnostic while being noninvasive.

REFERENCES

Alfirevic Z, Mujezinovic F, Sundberg K. Amniocentesis and chorionic villus sampling for prenatal diagnosis. Cochrane Database Syst Rev 2003:CD003252.

Beaudet AL. Using Fetal Cells for Prenatal Diagnosis: History and Recent Progress. Am J Med Genet C Semin Med Genet 2016; 172:123–127.

Bevilacqua E, Gil MM, Nicolaides KH, et al. Performance of screening for aneuploidies by cell-free DNA analysis of maternal blood in twin pregnancies. Ultrasound Obstet Gynecol 2015; 45:61–66.

Bianchi DW, Parker RL, Wentworth J, et al. DNA sequencing versus standard prenatal aneuploidy screening. N Engl J Med 2014; 370:799–808.

Bianchi DW. Should we 'open the kimono' to release the results of rare autosomal aneuploidies following noninvasive prenatal whole genome sequencing? Prenat Diagn 2017; 37:123–125.

Bunt CW, Bunt SK. Role of the family physician in the care of children with down syndrome. Am Fam Physician 2014; 90:851–858.

Dar P, Curnow KJ, Gross SJ, et al. Clinical experience and follow-up with large scale single-nucleotide polymorphism – based noninvasive prenatal aneuploidy testing. Am J Obstet Gynecol 2014; 211:e1–17.

Kotsopoulou I, Tsoplou P, Mavrommatis K, Kroupis C. Non-invasive prenatal testing (NIPT): limitations on the way to become diagnosis. Diagnosis 2015; 2:141–158.

Li Y, Zimmerman B, Rusterholz C, et al. Size separation of circulatory DNA in maternal plasma permits ready detection of fetal DNA polymorphisms. Clin Chem 2004; 50:1002–1011.

Liu L, Li K, Fu X, Chung C, Zhang K. A forward look at noninvasive prenatal testing. Trends Mol Med 2016; 22:958–968.

Lo YMD, Corbetta N, Chamberlain PF, et al. Presence of fetal DNA in maternal plasma and serum. Lancet 1997; 350:485–487.

Mackie FL, Hemming K, Allen S, Morris RK, Kilby MD. The accuracy of cell-free fetal DNA-based non-invasive prenatal testing in singleton pregnancies: a systematic review and bivariate meta-analysis. Br J Obstet Gynecol 2016; 124:32–46.

Masuzaki H, Miura K, Yoshiura S, Niikawa N, Ishimaru T. Detection of cell free placental DNA in maternal plasma: direct evidence from three cases of confined placental mosaicism. J Med Genet 2004; 41:289–292.

Newberger DS. Down syndrome: prenatal risk assessment and diagnosis. Am Fam Physician 2000; 62:825–832.

Taglauer ES, Wilkins-Haug L, Bianchi DW. Review: Cell-free fetal DNA in the maternal circulation as an indication of placental health and disease. Placenta 2014; 35:28:S64–S68.

Tang W, Wu Y, Liu J, Ren W. Research Letter: Prenatal diagnosis of low-level trisomy 3 mosaicism. Taiwanese J Obstet Gynecol 2017; 56:114–115.

Van Opstal D, Srebniak MI, Polak J, et al. False negative NIPT results: Risk Figures for Chromosome 13, 18 and 21 Based on Chorionic Villi Results in 5967 Cases and Literature Review. PLoS One 2016; 11:1–10.

Walknowska J, Conte FA, Grumbach MM. Practical and theoretical implications of fetal/maternal lymphocyte transfer. Lancet 1969; 1:1119–1122.

Wu J, Morris JK. Trends in maternal age distribution and the live birth prevalence of Down's syndrome in England and Wales: 1983-2010. Eur J Hum Genet 2013; 21:1032–1033.

Zelig CM, Knutzen DM, Ennen CS, Dolinsky BM, Napolitano PG. Chorionic Villus Sampling, Early Amniocentesis, And Termination Of Pregnancy Without Diagnostic Testing: Comparison of Fetal Risk Following Positive Non-invasive Prenatal Testing. J Obstet Gynaecol Can 2016; 38:441–445.

Chapter 17 Deriving oocytes from stem cells

Gustavo Tiscornia, Montserrat Barragán, Rita Vassena

INTRODUCTION

Infertility is a global disease that causes significant personal, financial and societal burdens. It is estimated that up to 15% of couples trying to conceive will have difficulties in doing so, and many of them will depend on assisted reproductive technologies (ART) to conceive.

The quality and quantity of oocytes available for reproduction is a major factor in determining the success of both ART treatments and natural conceptions. Despite the central role of oocyte developmental competence in this process, comparatively little is known about oocyte development and biology in the human species. This lack of knowledge is due to several factors: the impossibility of studying primordial germ cells (PGCs) and oocyte development during fetal life, the scarcity of postnatal oocytes available for research, and the technical challenges related to the study of small amounts of starting material.

The availability of large numbers of PGCs and oocytes at different stages of development would greatly advance our knowledge of the mechanisms involved in oocyte biology, including the genetic and biochemical sources of infertility. Moreover, large scale in vitro production of oocytes would increase our ability to develop effective drugs to address fertility preservation and contraception, to test gonadotoxicity of new molecules, and to screen for personalized reproductive therapy.

This chapter reviews the field of differentiation towards oocytes-from pluripotent cells, and highlights knowledge gaps which will need to be addressed move forward.

THE CONCEPT OF POTENCY

Self-renewal, potency and differentiation are crucial concepts in the fields of mammalian development and stem cell biology. Self-renewal, a fundamental characteristic of stem cell behavior , is the capability of a stem cell to undergo cell divisions that result in at least one daughter cell maintaining the potency level of initial cell. Differentiation, on the other hand, is the process by which a cell undergoes changes in structure and function that give rise to a different cell type of lower potency, more complex structure and more specialized functions. The expression 'developmental potency' (or simply 'potency') refers to a specific cellular phenotype: the capability of a cell type to differentiate. Potency can be considered a gradient that ranges from very high potency (totipotency) to no potency at all (nullipotency).

Totipotency is defined as the capability to differentiate into every cell type found in the organism, including extra-embryonic tissues that develop during the fetal period. Formally, the only cell type considered to be totipotent is the zygote created by fertilization. Early blastomeres (up to the 4-cell stage) can also show totipotent behavior under specific circumstances, as demonstrated by embryo splitting experiments in animals and births of healthy human babies after transfer of 4-cell embryos with only one blastomere intact (Van de Velde et al. 2008, Veiga et al. 1987).

Cell types can be positioned on this gradient according to their potency, and certain categories are commonly alluded to in the literature (pluripotent, multipotent, bipotent, monopotent, etc). At the blastocyst stage of early embryonic development, two cell populations can be distinguished: the inner cell mass (ICM), which will go on to develop the embryo proper; and the trophoblast, which will give rise to extra-embryonic tissues.

The term 'pluripotent' is commonly used to describe the ICM, as its cells will give rise to all the cell types of the adult organism. Since the cells in the ICM do not normally give rise to the trophoblast, they can no longer be considered totipotent. The cells in the ICM can be explanted, established and expanded in vitro, giving rise to embryonic stem cell (ESC) lines, which are also considered pluripotent.

Other classes of pluripotent stem cells are distinguished on the basis of their origin and the method used to establish them (**Table 17.1**). Parthenogenetic stem cells (PSCs), derived from oocytes induced to undergo parthenogenesis, and embryonic germ cells (EGCs), derived from PGCs, are established using approaches similar to those used to establish ESCs. Somatic cell nuclear transfer (SCNT) pluripotent cells are derived from oocytes after removal of the meiotic spindle, and substitution of the genetic material with the nucleus of a somatic cell. Finally, induced pluripotent stem cells (iPSCs) are obtained from somatic cells by over-expression of a small number of transcription factors such as Oct4, Klf4, Sox2 and c-Myc, a process called reprogramming.

In recent years, it has become increasingly clear that cellular potency is produced by an underlying regulatory state constituted by a specific transcriptional (mRNA, micro-RNAs) and proteomic profile, as well as defined epigenetic, metabolic, and signaling states. During the process of derivation, the underlying regulatory state of the in vivo cell population is said to be 'captured', and the regulatory state of the stem cell population established in vitro is considered to accurately reflect that of the original in vivo compartment.

However, the regulatory state of the in vitro cultured population may not be identical to that of the in vivo compartment. Both the derivation process and the culture conditions may result in alterations of the regulatory state. How different the resulting in vitro regulatory state is from the initial in vivo compartment may not be easy to determine,

Table 17.1 Different classes of pluripotency

Type of pluripotent cell	Source
Embryonic stem cells	Inner cell mass of a blastocyst stage embryo
Parthenogenetic stem cells	Parthenotes (activated oocytes)
Embryonic germ cells	Primordial germ cells
Somatic cell nuclear transfer embryonic stem cells	Embryos created following somatic cell nuclear transfer (cloning)
Induced pluripotent stem cells	Direct reprogramming of somatic cells

nor is it straightforward to define when the resulting regulatory state is different enough from the original regulatory state to consider the established population as a nonrepresentative cellular entity.

A regulatory state is not fixed or immutable; rather, it can be flexible, depending on the cell type, and may be departed from, or arrived at, through experimental manipulations such as reprogramming or SCNT.

REDUCTION OF POTENCY THROUGH DIFFERENTIATION

As embryonic development proceeds, cells gradually differentiate into types of cells of reduced potency. A strong potency reduction occurs during gastrulation, when the embryo reorganizes into the three germ layers (ectoderm, mesoderm and endoderm) and the germline; cells in each one these compartments will give rise to specific cell types.

Many of the tissues and organs that arise during organogenesis have an intense cellular turnover on which their functionality is crucially dependent (such as the blood, skin or gut). The cellular homeostasis of these systems depends fundamentally on a compartment of tissue specific adult stem cells. These cells are considered 'multipotent', as they are capable of differentiating into multiple cell types typical of their particular system. For example, hematopoietic stem cells (HSCs) are capable of generating the complete array of cell types that constitute the cellular fraction of the blood, but do not differentiate into cell types of other tissues or systems.

While HSCs are less potent than pluripotent stem cells, they maintain high potency within the context of their particular systems; HSC differentiation will produce either a 'common lymphoid progenitor' (CLP) or a 'common myeloid progenitor' (CMP), each of which is, in turn, the ancestor of several cell types and therefore also considered multipotent.

As the differentiation path proceeds, potency continues to decrease until 'bipotent' or 'unipotent' cell types are produced. Finally, terminally differentiated cells no longer capable of differentiation are referred to as 'nullipotent'. Other tissues and systems (including HSC, epidermal stem cells, muscle satellite cells and others) in which cellular turnover is lower also contain quiescent stem cell compartments that can be mobilized in response to injury (Arai et al. 2008, Lo Sicco et al. 2015, Rennert et al. 2012).

IN VIVO OOCYTE DEVELOPMENT

Differentiation toward the oocyte is particularly complex. In humans, PGCs can be observed in the posterior wall of the yolk sac around 24 days postconception. PGCs are monopotent, as they are fated to differentiate into either sperm or oocytes. However, it is only oocytes (not sperm) that conserve high levels of potency.

The PGCs can be cultured in vitro and established as EGCs, which are highly potent. The molecular and signaling determinants of germline specification are not well known. In mice, the bone morphogenetic protein 4 (BMP4) signaling pathway is known to be required for PGC specification. PGCs proliferate and migrate to the genital ridge while undergoing a complex differentiation program with expression of specific markers and a strong epigenetic component which involves global demethylation as well as histone mark modifications. Crucial interactions occur with somatic cells of the ovary.

In mammals, during late embryonic development, the oocyte initiates meiosis and arrests in prophase of the first meiotic division (prophase I; this arrest is not lifted until the beginning of menstruation after puberty). An oocyte then resumes meiosis during every menstrual cycle, resulting in maturation of a selected cohort of follicles and ovulation of an oocyte arrested at metaphase of the second meiotic division (metaphase II). Completion of meiosis and extrusion of the second polar body occur after fertilization (**Figure 17.1**).

DEMONSTRATION OF POTENCY

Demonstration of potency requires subjecting the cells to experimental manipulations in vitro or in vivo that result in differentiated progeny. In its most strict sense, the analysis must be clonal: a single cell must be capable of generating the entire range of cell types afforded by the potency claimed.

For example, for ESCs, pluripotency is demonstrated by a series of tests of increasing stringency:

- Cells must remain phenotypically stable over extended periods of culture
- A clonal population of ESCs (derived from a single cell) must be capable of differentiation in vitro toward the three germ layers and express markers of each compartment (ectoderm, mesoderm and endoderm)
- A clonal population should be able to form a benign tumor called a teratoma when injected in an immune deficient mouse. Histological analysis of the teratoma must show the presence of differentiated structures of a variety of systems, as well as markers for specific cell types of the three germ layers (Oh et al. 2009, Stachelscheid et al. 2013, Damjanov & Ahrlund-Richter 2007)

In the case of mouse embryonic stem cells (mESCs), the demonstration of pluripotency can be taken to a higher level of stringency by showing that:

- Labeled cells (e.g. expressing a fluorescent marker) can be injected into a blastocyst that is then transferred into a pseudopregnant female to test whether the marked cells can participate in normal development and be readily detected in newborn chimeric pups derived from the transferred embryo
- The chimeric animals obtained are capable of producing viable descendants (germline transmission)
- The demonstration of tetraploid complementation (the ability of mESC to give rise to viable and fertile offspring when injected into a 4N blastocyst, which is capable of forming extraembryonic tissues but not of sustaining development of the embryo past implantation)

IN VITRO DIFFERENTIATION TO OOCYTES

Several approaches have been taken to obtain oocytes. Important considerations in these methods are: the initial cell type (pluripotent cells, progenitors harvested from the germline at different stages of development), the final cell type sought (PGCs, oocyte-like cells at various stages of development, postmeiotic cells) and the culture methods used.

Importantly, key variables in the cell culture protocols are:

- The composition of the media (particularly growth factors and signaling molecules)
- Whether the cells are co-cultured with other cell types (organotypic cultures, use of feeder cell layers, aggregation with different cell types)
- Whether the protocol employs transgene overexpression to induce differentiation
- The culture protocol used (length of culture in a defined number of culture media)

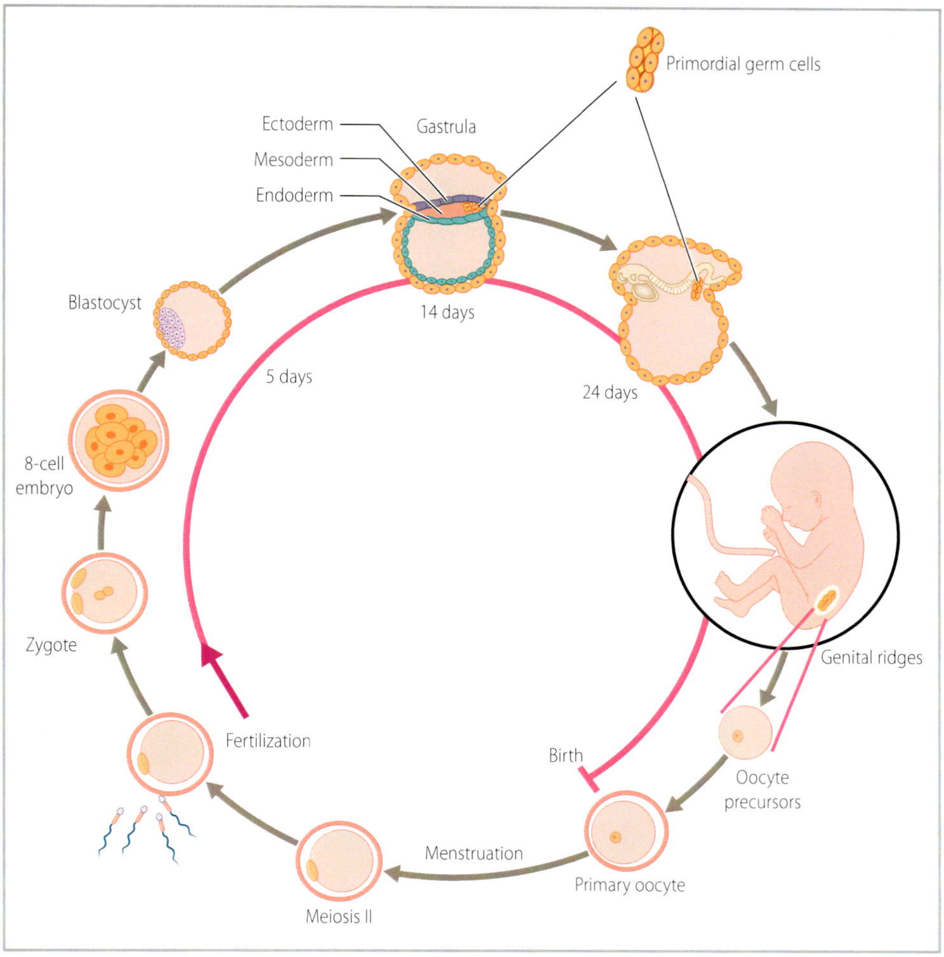

Figure 17.1 In vivo germline development.

- Whether the method involves a final in vivo differentiation stage to obtain mature and functional products (Ge et al. 2015)

Pluripotent stem cells could be a convenient starting population for an in vitro protocol for differentiation to oocytes due to their availability and high potency. The ideal protocol should be robust, result in a high yield of oocytes and reflect in vivo differentiation. Key factors in developing such a protocol are knowledge of the differentiation process in vivo, and an appropriate starting cell population.

Importantly, the resulting cells should be validated to check for expression of germ cell markers and that the cells have undergone the appropriate epigenetic changes associated with gamete determination. In mice, the generation of live offspring is also required. Most published studies have focused on the mouse system. For practical purposes, the process can be divided into two stages:

1. Differentiation of pluripotent cells to PGCs
2. Differentiation of PGCs to mature oocytes (female gametogenesis), a process that involves sex determination, meiosis and differentiation. While the first stage has been achieved in vitro, the second has not

DIFFERENTIATION OF MOUSE PLURIPOTENT CELLS TO OOCYTES

In mice, PGCs arise during gastrulation around embryonic day 6 (E6) from the postimplantation epiblast in response to BMP4 signaling from the neighboring extraembryonic ectoderm (Lawson et al. 1999). PGCs initially upregulate mesodermal genes such as T, Hoxa1 and Hoxb1, and later express transcription factors involved in PGC specification (Blimp1/Prdm1, Prdm14 and Tfap2c), of which Blimp1 is considered to be the main regulatory transcription factor (**Table 17.2**). By E8 (the eighth day of development of the mouse embryo), established PGCs express specific markers such as Sox2.

Shortly after specification, a small number of PGCs start migration along with the hindgut. During this process, proliferation occurs in response to still poorly understood signals and eventually, hundreds of cells exit the hindgut into the mesonephros and arrive at the genital ridges.

During this migration, PGCs undergo global demethylation, from an initial 70% of the genome on E6 to around 7% of the genome at E13.5 (Seisenberger et al. 2012). Imprinted genes are also completely demethylated by E13.5 (Hajkova et al. 2002, Kagiwada et al. 2013, Sato et al. 2003).

Global changes also occur in histone modifications, with a general decrease in histone H3 lysine 9 dimethylation (H3K9me2) and increase in histone H3 lysine trimethylation (H3K27me3). It is thought that these changes are related to the acquisition of high levels of latent potency by the terminally differentiated gametes.

Female PGCs at the genital ridge continue to proliferate. In response to retinoic acid (RA), produced in the adjacent mesonephros, the PGCs enter into meiosis. At around the time of birth, primary oocytes (arrested in prophase I) and somatic pregranulosa cells form the primordial follicle (Edson et al. 2009).

A number of approaches have been used to differentiate pluripotent cells to oocytes. Different groups have tested a range of parameters, including differentiation of pluripotent cells:

Table 17.2 Glossary of protein markers

Protein name	Full name	Class/molecular function	Developmental role
bFGF	Basic fibroblast growth factor	Cytokine	Differentiation of stem cells to germ-cell like
BLIMP1	PR domain zinc finger protein 1	Transcriptional repressor	PGCs specification
BMP4	Bone morphogenetic protein 4	Secreted polypeptide	Germ-line specification PGCs appearance
BOULE	Homolog of Boule (*Drosophila*)	RNA-binding protein	Late germ-cell marker
DAZ1	Deleted in azoospermia 1	RNA-binding protein	Late germ-cell marker
DAZL	Deleted in azoospermia-like	RNA binding protein	Late germ-cell marker
ERK	Extracellular signal-regulated kinases	Protein kinase	Differentiation of stem cells to germ-cell like
HOXA1	Homeobox protein Hox-A1	Homeodomain transcription factor	Early marker for PGCs
HOXB1	Homeobox protein Hox-B1	Homeodomain transcription factor	Early marker for PGCs
ITGB3	Integrin beta 3	Integrin	PGCs marker
KIT	Mast/stem cell growth factor receptor	Receptor tyrosine kinase protein	PGCs marker
KLF2	Kruppel-like factor 2	Transcription factor	Reprogramming
KLF4	Kruppel-like factor 4	Transcription factor	Reprogramming marker for established PGCs
LIF	Leukemia inhibitory factor	Cytokine	Inner cell mass differentiation
NANOG	Homolog of Nanog (*Drosophila*)	Transcription factor	Reprogramming marker for established PGCs
NANOS3	Homolog of Nanos3 (*Drosophila*)	RNA-binding protein	PGCs marker
OCT4	Octamer-binding transcription factor 4	Homeodomain transcription factor	Reprogramming marker for established PGCs
PRDM14	PR Domain-containing protein 14	Histone methyltransferase activity	PGCs specification
SCF	Stem cell factor	Cytokine	Induces PGCs proliferation
SOX17	SRY (Sex determining region Y)-Box 17	Transcription factor	PGCs specification
SOX2	SRY (Sex determining region Y)-Box 2	Transcription factor	Reprogramming marker for established PGCs
SSEA1	Stage-specific embryonic antigen 1	Carbohydrate adhesion molecule	PGCs marker
STELLA	Homolog of Stella (*Drosophila*)	Transcription repressor	PGCs marker
T	Brachyury	Transcription factor	Early marker for PGCs
TFAP2C	Transcription factor AP-2 gamma	Transcription factor	PGCs specification
TNAP	TRAFs and NIK-Associated Protein	Repressor of NF-κB	PGCs marker
VASA	Homolog of Vasa (*Drosophila*)	RNA binding protein	Late germ-cell marker

- As adherent monolayers (Hubner et al. 2003, Novak et al. 2006)
- In suspension as embryoid bodies (EBs) with the use of testicular cell conditioned media (Lacham-Kaplan et al. 2006)
- By use of retinoic acid and co-culture of EBs with ovarian granulosa cells (Kerkis et al. 2007, Qing et al. 2007)
- By use of oocyte specific promoters expressing fluorescent reporters (Salvador et al. 2008)
- By enrichment using biochemical methods (Saiti et al. 2008).

These reports have resulted in a variety of oocyte-like cells; however, in general these cells where not shown to enter meiosis or undergo maturation, and their functionality were not characterized. Importantly, their ability to produce healthy offspring was not demonstrated.

An important consideration for initial differentiation of ESCs or iPSCs to oocytes is the exact pluripotent state of the starting population and its responsiveness to BMP4 signaling as the first extrinsic trigger of the process. Two types of ESC lines can be established from the blastocyst in the mouse. ESC lines derived from the ICM are called naïve mESC, while ESC lines derived from the postimplantation epiblast are called epiblast stem cells (EpiSCs). Both types of lines differ significantly in their characteristics and behavior , e.g. they differ in response to leukemia inhibitory factor (LIF) or FGF/ERK signaling, marker profile, X-chromosome silencing and differentiation bias (Nichols et al. 2009).

Importantly, cells of either type show a degree of plasticity and can fluctuate between states depending on culture conditions. Naïve mESCs can be converted into EpiSc by culture in EpiSC medium, or can be completely blocked from transitioning to the EpiSC state by culture with specific growth factors and inhibitors (Weinberger et al. 2016). Conversely, EpiSC can revert to the naïve pluripotent state by forced expression of transcription factors such as Klf4 or Prdm14 and Klf2.

In particular, mESC and EpiSC react differently to BMP4 signaling. Exposure of mESC to BMP4 favors self-renewal (Qi et al. 2004), but EpiSC stimulated by BMP4 do not differentiate to PGCs (Richter et al. 2014). These results suggested that the ability of epiblast cells to give rise to PGCs in response to BMP4 signaling in vivo (PGC competence) originates in an intermediate cell type between mESC and EpiSC.

This rationale led Hayashi and colleagues (Hayashi et al. 2011) to differentiate mESC and then subject the differentiating cells to BMP4 stimulation at regular intervals. Remarkably, cells differentiated for 48 hours and subjected to BMP4 and stem cell factor (SCF; confirmed to induce proliferation in PGCs) stimulation gave rise to PGC-like cells (PGCLCs) which upregulated PGC-specific reporters, and expressed PGC markers such as Blimp1, Stella, SSEA1 and ItgB3. Further analysis revealed expression of other PGC markers, including Prdm14, Tfap2c, Hoxa1 and Hoxb1.

In addition, PGCLC had a specific transcriptional profile distinct from both mESC and EpiSC, and showed decreased and increased levels of H3K9me2 and H3K27me3 marks, respectively. This is similar to the behavior of in vivo PGCs. Transcriptional analysis suggest that 6-day-old PGCLC correspond to PGCs at E9.5 in vivo. PGCLCs cease to proliferate or thrive upon continued culture, suggesting that continued stimulation by SCF is insufficient to sustain proliferation. However, they resume proliferation when aggregated with E12.5 gonadal cells suggesting that gonadal cells provide an additional, yet unknown, PGC proliferation signal.

The PGCLC co-cultured with gonad cells resemble oogonia: they express late germ cell markers Dazl and Mvh, erase methylation in paternally imprinted genes, and undergo meiosis up to the prophase I stage. When aggregates were transplanted into the ovarian bursa of immunosuppressed adult female mice, oocyte-like cells at the germinal vesicle stage were recovered. These cells could be induced to resume meiosis to reach metaphase II, and resulted in healthy and fertile offspring after IVF and embryo transfer into recipient females (Hayashi et al. 2012).

Interestingly, PGCLC derived from iPSC behaved in a similar manner, although the percentages of normal fertilization and full-term development were lower than for PGCs and up to 50% of the zygotes had two maternal and one paternal pronuclei, suggesting iPSC derived PGCLCs have a defect in second polar body extrusion (Hayashi et al. 2012).

However, full in vitro differentiation from PGCLC to functional oocytes has not yet been achieved for any mammalian species, as the gonadal cues responsible for induction of primary oocytes from PGCs in vivo are still unknown.

DIFFERENTIATION OF HUMAN PLURIPOTENT CELLS TO OOCYTES

The study of human PGC specification has lagged behind that of mouse, mainly due to the impossibility of examining early human embryos. Despite general conservation of the germline differentiation pathway, significant differences between rodent and primate ESC and early embryonic development preclude direct extrapolation of mechanisms established in mice to human PGC specification (**Figure 17.2**) (De Felici 2013, Hackett et al. 2014, Irie et al. 2014,Nichols et al. 2009).

Initial studies determined that cells with germ cell markers arose spontaneously in human embryonic stem cell (hESC) differentiating in suspension, and that yields were increased in response to BMP4 signaling (Clark et al. 2004; Kee et al. 2006). Differentiation of hESC on fibroblast feeders in the presence of basic fibroblast growth factor (bFGF) resulted in 90% of germ-like cells expressing meiotic markers (West et al. 2008), and SSEA1+ cells showed partial imprint erasure and histone modifications consistent with PGC development (Tilgner et al. 2008).

Subtle alterations in the culture protocol, such as cell density and media change regime, resulted in differentiated cultures containing both germ cell-like and Sertoli-like cells (Bucay et al. 2009). While differentiation protocols based on BMP4-induced differentiation of hESC demonstrated an important role for genes such as Dazl, Daz and Boule, characterization of the resulting cells was incomplete (Kee et al. 2009).

More recently, the strategy followed by Hayashi and colleagues for differentiation of mESC to PGCLC has been reproduced with partial success in human pluripotent cells (Hayashi et al. 2011, Hayashi et al. 2012). The hESC were engineered to express a fluorescent reporter driven by the promoter of Nanos (a PGC specific marker) and differentiated towards a naïve pluripotent state (Gafni et al. 2013). When

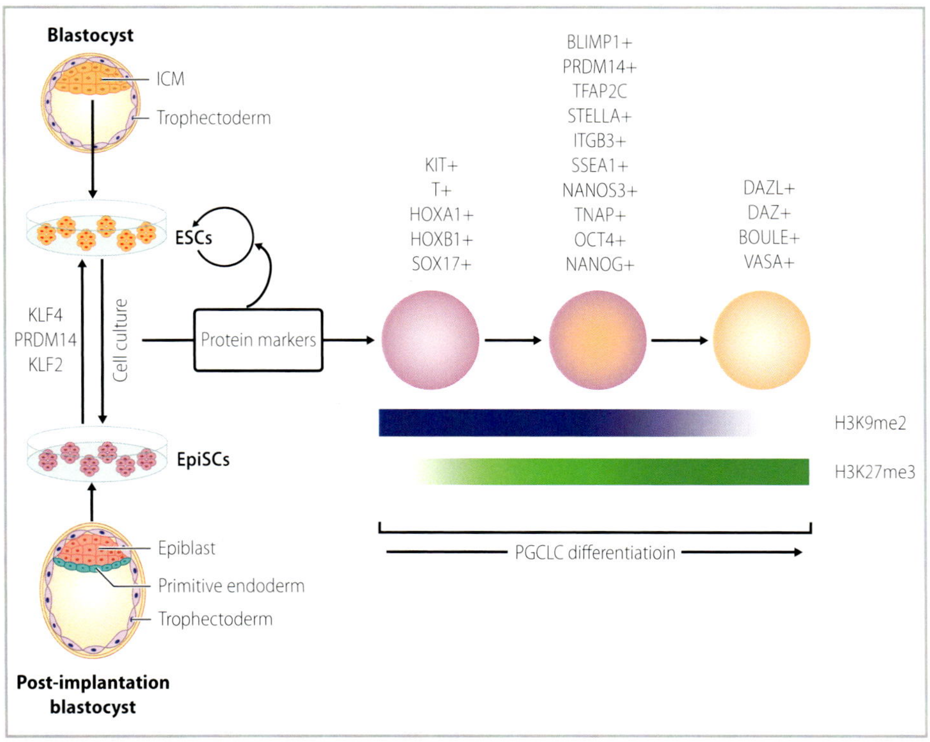

Figure 17.2 Mechanisms established in mice extrapolated to human primordial germ cell (PGC) specification. The more recent strategy for differentiation of human embryonic stem cells (hESC) into PGCLCs (PGC-like cells) is shown. Two types of ESC lines can be established: naïve embryonic stem cells (ESCs) derived from the blastocyst, and epiblast stem cells (EpiSCs) from the post-implantation epiblast. Naïve ESCs can be converted into EpiScs by cell culture and, conversely, EpiSCs can revert to the naïve pluripotent state by forced expression of transcription factors (Klf4 or Prdm14 and Klf2). Exposure of ESC to BMP4 favors self-renewal and the PGC competence originates in an intermediate cell type between ESC and EpiSCs. hESC differentiate while undergoing BMP4 signaling, and produce more protein markers as they do so. The resulting cells were shown to express key PGC marker genes (see **Table 17.2** for glossary of protein markers).

this reporter hESC line was differentiated while undergoing BMP4 signaling, up to 27% of cells upregulated the reporter. The resulting cells where shown to express key PGC marker genes such as Nanos3, Blimp1, Tfap2c, Stella, Tnap, Kit, Oct4 and Nanog, as well as Prdm14, and upon further differentiation, also late markers of PGCs such as Dazl and Vasa. In addition, Sox17 was shown to be an important, human specific, driver of PGC specification acting upstream of Blimp1 (Irie et al. 2014).

This recent breakthrough provides a robust paradigm for further characterization of the PGC differentiation pathway in humans.

CONCLUSION

Specification and differentiation of pluripotent cells to become oocytes is a complex process involving both genetic and epigenetic events. Intense effort has been devoted to studying this process in vivo and developing in vitro protocols to reproduce it in the laboratory by numerous research groups worldwide, both in mice and humans. Initial attempts resulted in cell types that were incompletely characterized and not demonstrated to be functional. Studies in the mouse (Hayashi et al. 2012) and in the human (Irie et al. 2014) constituted breakthroughs that have successfully achieved the differentiation of pluripotent cells to PGCLCs.

In the case of the mouse, the PGCLCs have been shown to be functional, although this has required a period of in vivo maturation However, despite their functionality, differences between the in vivo PGCs and PGCLC are evident. The availability of robust in vitro protocols to obtain PGCLC will undoubtedly allow thorough characterization of PGC specification, particularly in the human system where in vivo studies cannot be performed.

In vitro differentiation of mammalian PGCs or PGCLCs to competent metaphase II oocytes that can achieve fertilization and give rise to a viable organism has not yet been achieved in any system. Indeed, validation of PGCLC has only been possible by re-transferring PGCLC into an appropriate in vivo environment, underscoring the complexity of the cues required for completion of the differentiation program. In particular, entry into meiosis and the correct sequence of epigenetic changes during oogenesis seem particularly challenging. While there has been significant progress in our understanding of the initiation of the differentiation process to oocytes, much remains to be learned.

REFERENCES

Arai F, Suda T. Quiescent stem cells in the niche. StemBook. Cambridge (MA), 2008.

Bucay N, Yebra M, Cirulli V, et al. A novel approach for the derivation of putative primordial germ cells and sertoli cells from human embryonic stem cells. Stem Cells 2009; 27: 68–77.

Clark AT, Bodnar MS, Fox M, et al. Spontaneous differentiation of germ cells from human embryonic stem cells in vitro. Hum Mol Genet 2004; 13:727–739.

Damjanov I, Ahrlund-Richter L. Characterization of human embryonic stem cell-derived teratomas. In: Loring JF, Wesselschmidt RL, Schwartz PH, Human Stem Cell Manual: A Laboratory Guide. Cambridge, MA: Academic Press, 2007.

De Felici M. Origin, Migration, and Proliferation of Human Primordial Germ Cells (Oogenesis). Springer-Verlag London 2013:19–37.

Edson MA, Nagaraja AK, Matzuk MM. The mammalian ovary from genesis to revelation. Endocr Rev 2009; 30:624–712.

Gafni O, Weinberger L, Mansour AA, et al. Derivation of novel human ground state naive pluripotent stem cells. Nature 2013; 504:282–286.

Ge W, Chen C, De Felici M, Shen W. In vitro differentiation of germ cells from stem cells: a comparison between primordial germ cells and in vitro derived primordial germ cell-like cells. Cell Death Dis 2015; 6:e1906.

Hackett JA, Surani MA. Regulatory principles of pluripotency: from the ground state up. Cell Stem Cell 2014; 15:416–430.

Hajkova P, Erhardt S, Lane N, et al. Epigenetic reprogramming in mouse primordial germ cells. Mech Dev 2002; 117:15–23.

Hayashi K, Ogushi S, Kurimoto K, et al. Offspring from oocytes derived from in vitro primordial germ cell-like cells in mice. Science 2012; 338:971–975.

Hayashi K, Ohta H, Kurimoto K, et al. Reconstitution of the mouse germ cell specification pathway in culture by pluripotent stem cells. Cell 2011; 146:519–532.

Hubner K, Fuhrmann G, Christenson LK, et al. Derivation of oocytes from mouse embryonic stem cells. Science 2003; 300:1251–1256.

Irie N, Tang WW, Azim Surani M. Germ cell specification and pluripotency in mammals: a perspective from early embryogenesis. Reprod Med Biol 2014; 13:203–215.

Kagiwada S, Kurimoto K, Hirota T, et al. Replication-coupled passive DNA demethylation for the erasure of genome imprints in mice. EMBO J 2013; 32:340–353.

Kee K, Angeles VT, Flores M, et al. Human DAZL, DAZ and BOULE genes modulate primordial germ-cell and haploid gamete formation. Nature 2009; 462:222–225.

Kee K, Gonsalves JM, Clark AT, Pera RA. Bone morphogenetic proteins induce germ cell differentiation from human embryonic stem cells. Stem Cells Dev 2006; 15:831–837.

Kerkis A, Fonseca SA, Serafim RC, et al. In vitro differentiation of male mouse embryonic stem cells into both presumptive sperm cells and oocytes. Cloning Stem Cells 2007; 9:535–548.

Lacham-Kaplan O, Chy H, Trounson A. Testicular cell conditioned medium supports differentiation of embryonic stem cells into ovarian structures containing oocytes. Stem Cells 2006; 24:266–273.

Lawson KA, Dunn NR, Roelen BA, et al. Bmp4 is required for the generation of primordial germ cells in the mouse embryo. Genes Dev 1999; 13:424–436.

Lo Sicco C, Tasso R, Reverberi D, et al. Identification of a New Cell Population Constitutively Circulating in Healthy Conditions and Endowed with a Homing Ability Toward Injured Sites. Sci Rep 2015; 5:16574.

Nichols J, Smith A. Naive and primed pluripotent states. Cell Stem Cell 2009; 4:487–492.

Novak I, Lightfoot DA, Wang H, et al. Mouse embryonic stem cells form follicle-like ovarian structures but do not progress through meiosis. Stem Cells 2006; 24:1931–1936.

Oh SK, Chua P, Foon KL, et al. Quantitative identification of teratoma tissues formed by human embryonic stem cells with TeratomEye. Biotechnol Lett 2009; 31:653–658.

Qi X, Li TG, Hao J, et al. BMP4 supports self-renewal of embryonic stem cells by inhibiting mitogen-activated protein kinase pathways. Proc Natl Acad Sci USA 2004; 101:6027–6032.

Qing T, Shi Y, Qin H, et al. Induction of oocyte-like cells from mouse embryonic stem cells by co-culture with ovarian granulosa cells. Differentiation 2007; 75:902–911.

Rennert RC, Sorkin M, Garg RK, Gurtner GC. Stem cell recruitment after injury: lessons for regenerative medicine. Regen Med 2012; 7:833–850.

Richter A, Valdimarsdottir L, Hrafnkelsdottir HE, et al. BMP4 promotes EMT and mesodermal commitment in human embryonic stem cells via SLUG and MSX2. Stem Cells 2014; 32:636–648.

Saiti D and Lacham-Kaplan O. Density gradients for the isolation of germ cells from embryoid bodies. Reprod Biomed Online 2008; 16:730–740.

Salvador LM, Silva CP, Kostetskii I, et al. The promoter of the oocyte-specific gene, Gdf9, is active in population of cultured mouse embryonic stem cells with an oocyte-like phenotype. Methods 2008; 45:172–181.

Sato S, Yoshimizu T, Sato E, Matsui Y. Erasure of methylation imprinting of Igf2r during mouse primordial germ-cell development. Mol Reprod Dev 2003; 65:41–50.

Seisenberger S, Andrews S, Krueger F, et al. The dynamics of genome-wide DNA methylation reprogramming in mouse primordial germ cells. Mol Cell 2012; 48:849–862.

Stachelscheid H, Wulf-Goldenberg A, Eckert K, et al. Teratoma formation of human embryonic stem cells in three-dimensional perfusion culture bioreactors. J Tissue Eng Regen Med 2013; 7:729–741.

Tilgner K, Atkinson SP, Golebiewska A, et al. Isolation of primordial germ cells from differentiating human embryonic stem cells. Stem Cells 2008; 26:3075–3085.

Van de Velde H, Cauffman G, Tournaye H, et al. The four blastomeres of a 4-cell stage human embryo are able to develop individually into blastocysts with inner cell mass and trophectoderm. Hum Reprod 2008; 23:1742–1747.

Veiga A, Calderon G, Barri PN, Coroleu B. Pregnancy after the replacement of a frozen-thawed embryo with less than 50% intact blastomeres. Hum Reprod 1987; 2:321–323.

Weinberger L, Ayyash M, Novershtern N, Hanna JH. Dynamic stem cell states: naive to primed pluripotency in rodents and humans. Nat Rev Mol Cell Biol 2016; 17:155–169.

West FD, Machacek DW, Boyd NL, et al. Enrichment and differentiation of human germ-like cells mediated by feeder cells and basic fibroblast growth factor signaling. Stem Cells 2008; 26:2768–2776.

Chapter 18 Mitochondrial DNA disease

Louise Hyslop

INTRODUCTION

A mitochondrion is a cytoplasmic organelle which is bound by its own double membrane. Mitochondria are present in the majority of cells in eukaryotic organisms. They are responsible for generating most of the cell's supply of adenosine triphosphate (ATP), which is the source of chemical energy. The total number of mitochondria within a cell varies widely depending on the cell type. A human oocyte is estimated to contain around 200,000 mitochondria.

The shape of mitochondria is commonly depicted as bean-like (**Figure 18.1**) but mature oocytes contain predominantly spherical to oval mitochondria approximately 0.5–0.8 μm in diameter (see Motta et al. 2000, for review of mitochondrial morphodynamics in human oocytes and embryos). During preimplantation embryo development, the morphology of mitochondria starts to change after the 8-cell stage, with the most dramatic changes occurring at the early blastocyst stage of development (Sathananthan & Trounson 2000). This is in line with the increasing energy demands of the developing blastocyst, as it expands and hatches from the zona pellucida (ZP).

Mitochondria contain their own circular genome. The mitochondrial DNA (mtDNA) contains 37 genes that encode 13 proteins, 22 transfer RNAs and 2 ribosomal RNAs. The mitochondrial gene-encoded proteins are essential for the oxidative phosphorylation (OXPHOS) system that plays a key role in energy production.

The mtDNA is exclusively maternally inherited. Each fertilized oocyte is estimated to contain around 200,000 copies of mtDNA, and mutations can be present in all copies (homoplasmy) or only some of these copies (heteroplasmy). Pathogenic mtDNA mutations can cause a range of debilitating and life-threatening diseases if present above a certain threshold (see **Table 18.1**; DiMauro et al. 2013; Schon et al. 2013). The severity of the disease is often associated with the mutation load which is the ratio of mutated to wild-type mtDNA (Hellebrekers et al. 2012). Women with a heteroplasmic mtDNA mutation produce oocytes with varying mtDNA mutation loads. This is thought to be due to a phenomenon known as the mtDNA 'genetic bottleneck'. As a consequence, the transmission of mtDNA disease from mother to child is unpredictable for women with a heteroplasmic mtDNA mutation.

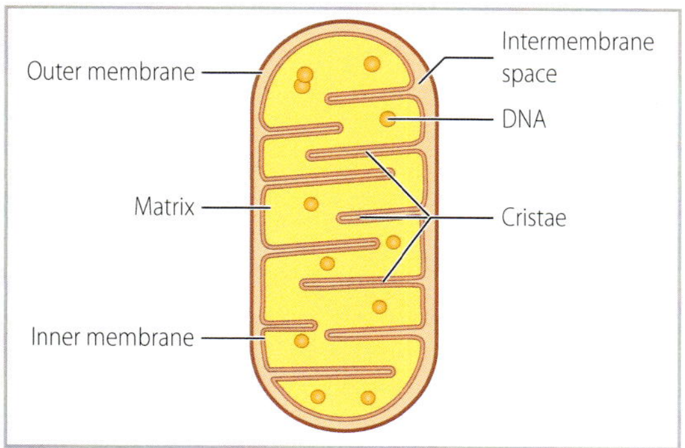

Figure 18.1 A mitochondrion.

HOMOPLASMY AND HETERPLASMY

Homoplasmy describes a cell where all copies of mitochondrial DNA are identical. Thus, a homoplasmic cell has a uniform collection of mtDNA: either every copy of mtDNA is wild-type or mutated. It is less common for patients with mtDNA disease to be homoplasmic for the pathogenic mtDNA mutation.

Heteroplasmy describes a cell with a mixture of wild-type and mutated mtDNA. When a heteroplasmic cell divides the mitochondria are randomly segregated so each daughter cell may receive different proportions of mutated mtDNA. The proportion of mutated mtDNA will determine the onset of clinical symptoms. The threshold level of mutated mtDNA for clinical symptoms varies for each mutation. An increasing proportion of mutated mtDNA is often associated with increasing severity of disease.

CURRENT OPTIONS

In most countries, current options for reducing or avoiding transmission of mtDNA disease are :

- genetic testing to determine whether the fetus is affected, with the option of termination,
- oocyte donation.

In a few countries, a recently developed method is becoming available: mitochondrial donation. This is sometimes referred to as having a 'three-parent baby' because the child has DNA from three people: the full mitochondrial genome from a donor, and the full set of 23 chromosomes from the mother and another set of 23 from the father.

Prenatal genetic diagnosis

Chorionic villus sampling (CVS) and amniocentesis are procedures in which cells originating from the developing fetus are sent for screening to determine the mutation load. Concern has been raised that the mutation load in the cells sampled does not reflect the mutation load in other fetal tissues. However, current evidence suggests this is not the case and prenatal testing remains an important option for couples (Nesbitt et al. 2014). CVS is performed at 10–12 weeks, whereas amniocentesis is performed at 14–20 weeks of pregnancy. Both procedures are considered to be safe but there is a small risk of miscarriage associated with each technique.

Noninvasive prenatal testing (NIPT) is an alternative method to prenatal genetic diagnosis which involves sampling the mother's blood (see Chapter 16). However, it should be noted that NIPT is not classed as a diagnostic test like CVS or amniocentesis, but rather it provides reassurance about the genetic health of the fetus. NIPT works by analyzing the DNA fragments, known as cell-free DNA, which is present in the maternal plasma during pregnancy. Most of the cell-free DNA comes from the mother (cell-free maternal DNA), but it is estimated that up to 15% of it comes from the unborn baby (cell-free fetal DNA). NIPT can be used to assess the sequences of DNA that are specific to a particular chromosome. Therefore, by analyzing and counting all the DNA sequences that link or map to each individual chromosome,

Table 18.1 Diseases caused by mutation of mitochondrial DNA. Each disease is summarized with the associated signs and symptoms

Disease	Mutation cause and description	Main signs and symptoms
Leber's hereditary optic neuropathy (LHON)	The majority of cases are caused by a mtDNA point mutation at positions 11778G>A, 3460G>A and 14484T>C respectively in the MT-ND4, MT-ND1 and MT-ND6 genes	Optic neuropathy
Leigh syndrome	Leigh syndrome can be caused by mtDNA or nuclear DNA mutations. mtDNA mutations cause between 20-25% of Leigh syndrome cases	Progressive neurodegenerative condition
Neuropathy, ataxia and retinitis pigmentosa (NARP)	Typically caused by mtDNA point mutation at position 8993T>G	Sensory neuropathy and ataxia beginning in childhood or early adulthood
Myoclonic epilepsy with ragged-red fibers (MERRF)	The majority of patients have a mtDNA point mutation at position 8344A>G	Myoclonic epilepsy and myopathy. Additional features can include dementia, peripheral neuropathy and bilateral deafness
Mitochondrial encephalomyopathy, lactic acidosis, stroke-like symptoms (MELAS)	Over 80% of patients have a mtDNA point mutation at position 3243A>G	Stroke-like episodes beginning before the age of 40. Additional features can include diabetes, lactic acidosis, bilateral deafness and cardiomyopathy
Kearns–Sayre syndrome (KSS)	Single, large scale mtDNA deletion	Retinitis pigmentosa and ophthalmoplegia Additional features can include bilateral deafness and diabetes
Chronic progressive external ophthalmoplegia (CPEO)	Single, large scale mtDNA deletion	Ophthalmoplegia, ptosis and myopathy
Pearson syndrome	Typically caused by single, large scale mtDNA deletions	Sideroblastic anemia and pancreatic dysfunction early in life Condition is often fatal in infancy

chromosomal conditions such as Down syndrome can be detected. However, NIPT cannot be used to assess mitochondrial mutations.

Preimplantation genetic diagnosis

Preimplantation genetic diagnosis (PGD) tests for genetic conditions within an embryo if the gene that causes the condition is known (see Chapter 15). PGD involves removal of one or two cells from cleavage stage embryos on day 3 of development (see Figure 15.8), or up to approximately four to six trophectoderm cells from blastocysts on day 5 or 6 of development (see Figure 15.9). These cells are sent for screening to determine which (if any) embryos are unaffected by the genetic condition.

PGD is currently offered to women who carry mtDNA mutations, to reduce the risk of transmitting mtDNA disease to the offspring. PGD is used to determine the mutation load of embryos, but this is only an effective option if there are also embryos produced with low mutation loads. Current evidence from a range of pathogenic mutations indicates the probability of developing mtDNA disease is low when the mutation load is <18% (Hellebrekers et al. 2012).

Oocyte donation

Currently, for women with homoplasmic mutation or high levels of mutated mtDNA, the only option to ensure the child is unaffected is by using donated oocytes.

MITOCHONDRIAL DONATION

An alternative strategy has been developed for women who consistently produce embryos with mutation levels above the threshold for mtDNA disease. This approach has focused on uncoupling the inheritance of nuclear and mtDNA by transplanting the nuclear DNA from either an oocyte or fertilized oocyte of an affected woman to that of an unaffected donor.

It should be noted that it is inevitable that some mitochondria will be carried over with the nuclear DNA. However, this approach would enable women with homoplasmic mutation or high levels of mutated mtDNA to have a genetically related child with a greatly reduced risk of transmitting mtDNA disease (Smeets et al. 2015).

Spindle transfer

Transplantation of the nuclear genome can be performed before the oocyte is fertilized (**Figure 18.2**). The most promising strategy is to perform the transfer when the oocytes are arrested at metaphase stage of the second meiotic division, i.e. the metaphase II (MII) stage. At this stage, the chromosomes are aligned on the MII spindle (**Figure 18.2**).

The chromosomes are not enclosed within a nuclear membrane, so conventional microscopy cannot be used to observe the transfer of the MII spindle. Therefore, advanced optics containing liquid crystal birefringence are used to enable spindle visualization. Such birefringence optics are well established in other micromanipulation technologies, such as cloning.

MII spindle transfer has been performed between rhesus macaque oocytes. The transfer of the resulting embryos resulted in the birth of healthy monkeys with undetectable mtDNA carryover (Tachibana et al. 2009).

Low level mtDNA carryover has also been achieved following MII spindle transfer between human oocytes (Paull et al. 2013, Tachibana et al. 2013). Whilst the fertilization rate of the resulting MII spindle transfer oocytes was similar to that of control oocytes (73% versus 75%), there was a high incidence of abnormal fertilization with 25% of fertilized MII spindle transfer oocytes containing three pronuclei (PN) with a single polar body (Tachibana et al. 2013). As far as we are aware, no data has yet been presented on blastocyst morphology and quality to provide an indication of efficacy.

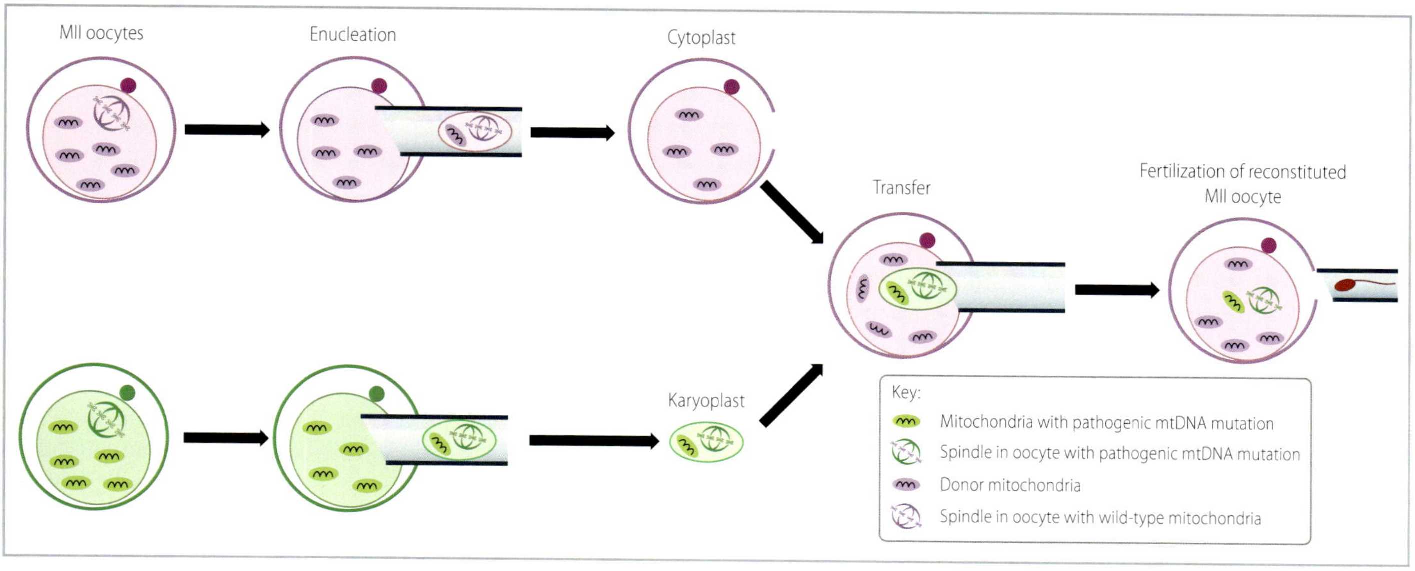

Figure 18.2 Maternal spindle transfers. The mother's cells have mitochondria with a pathogenic mitochondrial DNA mutation (green). The spindle is removed from the affected oocyte (green) to become the karyoplast. The spindle from the mitochondrial donor's oocyte (purple) is removed so that this oocyte, which has wild-type mitochondria (purple), has no spindle and is known as a cytoplast. The karyoplast and cytoplast are then combined, so that the reconstituted metaphase II oocyte can now be fertilized.

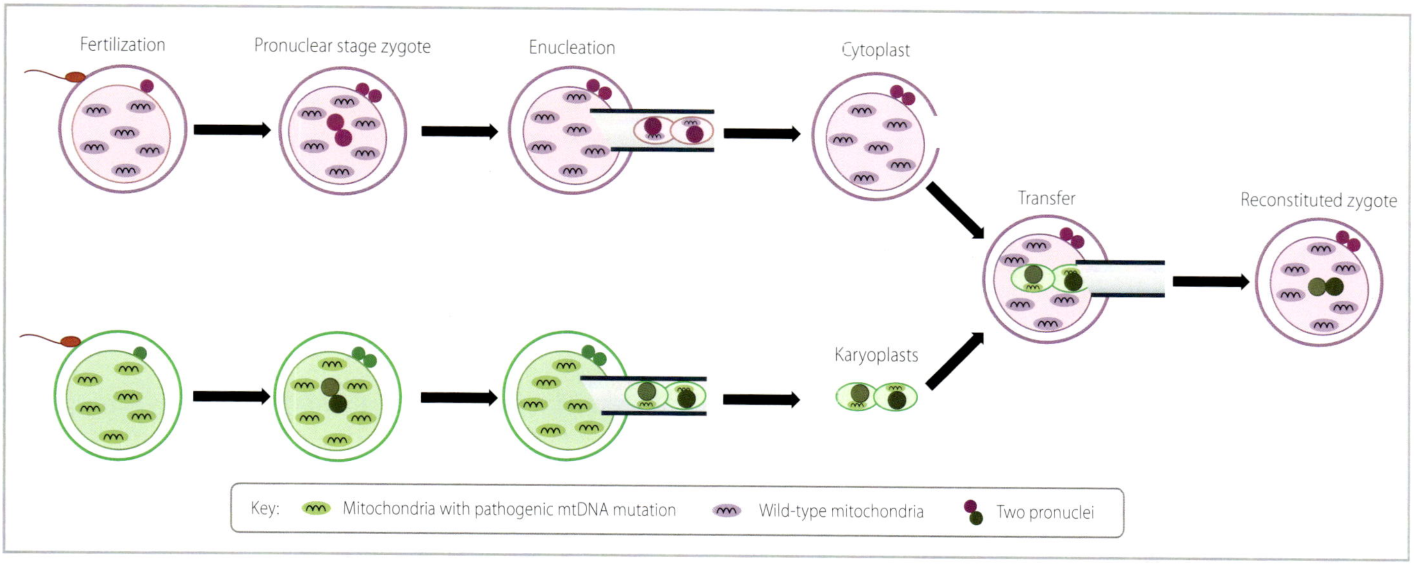

Figure 18.3 Pronuclear transfer. Green represents mitochondria with a pathogenic mitochondrial DNA mutation whereas purple represents wild type mitochondria. Both the affected oocyte (the mother's) and the unaffected oocyte (the mitochondrial donor's) are independently fertilized, and monitored for the appearance of two pronuclei (2PN). The 2PN are removed from the affected oocyte (green) to become the karyoplast. The 2PN from the recipient zygote (purple) are removed so that the recipient oocyte has no PN and is known as a cytoplast. The karyoplast and cytoplast are then combined, so that the reconstituted 2PN zygote can now undergo syngamy and develop into a healthy embryo.

Pronuclear transfer

Transplantation of the nuclear genome can be performed provided the oocyte has fertilized and the PN are visible (**Figure 18.3**). The technique of PN transfer (PNT) requires the use of reversible microtubule and actin depolymerizing drugs to facilitate PN removal without the need to penetrate the plasma membrane with the removal pipette. The PN are then 'pinched-off' with a minimal amount cytoplasm to form a membrane-enclosed karyoplast (**Figure 18.4**).

Fusion of the karyoplast with an enucleated zygote (cytoplast) is facilitated by the use of 'hemagglutinating virus of Japan envelope (HVJ-E). Electrical fusion is not well tolerated by human zygotes, whereas HVJ-E fuses the karyoplast and enucleated zygote membranes with high efficiency (Craven et al. 2010).

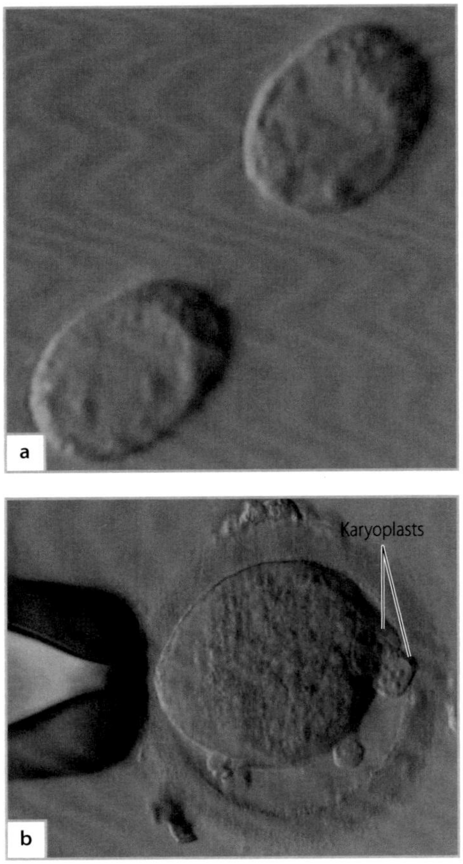

Figure 18.4 Reconstitution of the human zygote. (a) Two karyoplasts with minimal cytoplasm around each pronucleus. (b) Cytoplast with two karyoplasts immediately after transfer.

HEMAGGLUTINATING VIRUS OF JAPAN (HVJ)

The HVJ is a single-stranded RNA virus and a member of genus *Respirovirus*, which mainly infects mammals. HVJ is also called the *Sendai* virus.

The HVJ envelope (HVJ-E) is a nonproliferative and noninfectious vesicle purified after complete inactivation of HVJ. HVJ-E is therefore called the inactivated Sendai virus. The HVJ-E has a high membrane-fusing potential comparable to that of live virus, and is therefore utilized in embryology to assist the fusion of biopsied pronuclei into enucleated zygotes.

In the early 1980s, PNT between mouse zygotes resulted in the birth of live offspring (McGrath and Solter 1983). More recently, PNT was performed with zygotes of transmitochondrial mice (mito-mice) that were heteroplasmic for wild-type and pathogenically deleted mtDNA (Sato et al. 2005). The PN from mito-mouse zygotes were fused with enucleated normal zygotes, and the resulting offspring did not express the respiration defects throughout their lives, indicating the technique was successful in preventing the mitochondrial disease. Detailed carryover analysis has been performed on offspring following PNT between mouse zygotes of different mouse strains with sequence differences in mtDNA (Meirelles and Smith 1997). These studies revealed a high average mtDNA carryover of 24% in the pups but this could reflect the large size of the PN.

Proof of concept experiments with abnormally fertilized human oocytes have demonstrated that the transplantation of the nuclear DNA was technically feasible and compatible with onward embryo development (Craven et al. 2010). Following modifications to the technique, the average mitochondrial carryover reported was <2%. Preclinical studies have been conducted to optimize the technique with normally fertilized human oocytes and investigate the likely safety and efficacy (Hyslop et al. 2016).

Surprisingly, the technique used for abnormally fertilized human zygotes was not well tolerated by normally fertilized zygotes, so an alternative approach was developed. The PN were transferred shortly after their appearance rather than just prior to syngamy. This simple modification improved the survival and blastocyst development rate of PNT zygotes. Blastocyst quality was improved by switching to Ca^{2+} and Mg^{2+} free manipulation medium and reducing the HVJ-E concentration.

Following introduction of all four further modifications to minimise carryover of mitochondria (see Box), analysis of control and PNT blastocysts revealed the optimized PNT procedure had no detectable effect on gene expression and the incidence of aneuploidy. Evaluation of carryover revealed that PNT has the potential to reduce the risk of mtDNA disease but further modifications may be required to eradicate the disease in all cases.

Procedure

Synchronization of the patient and donor cycles can be challenging, so oocyte vitrification is a useful option to consider. During preclinical studies, it was shown that the mitochondrial carryover was lower if the cytoplast originated from fresh rather than vitrified oocytes. Vitrification of the patient's oocytes, rather than donor oocytes, may minimize mtDNA carryover and has the additional benefit of stockpiling patient's oocytes before they become susceptible to maternal age-related aneuploidy.

MINIMIZING MITOCHONDRIA CARRYOVER DURING PN TRANSFER

Four modifications to minimize carryover of mitochondria during pronuclei (PN) transfer:

- Removal of the PN separately rather than together in a single karyoplast.
  It is difficult to minimize the amount of cytoplasm between the PN when removed together
- Sucrose was used to shrink the zygotes prior to the procedure to facilitate enucleation and fusion.
  However, the mtDNA carryover was higher when the procedure was performed with sucrose. Exclusion of sucrose reduced the carryover and had a minimal effect on survival
- Shearing of excess cytoplasm between the pipette and zona pellucida (ZP).
  If a karyoplast contains excess cytoplasm it should be aspirated into the pipette by the excess cytoplasm before aspiration of the PN. Once the PN has been expelled during the transfer, the excess cytoplasm can be sheared away between the pipette tip and ZP
- For the preclinical studies, the transfers were performed between normally fertilized zygotes from fresh and vitrified/warmed oocytes.
  The carryover was lower if the cytoplast originated from fresh rather than vitrified oocytes

The PNT procedure is performed shortly after PN appearance. Intracytoplasmic sperm injection (ICSI) is performed to synchronize the PN appearance in a narrower time frame and allow transfer between zygotes at a similar stage.

Removal of the PN then takes place via the following steps:

1. The zygotes are placed in a medium containing reversible microtubule and actin depolymerizing drugs. Nocodazole reversibly interferes with the polymerisation of microtubules by binding to tubulin. Drugs like cytochalasin B and latrunculin A inhibit new actin polymerization but have different mechanisms of action
2. The zygote is immobilized by gentle suction with a holding pipette. To minimize carryover, it is critical that the zygote is positioned with both PN in the same plane of focus. In addition, the polar bodies should be distant from the location of biopsy pipette insertion
3. A breach is created in the zona pellucida (ZP) using a laser to facilitate insertion of the biopsy pipette
4. The biopsy pipette is inserted and positioned with minimal cytoplasm between the PN and the opening of the pipette
5. The PN is gently aspirated into the pipette and the biopsy pipette slowly removed to facilitate separation
6. The karyoplast is expelled from the biopsy pipette before the removal of the second PN

Procedure troubleshooting

Karyoplast lysis

The karyoplasts can be prone to lysis so minimal manipulation is recommended, particularly after exposure to HVJ-E. Karyoplasts must not be completely expelled into the HVJ-E drop but stopped as soon as the leading karyoplast reaches the opening of the biopsy pipette. The small amount of HVJ-E taken up into the pipette is sufficient for efficient fusion of both karyoplasts with the cytoplast.

The procedure for fusion of the cytoplast with the karyoplasts is:

1. The karyoplasts are transferred in the biopsy pipette to the hemagglutinating virus of Japan envelope (HVJ-E) solution. It is important that the karyoplasts are not expelled into the HVJ-E and only a small amount of HVJ-E is aspirated into the pipette
2. The cytoplast is immobilized by the holding pipette with the hole in the zona pellucida (ZP) positioned to allow easy insertion of the biopsy pipette containing the karyoplasts
3. The karyoplasts are slowly expelled beneath the ZP. Any excess cytoplasm in the karyoplast can be sheared between the ZP and tip of the biopsy pipette
4. The reconstituted zygote is washed with culture medium before overnight culture

Cytoplast lysis

If the removal of the karyoplast is performed too quickly the cytoplast may lyse.

Karyoplast(s) don't remain inside the ZP after transfer

It is important to ensure both karyoplasts are not deposited just beneath the breach in the ZP. When transferring the reconstituted zygote to a new dish for onward culture, it is important to ensure a large embryo handling pipette is used to reduce the risk of the karyoplasts getting pushed out of the breach in the ZP.

Training

New operators should be familiar with the micromanipulation equipment and experienced in oocyte and embryo manipulation. During training in the procedure, the trainee should perform technical controls in which the PN are removed and replaced in the same zygote (autologous transfer). Technical competence can then be assessed by comparing blastocyst development following autologous transfer to unmanipulated controls. Blastocyst formation and quality of the technical controls should not differ from unmanipulated controls. In addition, it is critical that competence in minimizing carryover is assessed.

In the UK, only embryologists who have been assessed as competent by the Human Fertilization and Embryology Authority (HFEA) and subsequently named on the clinic's HFEA licence are allowed to perform maternal spindle transfer or PNT. The application for competency assessment should contain the evidence of the embryologists experience in the techniques and include the embryo survival rate, blastocyst development and rate of mtDNA carryover. Quantitative pyrosequencing is used to measure mtDNA carryover; embryo biopsy would then be required and the cells sent for analysis by an accredited mitochondrial diagnostic laboratory.

Regulation

In 2015, the legislation was put in place to make the UK the first country in the world to allow the use of mitochondrial donation (Craven et al. 2016). Alongside this, the HFEA have developed a licensing framework specifically for mitochondrial donation.

Firstly, a licence variation application must be submitted, so that the HFEA's Licence Committee can then assess:

- Suitability of the clinics processes and equipment
- Competence of the embryologist(s) in performing the technique(s)
- Documented process for follow-up of children born as a result of the treatment where patients have consented
- Patient and donor information

If the application is successful, a variation will be made on the clinic's HFEA licence and the second stage of the application process can begin. A patient-specific application must be submitted by the clinic to the HFEA when mitochondrial donation is assessed as a suitable treatment. The regulations only permit the use of mitochondrial donation for the avoidance of serious mitochondrial disease. The HFEA's Statutory Approvals Committee will assess the evidence that without mitochondrial donation there would be a significant risk that a child will have or develop serious mitochondrial disease.

It is anticipated that other countries are likely to follow suit, but in 2015 the UK was the only country to have approved regulations. The US Food and Drug Administration (FDA) reported they would be reviewing recommendations made by a committee convened by the National Academy of Science, Engineering and Medicine but at time of press was on hold due to the latest federal budget preventing funds to be spent on evaluating applications for mitochondrial donation research and clinical application.

SUMMARY

Preclinical studies indicate that PNT will reduce the risk of transmitting mtDNA disease; however, at this time there is no guarantee that it will eliminate the risk. Further refinement of the procedure is required to ensure the carryover of mutated mitochondria is consistently minimal.

REFERENCES

Craven L, Tuppen HA, Greggains GD, et al. Pronuclear transfer in human embryos to prevent transmission of mitochondrial DNA disease. Nature 2010; 465:82–85.

Craven L, Herbert M, Murdoch A, et al. Research into Policy: A Brief History of Mitochondrial Donation. Stem Cells 2016; 34:265–267.

DiMauro S, Schon EA, Carelli V, et al. The clinical maze of mitochondrial neurology. Nat Rev Neurol 2013; 9:429–444.

Hellebrekers DM, Wolfe R, Hendrickx AT, et al. PGD and heteroplasmic mitochondrial DNA point mutations: A systematic review estimating the chance of healthy offspring. Hum Reprod Update 2012; 18:341–349.

Hyslop LA, Blakeley P, Craven L, et al. Towards clinical application of pronuclear transfer to prevent mitochondrial DNA disease. Nature 2016; 534:383–386.

McGrath J, Solter D. Nuclear transplantation in the mouse embryo by microsurgery and cell fusion. Science 1983; 220:1300–1302.

Meirelles FV, Smith LC. Mitochondrial genotype segregation in a mouse heteroplasmic lineage produced by embryonic karyoplast transplantation. Genetics 1997; 145:445–451.

Motta PM, Nottola SA, Makabe S, Heyn R. Mitochondrial morphology in human fetal and adult female germ cells. Hum Reprod 2000; 15:129–147.

Nesbitt V, Alston CL, Blakely EL, et al. A national perspective on prenatal testing for mitochondrial disease. Eur J Hum Genet 2014; 22:1255–1259.

Paull D, Emmanuele V, Weiss KA, et al. Nuclear genome transfer in human oocytes eliminates mitochondrial DNA variants. Nature 2013; 493:632–637.

Sathananthan AH, Trounson AO. Mitochondrial morphology during preimplantation human embryogenesis. Hum Reprod 2000; 15:148–159.

Sato A, Kono T, Nakada K, et al. Gene therapy for progeny of mito-mice carrying pathogenic mtDNA by nuclear transplantation. Proc Natl Acad Sci USA 2005; 102:16765–16770.

Schon EA, DiMauro S, Hirano M. Human mitochondrial DNA: Roles of inherited and somatic mutations. Nat Rev Genet 2013; 13:878–890.

Smeets HJ, Sallevelt SC, Dreesen JC, de Die-Smulders CE, de Coo IF. Preventing the transmission of mitochondrial DNA disorders using prenatal or preimplantation genetic diagnosis. Ann NY Acad Sci 2015; 1350:29–36.

Tachibana M, Sparman M, Sritanaudomchai H, et al. Mitochondrial gene replacement in primate offspring and embryonic stem cells. Nature 2009; 461:367–372.

Tachibana M, Amato P, Sparman M, et al. Towards germline gene therapy of inherited mitochondrial diseases. Nature 2013; 493:627–631.

Chapter 19 Uterine transplantation

Benjamin P Jones, Srdjan Saso, J Richard Smith

INTRODUCTION

Uterine transplantation (also called UTx) is a potential therapeutic modality for women with absolute uterine factor infertility (AUFI), a condition that affects 1 in 500 women of childbearing age (Hellström et al. 2014). AUFI refers to women with infertility secondary to either the absence of a uterus or the presence of an anatomically or physiologically nonfunctioning uterus, the causes of which can be congenital or acquired (**Figure 19.1**).

The current options for women with AUFI to become mothers include adoption or surrogacy. Not only are these options associated with complex legal, financial, cultural, ethical and religious factors, but a woman's inability to conceive, carry pregnancy and ultimately bear children negatively affects the perception of her own femininity and quality of life (Laggari et al. 2009).

More than a third of women with infertility suffer severe symptoms of depression and have a 2-fold increased risk of suicide (Kjaer et al. 2011). See Chapter 13 for an in-depth description of the role of counseling for infertile couples.

Uterine transplantation gives women with AUFI the opportunity to conceive and carry pregnancy, and may also improve their psychological well-being.

CONDITIONS WHICH BENEFIT FROM UTERINE TRANSPLANTATION

Mayer–Rokitansky–Küster–Hauser syndrome

The most common form of congenital AUFI is linked to women with Mayer–Rokitansky–Küster–Hauser syndrome (MRKH), otherwise known as uterine agenesis. This accounts for approximately 75% of the women in the UK requesting UTx.

MRKH has an approximate incidence of 1 in 5000 (Folch et al. 2000). The syndrome arises due to failure of the Müllerian ducts to develop, resulting in an absence of the uterus and fallopian tubes, with a varying degree of vaginal shortening. Women with MRKH are genotypically and phenotypically female, with normally functioning ovaries and a normal hormone profile.

Inheritance is mostly sporadic, although familial cases have been reported. There have been no reported inherited cases where women with MRKH have commissioned surrogates using their own oocytes.

There are two subtypes that are typically considered in MRKH. Type 1, or typical MRKH, incorporates isolated uterovaginal aplasia or hypoplasia; whilst type 2, or atypical MRKH, additionally has associated renal, ovarian, skeletal or hearing abnormalities.

In developed societies, women with MRKH are generally diagnosed at a young age, which understandably can create psychological implications relating to body image, psychosexual development, identity and femininity.

The treatment of MRKH should be holistic, including appropriate psychological counseling , and either dilator therapy or surgical intervention in women whose vaginal length is suboptimal.

Hysterectomy

The most common cause of AUFI is hysterectomy, although conversely such women only constitute approximately 20% of the women requesting UTx in the UK. Most women undergo a hysterectomy to treat gynecological cancer. Less commonly, hysterectomies take place due to postpartum hemorrhage or benign gynecological disease.

From an oncological perspective, more than 1000 women with cervical cancer, 500 with ovarian cancer and 120 with endometrial cancer present in the UK annually under the age of 45 years (Farthing. 2006). With this in mind, there is increasing consideration for fertility preserving therapeutic modalities in individually selected cases, where ongoing fertility is desired and this is considered oncologically safe.

Early stage cervical cancer can be safely managed by radical abdominal or vaginal trachelectomy; endometrial cancer can be managed with progestogens; borderline ovarian tumors can be managed with ovarian cystectomy; and placental site trophoblastic tumors can be managed using the modified Strassman procedure. When considering cervical cancer, Sonoda et al. (2004) found that 48% of patients under the age of 40 years, who underwent radical surgery for early-stage cervical cancer, were suitable for fertility preserving treatment, highlighting the potential number of cases that could be considered, should fertility still be desired.

MODIFIED STRASSMAN PROCEDURE

The modified Strassman procedure is a surgical procedure to unify a bicornuate uterus or a didelphys uterus in order to provide reproductive capability. Metroplastic surgery was described by Strassman in 1952 for class III, IV and V anomalies, and it was subsequently modified and simplified by Jones in 1953 (wedge excision of the septum) and Tompkins in 1962 (incision of the septum).

With respect to benign gynecological disease, hysterectomy is predominantly performed in women of reproductive age for severe, refractory chronic pelvic pain. Pain is reported as the primary reason for hysterectomy in 10–40% of cases (Mowers et al. 2016). However, following hysterectomy for chronic pain, 20–40% of women experience persistent pain postoperatively. Therefore, it is vital that hysterectomy should only be considered as a last resort, as part of multidisciplinary management with pain specialist input, once all conservative options have been exhausted.

From an obstetric perspective, hysterectomy is only performed as last-line, life-saving management of uncontrolled, severe hemorrhage. Risk factors associated with cesarean hysterectomy include cesarean section, multiparity, uterine atony and placental adherence. Given that the rate of cesarean section continues to steadily increase globally, it is predicted that the rate of cesarean hysterectomy will increase in a similar fashion, from the present rate of approximately 1 in 2000 deliveries.

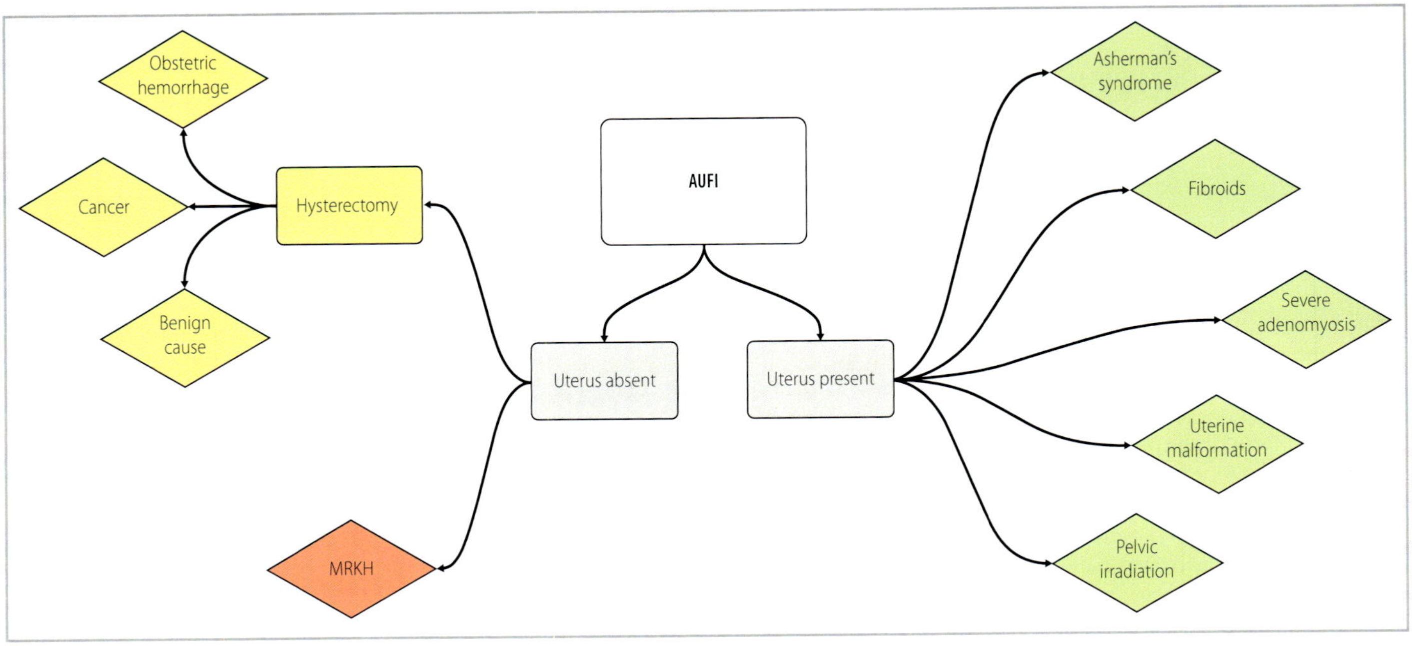

Figure 19.1 Causes of absolute uterine factor infertility (AUFI).

Asherman's syndrome

The main cause of AUFI where the uterus is present, but not functional, is Asherman's syndrome. This syndrome relates to intrauterine synechia, and is an acquired uterine condition, characterized by the formation of adhesions (scar tissue) inside the uterus and/or the cervix. This often causes the front and back walls of the uterus stick to one another. In such cases, the intrauterine adhesions cause amenorrhea , recurrent miscarriage and infertility. Whilst the pathophysiology remains poorly understood, it most commonly arises as a consequence to endometrial curettage following miscarriage or postpartum and less frequently after myomectomy, cesarean section or pelvic infection. Pregnancy-related dilation and curettage have been shown to account for 90% of Asherman's syndrome cases (Schenker and Margalioth 1982).

Fertility restoration can sometimes be achieved using hysteroscopic adhesiolysis. However, infertility rates can be as high as 50%., and in those patients who do become pregnant, up to 40% miscarry. In some severe cases, where hematometra results in severe cyclical pain and retrograde menstruation, hysterectomy is performed for symptomatic relief.

HISTORY

Organ transplantation is a medical procedure whereby an organ is removed from one body and placed in the body of a recipient, to replace a damaged or missing organ. Transplants that are performed between two different people are called allografts. Allografts can either be from a living or cadaveric source.

Organ transplantation has traditionally been reserved for life-saving operations where no other treatment option is available. Transplantation surgery has transitioned in recent years to include quality of life improving procedures, including face, hand, intestine and cornea transplantation.

Whilst the concept of UTx was considered in the 1960s as a therapeutic option for women with uterotubal factor infertility, the advent and subsequent success of IVF treatment halted progression. It wasn't until the late 1990s, during the development of the radical abdominal trachelectomy, when the possibility of UTx was re-evaluated, once it was realized the uterus remained viable if it was supplied by just two of its six vessels (Smith et al. 1997).

Following this, a series of interlinked animal studies were undertaken to assess vital surgical, immunological and fertility aspects of UTx. At the time of writing 14 UTx cases have been performed in humans. A number of important lessons can be taken from these studies and provide a framework for future cases.

Lessons from animal models

Surgical considerations

Determining the optimal surgical technique, with particular consideration given to the vascular anastomosis, is important. The first study reporting UTx was by Zhordania and Gotsiridze (1963) utilizing both small and large animals including 20 dogs, 10 rabbits and 18 ewes. Autotransplantation procedures were undertaken using a graft containing the uterus, fallopian tubes and ovaries. The graft was subsequently placed within the omentum for revascularization , introducing the concept of an omentopexy. The results were surprisingly impressive with no reported complications and a 62.5% spontaneous pregnancy rate in the ewes, all of which underwent vaginal deliveries.

Subsequent UTx studies using the omentopexy technique, predominantly in canine models, were not as effective. This therefore led to consideration of other methods of revascularization .

Due to the small size of the uterine vessels in small animal models such as rabbits and rats, a large vessel patch incorporating the aorta and vena cava vessels was used. Whilst this method proved successful in a variety of models including dog, rat, rabbit and mouse, it was not a method that could be extrapolated to the human model.

Studies in larger animals ensued, which allowed a microvascular vessel anastomosis, using the uterine vessels, to be attempted in the porcine model (Sieunarine et al. 2005). A supracervical hysterectomy was performed on eight sows of proven fertility. After 1 hour of cold storage in a transplant solution, the graft was reintroduced, using a uterine vessel anastomosis. Postoperatively, one sow survived to 3 months with no signs of estrus, whilst three sows were killed on days 6, 33, and 54, respectively, due to pelvic infection. Histopathology of the uterine grafts revealed gradual vessel thromboses. This was suggestive that a microvascular anastomosis is unlikely to be successful and that a larger vessel patch would be necessary.

Subsequently a macrovascular patch, utilizing an internal iliac to external iliac anastomosis, was trialed in larger animals including sheep, pigs and primates with established viability postoperatively (Saso et al. 2014). This established a viable, and importantly achievable anastomosis, in an animal model that largely resembles the human pelvis, clarifying an essential aspect of the UTx procedure.

Immunological considerations

The immune response of a host toward a uterine graft can be just as deleterious as the host response toward other transplanted organs. Rejection can be defined as destruction of the donor graft by the host's immune response, activated against the graft's alloantigens because of a difference in the genetic make-up of the two individuals.

Tremendous advances have been made in the field of solid-organ transplantation, which has led to increased survival in patients with pathologies that had previously been considered terminal. A key discovery was the introduction of the calcineurin inhibitors, cyclosporin A (CsA) and tacrolimus, in the 1980s. These immunosuppressive drugs agents exert their action by blocking the phosphatase activity of calcineurin, which leads to inhibition of lymphocytic interleukin-2 production.

It is key in organ transplantation, particularly in quality of life improving transplant, that the 'burden' of immunosuppressive medications is offset by overall improvement in quality of life. To achieve this, the minimum number of agents should be used at the smallest dose possible, to achieve the immunosuppressive effect whilst avoiding use of steroids where possible.

The first UTx study to be published after the implementation of CsA was by Confino and colleagues (1986) using a rabbit model. Ten allogeneic transplants were performed, six of which were treated with CsA, whilst four were not given any immunosuppression. Those rabbits without immunosuppression all revealed rejection, supporting the hypothesis that a uterine graft behaves in a similar manner to the kidney, liver and cardiac grafts. In the six rabbits that were given CsA, four survived for only 1 month, of which 75% of these developed pelvic abscesses. This highlighted the risk of infection with the use of immunosuppressive agents. Other complications that can occur as a consequence to long-term immunosuppression include hypertension, diabetes, anemia and oncological change.

A unique advantage of UTx over other transplants is that once the uterus has served its purpose and the woman's family is complete, the graft can be removed allowing cessation of all immunosuppressive medications, thus negating the risks associated with long term use. Further interlinked studies were subsequently undertaken to characterize the rejection response and demonstrated the effective use of calcineurin inhibitor monotherapy in both small (using tacrolimus in rats) (Diaz-Garcia et al. 2010) and large animals (using CsA in sheep) (Ramirez et al. 2011).

Another key immunological aspect to consider was the ability to detect rejection in the recipient graft. Whilst symptoms of rejection may include abdominal pain or vaginal discharge/bleeding, such symptoms would only become apparent once rejection had been firmly established. Johannesson et al. (2013) demonstrated that early rejection was not detectable on serum markers, but could be accurately determined through the use of cervical biopsies. This method negates the need to take endometrial biopsies and allows the detection of early graft dysfunction and the ability to take action before irreversible damage is caused.

With regard to the effect of immunosuppression on pregnancy, UTx has the luxury of data from over 14000 post-transplantation live births, since the first birth to a transplant recipient occurred in 1963 (Davision and Baylis. 2002). Initial observations on post-transplant pregnancies indicated a higher incidence of preterm deliveries, low birth weights, and maternal hypertension; however, there was no rise in the rate of structural malformations.

It should be noted that this data was taken from transplants performed for life-threatening conditions, not in women who are otherwise healthy, as would be the case in UTx. Thus, it would be unfair to directly extrapolate from these findings. This is reaffirmed by the fact that when pregnancy outcomes are compared before and after organ transplantation, the odds of preeclampsia, fetal growth restriction, preterm birth, and the risk of miscarriage were all statistically similar both pre- and post-transplantation (Kallen et al. 2005).

Lessons from human cases

First human uterine transplantation

The first human UTx procedure took place in 2000, in Saudi Arabia, using a living donor (Fageeh et al. 2002). The recipient was a 20-year-old woman who had previously undergone an emergency hysterectomy to treat postpartum hemorrhage. The donor was a 46-year-old woman with benign multiloculated ovarian cysts.

The graft included the uterus, cervix, fallopian tubes and surrounding ligamentous tissue. The uterine vessels were divided 25 mm from the uterus and extended using 60–80 mm lengths of saphenous vein. The graft was fixed anatomically in the recipient's pelvis, connected laterally to the pelvic side wall and inferiorly the cervix was anastomosed to the recipient's vagina. The extended uterine vessels were anastomosed to the recipient's external iliac vessels. Immunosuppression was provided in the form of cyclosporin, azathioprine and prednisolone.

Postoperatively, ultrasound Doppler (to see how blood flows through the blood vessels), MRI (to provide detailed images of the organs), and serum CD4/CD8+ cell ratios (to check the immune system) were all used to detect rejection. One episode of rejection was noted on the ninth postoperative day and was promptly treated with antithymocytic globulin (ATG) and increased doses of steroid and azathioprine. Combined estrogen and progestogen hormonal therapy was initiated, despite the presence of normally functioning ovaries. The uterus appeared functional by demonstrating endometrial proliferation ultrasonographically and the recipient experienced two withdrawal bleeds following cessation of the hormone therapy.

Unfortunately, 99 days postoperatively the woman developed acute vascular thrombosis, with the uterus appearing dusky colored and prolapsed. She had an emergency hysterectomy. On reflection this case provided hope that UTx may be feasible in the human setting. However, the general consensus was that it was undertaken prematurely, by a team with no previous research experience in UTx, at a time when important animal studies were still ongoing. It also highlighted the risks of vascular thrombosis, which were subsequently shown in animal models, and the need to ensure the graft is sufficiently supported anatomically to reduce the risk of torsion. The decision to transplant the fallopian tubes is also questionable, owing to the significant risks of ectopic pregnancy from spontaneous conception following radical pelvic surgery.

Second human uterine transplantation

The second human UTx was performed in 2011 in Turkey, using a deceased 22-year-old, nulliparous donor (Akar et al. 2013). The term 'deceased' in the context of UTx, refers to brain stem dead, heart beating donors. The recipient was a 21-year-old woman with MRKH who had been previously undergone vaginal reconstruction with an intestinal neovagina. The retrieval graft included uterus, proximal vagina and the internal iliac vessels as well as a wide excision of broad ligament, round ligament, and the vesicouterine and sacrouterine peritoneum. The uterus was implanted in an orthotopic position, fixed using the surrounding ligamentous support and revascularized using internal iliac to external iliac anastomoses.

Immunosuppression was commenced using an induction regimen of thymoglobulin for the first 10 days along with high dose prednisolone (1000 mg/day). Tacrolimus (0.2 mg/kg with plasma levels 15–20 ng/mL) was commenced after 7 days and continued as maintenance immunosuppression along with mycophenolate mofetil (MMF; 2 g/day) and a smaller dose of prednisolone (20 mg/day).

The recipient recovered postoperatively and the uterus appeared functional clinically, after the onset of menstruation 20 days later, and radiologically after the visualized of cyclical endometrial proliferation. Rejection was monitored using vaginal biopsies every 2 weeks for the first 3 months and endometrial biopsies were taken every 3 months. Whilst the transplanted graft has remained in situ, the recipient has yet to bear a child after multiple embryo transfers and early miscarriages.

The most important lesson taken from this case was the decision to use a nulliparous donor. Whilst the uterus may have appeared macroscopically and radiologically normal, the only way to truly determine functionality is following childbirth.

Another important consideration in the recipient selection process was the decision to use a woman who had previously undergone reconstructive vaginal surgery with the creation of a neovagina using intestinal tissue. It is likely that nonphysiological discharge in the distal vagina may create a hostile environment for conception and the maintenance of pregnancy. This may have contributed to the poor obstetric outcome.

The use of vaginal biopsies to detect rejection was novel, with no previous evidence of a correlation between such biopsies and rejection. Furthermore, the use of endometrial biopsies, in the context of an immunosuppressed woman, risks the introduction of unwanted pathogens and should be avoided where possible.

Human uterine transplantation in Sweden

The following nine UTx procedures were undertaken by the Swedish team, led by Professor Brännström between 2012 and 2013, using living donors (Brännström et al. 2014). The living donors were aged between 39 and 62, did not suffer with any significant medical comorbidity and were vitally all multiparous. The recipients were mostly related to the donors, were of normal body habitus and did not smoke. Eight of the women had MRKH and the other recipient had previously undergone hysterectomy for cervical cancer. All the women underwent a 12-month counseling and investigation period preoperatively.

The donor graft included the uterus, cervix, surrounding ligamentous tissue and the internal iliac vessels. The implantation operations saw the uterus aligned in the normal anatomical position, secured with surrounding ligamentous support with a vascular anastomosis between the internal iliac vessels and the external iliac vessels.

Induction immunosuppressive was given in the form of methylprednisolone and ATG with maintenance tacrolimus (plasma trough levels 10–15 ng/mL) and MMF (50–60 mg h/L) for the first 6 months. The MMF was stopped prior to embryo transfer due to its potential teratogenic effect in pregnancy.

Two recipients experienced complications that necessitated emergency hysterectomy. One recipient, who had heterozygous protein C deficiency, developed acute uterine artery thrombosis despite prophylactic low molecular weight heparin, on the third postoperative day. Another recipient re-presented with recurrent pelvic infections and, despite multiple courses of antibiotics, developed a pelvic abscess and early signs of sepsis. She subsequently underwent hysterectomy 105 days postoperatively. This recipient in particular had a short vaginal cuff, which was thought to be a contributory factor, owing to the risk of vertical transmission of bacteria.

On reflection, it is important that women are selected appropriately, and women who are not suitable (e.g. carriers of thrombophilias or women with short vaginas) are not selected in the first instance for quality of life improving transplants such as UTx.

With consideration for the donors, two ureteric injuries were sustained; one was noted and repaired intraoperatively, whilst another reattended with a uretovaginal fistula which required treatment with an initial pyelostomy before definitive reimplantation of the ureter 5 months later.

Rejection in the remaining seven recipients was monitored using cervical biopsies. Subclinical episodes of mild rejection were noted in four women, which were successfully treated with corticosteroids in most cases, with the addition of prednisolone and azathioprine in the maintenance immunosuppression. Embryo transfer was undertaken from 12 months onwards.

In September 2014, the first live birth after UTx was announced, demonstrating that UTx could be a suitable treatment for women with AUFI. The Swedish team have since declared that four further babies have been born following UTx, resulting in an impressive live birth rate of 71%.

The great success of this Swedish trial has set the benchmark for future UTx programs . Furthermore, the association between the use of multiparous donors and exceptional fertility rates reaffirms the need to use donor uteri of proven functionality. From an obstetric perspective, it is of interest the pregnancy resulting in the first child born following UTx was complicated by severe pre-eclampsia. The recipient had atypical MRKH, with unilateral renal agenesis. Given the relationship between chronic kidney disease and hypertensive disorders of pregnancy, as well as the increased risk of gestational diabetes, women with significant kidney pathology should not routinely be considered for UTx.

Subsequent human uterine transplantations

Three further UTx procedures have been carried out since: in China, the USA and most recently the Czech Republic. Whilst they have not been officially reported, lessons can be learned from what is known about the former two cases.

1 The UTx undertaken in China, used a living donor, and performed a robotic assisted uterine graft retrieval. If living donors are being used, then minimal access surgical techniques, with the appropriate expertise, should be used to minimize surgical morbidity to the donor.
2 The case in the USA, using a deceased donor, was unsuccessful, with hysterectomy being performed due to candidal vasculitis, which resulted in intra-abdominal hemorrhage. Invasive candidiasis is an established complication in solid organ transplantation (Silveira et al. 2013), being particularly prevalent in small bowel and lung transplants, but least common in kidney transplants.

UTx requires particular consideration since candida is a commensal organism in the vagina, and the distal part of the vagina is commonly included in the transplant graft. The Swedish trial did not report any complications related to fungal infections, which suggests it may be more prevalent in deceased donor models. It is therefore essential to screen both recipients and donors, as well as sending a sample of the preservation solution the graft is stored in for microbiological assessment.

The latter sample is essential as this is where the opportunity arises for pathogens from the nonsterile vaginal cuff to infiltrate the sterile areas of the graft such as the vital blood vessels that will eventually be used for the anastomosis. Appropriate preoperative vaginal cleansing in both donor and recipient is essential with further intraluminal cleansing of the vaginal cuff prior to placing the graft in the cold preservation solution. Empirical antifungal treatment should be given, which should be tailored accordingly depending on the subspecies isolated.

FUTURE PROSPECTS

Recent years have seen prolific developments in UTx, but it is still in its experimental phase, and we eagerly await the outcomes of further human trials. UTx research teams have been established globally, and the International Society for Uterine Transplantation (ISUTx) has now been established, with its inaugural meeting held in Gothenburg in January 2016. With 21 UTx teams, based across 18 countries, a collaborative approach within this society should accelerate progress. Furthermore, the creation of official guidelines and recommendations, along with the institution of an international registry should optimize safety and performance monitoring.

The immediate future in the UK sees the first trial of UTx which is expected to commence in 2018 with the anticipation that ten UTx procedures will be performed over a 2-year period. All potential recipients will undergo a period of between 6–12 months of counseling and preoperative investigation (**Table 19.1**). The selection criteria for potential recipients are summarized in **Table 19.2**. Fertility treatment including embryo cryopreservation of at least ten embryos will subsequently be undertaken and the recipient would undergo a detailed consent process prior to being placed on a waiting list until a suitable brain stem dead, heart being donor becomes available.

The selection criteria for donors are listed in **Table 19.3**. Once such a donor is identified, the transplant will take place using an external iliac to internal iliac anastomosis. The donor surgery incisions are pictorially demonstrated in **Figure 19.2**. The graft will then be removed, positioned in a sterile bowl containing cold preservation solution, before being placed in a series of three plastic bags (**Figure 19.3**). It will then be transported in an organ transport box to the implantation hospital.

The recipient surgery, including vascular and vaginal anastomoses is depicted in **Figure 19.4**. The ligamentous and soft tissue support will be provided anteriorly with bladder peritoneum, laterally to the broad and uterosacral ligaments and inferiorly to the vagina and paravaginal tissues. Post-transplant, the recipient will be required to take aspirin and immunosuppressive therapy whilst the graft remains in place. Embryo transfer, using a single embryo only, will commence 6 months after transplantation, subject to an uncomplicated course. Following successful conception, high risk antenatal care would ensue with delivery by cesarean section between 35–37 weeks gestation, unless clinically indicated sooner. In the absence of complications, the process could be repeated for another child if desired by the recipient.

Hysterectomy is planned for 3–6 months following the completion of the woman's family. If the trial is successful, we feel that a national program could be set up in the UK from 2020 onwards, offering between 5–10 women a year with AUFI the chance to undergo UTx.

Table 19.1 Recipient preoperative counseling and investigations

Inclusion criteria	Exclusion criteria
Surgical team review	• History • Examination: Ensure vaginal length >6 cm • Blood tests – Hematology: Full blood count, clotting, thrombophilia screen – Biochemistry: Urea and electrolytes, liver function tests, – Infection screen: HBV, HCV, EBV, TORCH, syphilis • Genitourinary medicine (GUM) screen: Chlamydia, gonorrhea, Trichomonas vaginalis, Candida • Radiology: Chest X-ray, pelvic ultrasound, MRI abdomen/pelvis • Electrocardiogram (ECG)
Clinical psychologist	• Initial interview and separate interview with partner • Structured clinical interview for DSM (SCID-RV) • Marital taxon interview measure • The World Health Organization Quality of Life BREF (WHOQOL-BREF) • Fertility quality of life tool (FertiQoL) • Hospital anxiety and depression scale (HADS) • Dyadic adjustment scale (DAS) • 36 item short form health survey (SF-36) • Modified medical outcomes study social support survey (mMOS-SS) • Beliefs about medicines questionnaire – general (BMQ-General) • Immunosuppressant treatment adherence scale (ITAS) • Pictorial representation of illness and self-measure (PRISM) • Rosenberg's self-esteem scale • Cognitive fusion scale • Engaged living questionnaire • Multidimensional body-self relations questionnaire (MBSRQ)
IVF team review	• Blood tests: Follicle-stimulating hormone, luteinizing hormone, progesterone, anti-Mullerian hormone, estradiol • Male partner semen analysis • Egg collection and ICSI • Embryo freezing day 5 (minimum number of 10 sufficient quality needed)
Transplant team review	• Group and screen • Tissue typing
Partner testing	• Infection screen: HBV, HCV, EBV, • TORCH, syphilis • GUM screen: Chlamydia, gonorrhea, *Trichomonas vaginalis*

TORCH (Toxoplasma gondii, other viruses, rubella, cytomegalovirus, herpes simplex): blood test designed to screen for a group of infectious agents.

DSM (SCID-RV): an interview process to assess a person's mental state in accordance with the Diagnostic and Statistical Manual of Mental Disorder (DSM). This manual is published by the American Psychiatric Association (APA).

World Health Organization Quality Of Life BREF (WHOQOL-BREF): assesses a person's perceptions in the context of their culture and value systems, and their personal goals, standards and concerns.

Table 19.2 Recipient inclusion and exclusion criteria

Inclusion criteria	Exclusion criteria
• Female • Absolute uterine factor infertility • Proven functioning ovaries (antral follicle count and anti-Müllerian hormone level) • Aged 24–38 years (40 years if eggs were frozen at <38 years) • Normal length vagina – no skin/intestinal neovagina • BMI <30 kg/m2 • Lives in UK as a resident • Fluent in the English language • Sufficient embryo quality/quantity (<10 satisfactory embryos)	• Previous children – including adopted or born through surrogacy • Previous multiple major abdominal/pelvic surgery • Premature ovarian failure with no frozen mature eggs/embryos • Severe endometriosis • Significant medical problems including: – renal pathology – thrombophilia • Previous cancer <5 years in remission • History of significant psychiatric illness

Table 19.3 Donor inclusion and exclusion criteria

Inclusion criteria	Requirements
Pre-menopausal	>16 years
Multiparous	< 4 deliveries
ABO compatible and no antibodies	HLA compatibility not essential but preferred
Normal pelvic ultrasound	Myoma <1 cm acceptable but not submucosal • Submucous fibroid(s) • Moderate to severe adenomyosis • Congenital uterine anomalies
Macroscopically normal cervix	Benign appearing polyp acceptable but send for urgent histology
HPV negative	Urgent swab to be sent prior to retrieval
Negative GUM screen	Chlamydia, gonorrhoea, trichomonas vaginalis
Negative infection screen	HIV, Hepatitis B, Hepatitis C, syphilis
Exclusion criteria	**Further information**
History of cancer	
Significant systemic disease	Diabetes, SLE etc
Previous multiple / significant uterine surgery	• 2 × Caesarean section acceptable • No previous myomectomies
Previous significant cervical surgery	Cone biopsy or LLETZ
Previous preterm delivery	<37 weeks' gestation
Previous recurrent miscarriages	≥ 3 Live birth to miscarriage ratio >1
Current intravenous drug abuse	
Active bacteremia / fungemia	

Abbreviations: HLA, human leukacyte antigen; GUM, genitourinary medicine; SLE, systemic lupus erythematosus; LLETZ, large loop excision of the transformation zone.

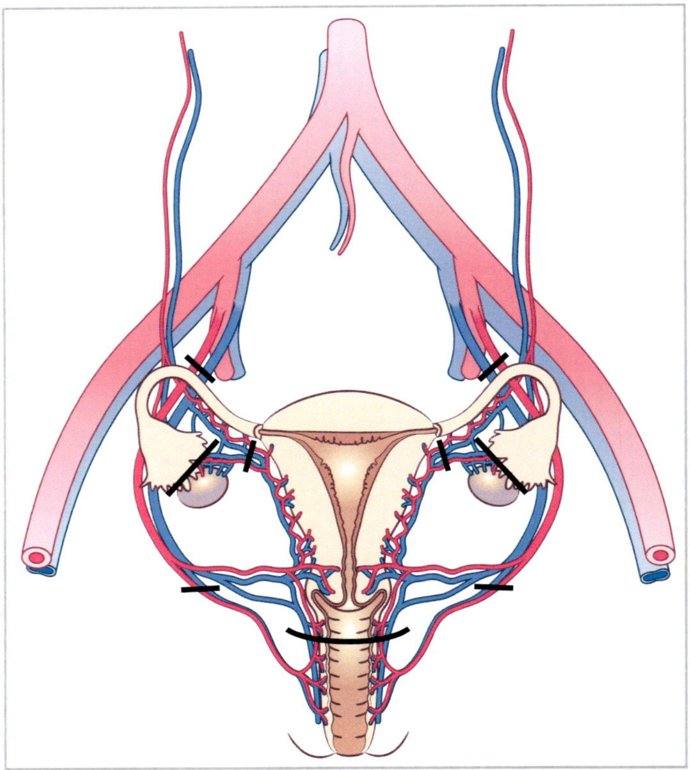

Figure 19.2 Anatomy and incision points for uterine transplant retrieval.

Donors

Should the donor be living?

Perhaps, the biggest uncertainty regarding UTx at present is the choice of using deceased or living donors. Although 12 of the 14 cases to date have been living donors, the future cases planned are divided more equally. Some argue that the use of living donors is unacceptable owing to the intraoperative and immediate postoperative risk to the donor. Given the average length of donor retrieval operation in the Swedish study was over 11 hours, the risk of venous thromboembolism is significant, and one that is difficult to justify with the current operative times.

Furthermore, major pelvic surgery has significant associated intraoperative risk. Two donors (14%) have so far suffered ureteric injuries, one which was noted intraoperatively and immediately repaired, whilst the other re-presented postoperatively with an uretovaginal fistula. (Johannesson and Järvholm, 2016). Not only is the risk to the donor negated, but the use of deceased donors also allows a more radical dissection, which enables greater caliber vessels to be taken, theoretically reducing the risk of graft thrombosis, whilst a longer vaginal cuff could be taken to reduce the risk of ascending bacterial infection.

Conversely, the use of living donors has a number of advantages. Logistically, planning an elective surgery using living donors is straightforward, and given the expertise required from multiple disciplines, is organizationally superior to the on-call arrangement

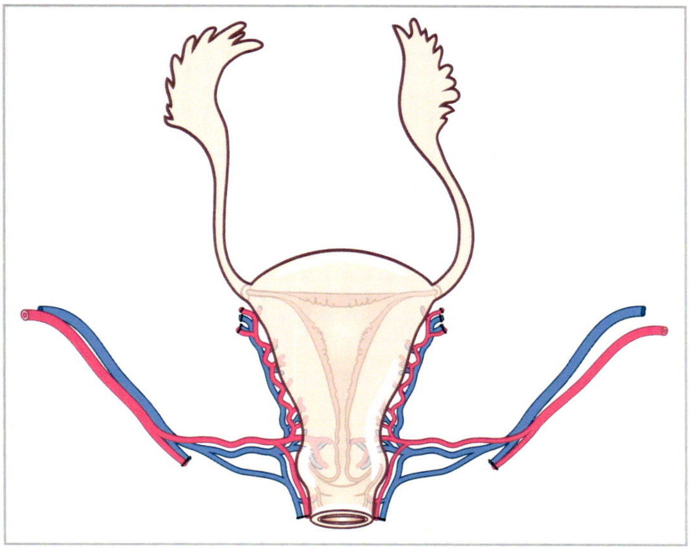

Figure 19.3 Uterine transplant graft following retrieval.

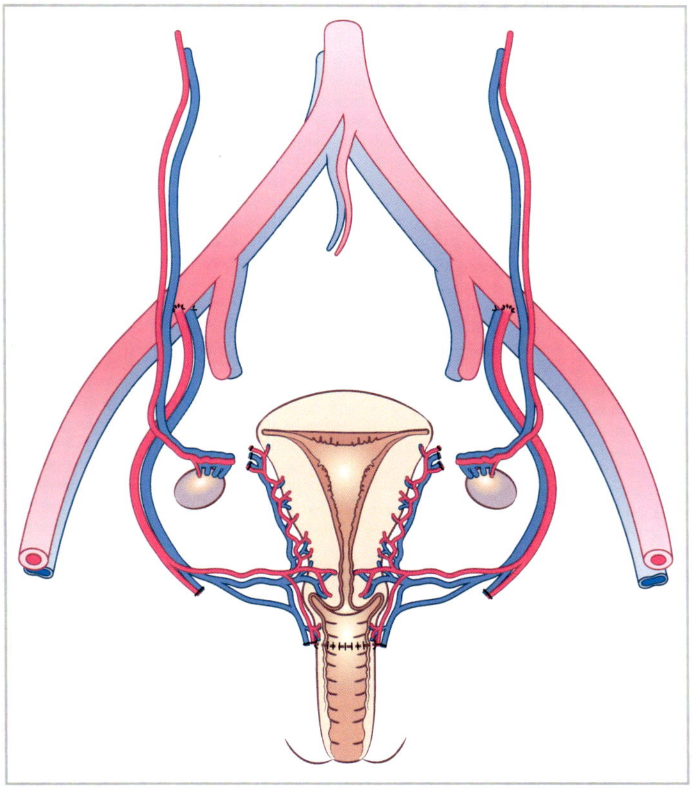

Figure 19.4 Recipient anatomy following uterine transplantation demonstrating vascular and vaginal anastomoses.

necessitated by using deceased donors. However, the success of multiorgan retrievals, orchestrated by National Health Service Blood and Transplant (NHSBT) in the UK, involving heart, lung, liver, kidney and small bowel transplants, demonstrates that such a system is feasible. An on-call rota, made up of individual teams with the necessary expertize, allows sufficient cross-cover to prevent interference with everyday schedules.

Using living donors also allows a greater time to investigate the donor. At a minimum, these should include a cervical smear +/- HPV testing, a genitourinary medicine (GUM) screen including chlamydia, gonorrhea and Trichomonas vaginalis testing and a vaginal culture to exclude candidal infection and bacterial vaginosis. An ultrasound scan, preferably performed transvaginally, should also be undertaken to exclude structural abnormalities. This array of investigations can however be performed in the deceased donor model, with the results expedited to ensure results are available within the 12–24-hour window preretrieval. In this time, the donor is physiologically optimized, family members are counseled and consented, and other retrieval teams perform their preliminary investigations. The use of living donors allows further investigation such as MRI, which whilst not essential, would potentially enable greater diagnostic accuracy with conditions such as adenomyosis.

The use of CTA and MRA is also beneficial to assess vessel morphology, calibre and patency.

It is anticipated that there is a role for both deceased and living donors in the future. While the feasibility of living donors has been demonstrated following successful live births, evolution of the surgical technique is needed to reduce donor risk to ensure long-term sustainability. Moreover, we still await a successful live birth following UTx using a deceased donor. Only when more cases have been performed using both donor types can efficacy be compared to determine if one donor type is superior.

Intrafamilial donation

Immunologically, the use of living donors would most likely lead to trend of close family members donating their wombs, as opposed to entirely altruistic acts from strangers. This may have benefit immunologically with a closer tissue match, which in turn may reduce the likelihood of acute rejection episodes and potentially reduce immunosuppressant exposure. Interestingly from the Swedish trial, the three women who did not experience rejection episodes all received donor uteri from their mothers.

However, finding a family member to donate a uterus may not always be possible. In this event it is unlikely that strangers acting altruistically would create a large enough pool of donors for a long term sustainable program.

Transgender donors

Consideration could be given to female to male transgender patients who plan to undergo gender reassignment surgery including hysterectomy. Whilst idealistic, the hysterectomy would need to be more radical than a standard hysterectomy, highlighting a potential drawback.

Radical hysterectomy

Johannesson et al. (2012), compared postoperative outcomes in radical hysterectomy patients and women undergoing a modified radical hysterectomy with vascular dissection of the uterine vessels away from the anterior division of the internal iliac vessels. The median lengths of the free portions of the uterine arteries were 68 mm (left) and 65 mm (right), whilst the venous lengths were 55 mm (left) and 50 mm (right). Given the internal-external iliac artery distance, which corresponds to the distance between the proposed anastomosis sites, was 90 mm, these distances demonstrate there would be sufficient length to undertake the anastomosis required in UTx. Importantly there was no significant difference in pre-operative or postoperative complications, compared with a standard radical hysterectomy control group. It is likely that if the uterine vessels are excised this laterally, that there would not be an associated increased risk of thrombosis although further studies would be needed to clarify this.

Bioengineered uterine patch

The long-term future of UTx will undoubtedly focus around the development of a bioengineered uterine graft, the use of which would negate surgical risk to the donor as well as the need for immunosuppression. Hellström et al. (2016) demonstrated the ability to repair a rat uterus using a bioengineered uterine patch. Three different uterine scaffolds were created following a decellularization process. Following the isolation of uterine cells and green fluorescent protein labeled bone marrow-derived mesenchymal stem cells, the scaffolds were used to develop a uterine tissue construct. A 5 mm × 10 mm full thickness segment from the uterine horn of a recipient rat was then excised, and subsequently repaired using the bioengineered graft. Two control groups were included who underwent autotransplantation procedures or were no operated on. Following mating, two out of the three scaffolds had both similar pregnancy rates and similar numbers of fetuses to the control groups, with fetal development clearly seen in the areas where the patches were located. This remarkable progress has set the benchmark high for the future of UTx and with ongoing innovation, a truly viable treatment option for women with AUFI may develop.

ACKNOWLEDGEMENTS

The authors would like to thank Dee McLean for providing the artwork for this chapter.

REFERENCES

Akar ME, Ozkan O, Aydinuraz B, et al. Clinical pregnancy after uterus transplantation. Fertil Steril 2013; 100:1358–1363.

Brännström M, Johannesson L, Dahm-Kähler, P, et al. First clinical uterus transplantation trial: a six-month report. Fertil Steril 2014; 101:1228–1236.

Brännström M, Johannesson L, Bokström H, et al. Livebirth after uterus transplantation. Lancet 2014; 385 607–616.

Confino E, Vermesh M, Thomas W, Jr, Gleicher N. Non-vascular transplantation of the rabbit uterus. Int J Gynaecol Obst 1986; 24:321–325.

Davision JM, Baylis C. Renal disease. In: de Swiet M, (edn). Medical disorders in obstetric practice. 4th ed. Malden, Mass: Blackwell Science 2002:198–266.

Diaz-Garcia C, Akhi SN, Wallin A, et al. First report on fertility after allogeneic uterus transplantation. Acta Obstet Gynecol Scand 2010; 89:1491–1494.

Fageeh W, Raffa H, Jabbad H, Marzouki A. Transplantation of the human uterus. Int J Gynaecol Obstet 2002; 76:245–251.

Farthing A. Conserving fertility in the management of gynaecological cancers. BJOG 2006; 113:129–134.

Folch M, Pigem I, Konje JC. Mullerian agenesis: etiology, diagnosis, and management. Obstet Gynecol Surv 2000; 55:644–649.

Hellström M, El-Akouri RR, Sihlbom C, et al. Towards the development of a bioengineered uterus: Comparison of different protocols for rat uterus decellularization. Acta Biomaterialia 2014; 10:5034–5042.

Hellström M, Moreno-Moya JM, Bandstein S, et al. Bioengineered uterine tissue supports pregnancy in a rat model. Fertil Steril 2016; 106:487–496.

Johannesson L, Diaz-Garcia C, Leonhardt H, et al. Vascular pedicle lengths after hysterectomy: toward future human uterus transplantation. Obstet Gynecol 2012; 119:1219–1225.

Johannesson L, Järvholm S. Uterus transplantation: current progress and future prospects. Int J Women's Health 2016; 8:43–51.

Kallen B, Westgren M, Aberg A, Olausson PO. Pregnancy outcome after maternal organ transplantation in Sweden. BJOG 2005; 112:904–909.

Kjaer TK, Jensen A, Dalton SO, et al. Suicide in Danish women evaluated for fertility problems. Hum Reprod 2011; 26:2401–2407.

Laggari V, Diareme S, Christogiorgos S, et al. Anxiety and depression in adolescents with polycystic ovary syndrome and Mayer-Rokitansky-Kuster-Hauser syndrome. J Psychosom Obstet Gynaecol 2009; 30:83–88.

Mowers EL, Lim CS, Skinner B, et al. Prevalence of Endometriosis During Abdominal or Laparoscopic Hysterectomy for Chronic Pelvic Pain. Obstet Gynecol 2016; 127:1045–1053.

Ramirez ER, Ramirez DK, Nessetti MB, et al. Pregnancy and outcome of uterine allotransplantation and assisted reproduction in sheep. J Minim Invasive Gynecol 2011; 182:238–245.

Saso S, Petts G, Thum MY, et al. Achieving uterine auto-transplantation in a sheep model using iliac vessel anastomosis: a short-term viability study. Acta Obstet Gynecol Scand 2014.

Schenker JG, Margalioth EJ. Intra-uterine adhesions: an updated appraisal. Fertil Steril 1982; 37:593–610.

Sieunarine K, Zakaria FB, Boyle DC, et al. Possibilities for fertility restoration: a new surgical technique. Int Surg 2005; 90:249–256.

Smith JR, Boyle DC, Corless DJ, et al. Abdominal radical trachelectomy: a new surgical technique for the conservative management of cervical carcinoma. Br J Obstet Gynaecol 1997; 104:1196–1200.

Silveira FP, Kusne S. Candida infections in solid organ transplantation. Am J Transplant 2013; 13:220–227.

Sonoda Y, Abu-Rustum NR, Gemignani ML, et al. A fertility-sparing alternative to radical hysterectomy: how many patients may be eligible? Gynecol Oncol 2004; 95:534–538.

Zhordania IF, Gotsiridze OA. Autotransplantation of the uterus into the omentum. Int J Fertil 1963; 8:849–857.

Chapter 20 Fertility preservation: oocytes

Greta Verheyen, Ingrid Segers, Neelke De Munck, Dominic Stoop, Michel De Vos

INTRODUCTION

Despite successful pregnancies using thawed human oocytes after slow freezing in the late 1980s and 1990s, the introduction of vitrification for human oocytes in the late 1990s was highly successful. Compared to slow freezing, vitrification is associated with higher survival when oocytes are warmed, and also with high fertilization and pregnancy rates.

Advances in the field of oocyte cryopreservation techniques have created a wide range of indications for oocyte storage. With regard to the practice of oocyte donation, many IVF centers have switched from fresh oocyte donation to use of cryopreserved oocytes stored in a donor oocyte bank. This solves the problem of donor-recipient synchronization and allows a more efficient oocyte distribution among different recipients.

The success of oocyte vitrification has also opened the door for female fertility preservation (FP). For females who need to undergo gonadotoxic treatment, adult women, adolescents and even prepubertal girls now have the option to counteract fertility loss through cryostorage of oocytes, either as a stand-alone approach or in combination with ovarian tissue freezing. This strategy can also be applied for patients with a non-cancerous condition and a risk of premature ovarian failure. Moreover, age-related fertility decline is becoming increasingly popular as an indication for oocyte vitrification.

This chapter covers the clinical and laboratory aspects of female FP by means of oocyte and ovarian tissue banking.

OOCYTE CRYOPRESERVATION FOR ONCOFERTILITY: CLINICAL ASPECTS

Oocyte banking

Cycles with super-ovulation

The significantly better survival rate of vitrified-warmed oocytes, compared to their slow frozen-thawed counterparts, holds huge promise for cancer patients who have chemotherapy-naive oocytes vitrified for future use. Cryopreservation of mature oocytes and embryos following controlled ovarian stimulation (COS) in women is currently the only technique endorsed by the American Society for Reproductive Medicine (ASRM) (The Practice Committee of the ASRM, 2013).

Indeed, clinical trials in infertile patients have shown that standard hormone driven procedures are more efficacious than treatments that are based on the collection of immature oocytes from small antral follicles after low-dose stimulation or no hormone treatment at all (Walls et al. 2015). Therefore, use of COS to obtain mature oocytes should be recommended as the optimal FP method, unless the patient's medical condition requires an urgent start of chemotherapy.

In order to facilitate timely initiation of ovarian stimulation, prompt referral of the patient to a reproductive clinic with an integrated FP service is mandatory. Upon referral, ovarian reserve assessment based on antral follicle count (AFC) and serum anti-Müllerian hormone (AMH) analysis should guide the selection of the gonadotropin starting dose, in order to obtain optimal ovarian response.

Overall, cancer patients referred for FP, especially those with a BRCA1 (breast cancer 1) mutation, have lower numbers of oocytes retrieved after COS compared with healthy age-matched controls. Although the use of a higher dose of gonadotropins may be an appealing strategy to enhance oocyte yield, this may not necessarily lead to a higher number of oocytes. Furthermore, increased doses of gonadotropins may result in higher rates of chromosomally abnormal oocytes (Baart et al. 2007).

Letrozole, an aromatase inhibitor, is added to the stimulation protocol in women with estrogen receptor positive breast cancer, to avoid high serum E2 levels. This approach yields similar oocyte numbers compared to standard COS protocols and has not been shown to raise the risk of breast cancer recurrence. Gonadotropin-releasing hormone (GnRH) antagonist stimulation protocols followed by a GnRH agonist ovulation trigger are generally recommended for FP, to avoid ovarian hyperstimulation syndrome (OHSS), the most serious complication of COS.

Further modifications of ovarian stimulation protocols, established to optimize oocyte retrieval within the limited time-frame of FP, include the initiation of ovarian stimulation irrespective of the menstrual phase (so-called 'random-start', Cakmak et al. 2013) and repeated oocyte retrieval after consecutive rounds of ovarian stimulation (Turan et al. 2013).

Cycles without super-ovulation

When conventional hormonal stimulation of the ovaries is not a suitable approach because of a cancer type that requires an urgent start of chemotherapy, alternative FP methods should be considered, including cryopreservation of ovarian cortex and in vitro maturation (IVM) of oocytes. For the latter, conventional hormonal stimulation may be possible, but this could delay the start of chemotherapy. In contrast to the established method of oocyte vitrification after COS, this approach is still considered experimental, since the follow-up of children resulting from these methods is currently limited.

Oocyte IVM does not require ovarian stimulation with gonadotropins and is based on the potential of immature oocytes from small antral follicles to resume meiosis spontaneously upon release from the follicular environment. IVM has been applied in human reproduction since the early 1990s, most commonly in women with polycystic ovaries (PCO), because of their high AFC. The efficiency of IVM has steadily increased over the past decade, and IVM children do not appear to have a higher risk of congenital malformations compared with children conceived after standard COS and ICSI (Fadini et al. 2012). However, few live births have so far been reported following both warming of vitrified oocytes after IVM in healthy patients, and after embryo vitrification following IVM in a cancer patient (Zhang et al. 2010).

Immature oocytes can be harvested transvaginally from ovaries of cancer patients without hormonal pretreatment at any stage of the menstrual cycle, and similar oocyte numbers are retrieved during the luteal and follicular phase cycle (Grynberg et al. 2016). Therefore, this technology is highly suitable for patients with a cancer type that requires very urgent (<2 weeks) initiation of systemic therapy. Research in infertile women has shown that the yield of IVM oocytes, and as a consequence the clinical performance of the technique, is correlated with AFC and AMH (Guzman et al. 2013). This observation has been confirmed in the FP setting, where an AFC of 20 follicles and serum AMH level of 3.7 ng/mL were found to be required for the cryopreservation of at least ten IVM oocytes (Sonigo et al. 2016).

Nevertheless, in view of the limited experience with vitrified-warmed IVM oocytes and the reduced potential of IVM oocytes as obtained from studies in women with PCO, it is recommended to combine IVM with ovarian tissue cryopreservation (OTC) when predicted gonadotoxicity is high and when ovarian stimulation is not possible.

Ovarian tissue banking

For patients with a cancer type that precludes a delay of the start of chemotherapy, and for prepubertal children, in whom ovarian stimulation is not feasible because of immaturity of the hypothalamo-pituitary-ovarian axis, OTC has been the option of choice for more than a decade (Donnez et al. 2006).

Depending on the size of the ovaries, either a unilateral oophorectomy can be performed or a number of ovarian cortical biopsies can be taken, although there is no evidence as to which approach is preferable. Indeed, oophorectomy will reduce the functional ovarian reserve of a patient by 50% and is therefore only performed in cases at high risk of chemotherapy induced gonadal damage. Nevertheless, oophorectomy generally leads to an earlier menopause, but not to premature ovarian insufficiency.

In a plea to have the procedure endorsed as an established rather than investigational approach, one specialist center reviewed the outcome of 111 infertile women who underwent ovarian cortex transplantation following OTC, and reported that 32 women (29%) had a live birth (Donnez et al. 2015). Furthermore, the potential of OTC in young girls has been illustrated by a reported live birth after an autograft of ovarian tissue that had been cryopreserved during childhood (Demeestere et al. 2015).

Following advances in IVM, OTC is increasingly combined with IVM following direct aspiration from small antral follicles during the processing of ovarian cortex or found in the dissection medium. This procedure, i.e. retrieval of immature oocytes from extracorporeal ovarian tissue followed by IVM, is referred to as IVM 'ex vivo' and has the potential to further increase the chances of a live birth after OTC. Although this novel approach of IVM 'ex vivo' has so far only resulted in two reported live births, it holds promise especially for the reproductive future of young women with a hematological cancer type, in whom ovarian tissue grafting confers a high-risk of malignant cell reintroduction (Rosendahl et al. 2013).

OOCYTE PRESERVATION FOR ANTICIPATION OF GAMETE EXHAUSTION

The average age at which women give birth to their first child has increased in recent decades (Lockwood 2011). Multiple factors have contributed to this evolution, such as better access to contraception and also the pursuit of personal ambitions in education and career. Also, women with a desire for children may be forced to postpone motherhood because of the lack of a partner or because they may have a partner who is not ready to have children. This social-economic revolution has led to an increasing number of women confronted with age-related fertility loss.

The introduction of efficient oocyte cryopreservation methods enables women to have oocytes cryopreserved and to use them later when they are confronted with age-related infertility. This technique is often referred to as nonmedical, social freezing, elective freezing or anticipated gamete exhaustion (AGE) banking (Van Loendersloot et al. 2011, Stoop et al. 2014).

Several surveys have been performed in order to assess the profiles of the women who elect to cryopreserve oocytes. Most women are between 35 and 40 years old, single and well-educated (Baldwin et al. 2015, Hodes-Wertz et al. 2013, Stoop et al. 2015). However, few studies have been published so far on the outcome of treatments with warmed oocytes after the women return to use them. Knopman and co-workers (2010) first reported a pregnancy at the age of 41 years, with the use of oocytes cryopreserved at the age of 38 years. More recently, a Spanish group reported on the outcome of 137 women who returned after elective oocyte cryopreservation for nononcological reasons (Cobo et al. 2016). Acceptable outcomes were obtained if at least eight to ten mature oocytes were cryopreserved in women under the age of 35 years. A significantly poorer outcome, however, was observed in women banking after the age of 36 years. The authors therefore concluded that women should ideally have their oocytes cryopreserved at younger ages in order to increase future outcome success.

Van Loendersloot and colleagues (2011) compared the cost-efficiency of AGE banking at the age of 35 years followed by the use of these oocytes at the age of 41 years, with a strategy of either natural conception or with ART using fresh oocytes in women without preventive oocyte banking. Preventive oocyte cryopreservation appeared to be cost-efficient provided that at least 61% of the women returned to use their cryopreserved oocytes.

More recent studies have attempted to identify the most cost-efficient age when oocytes cryopreservation should be undertaken (Baldwin et al 2015, Hodes-Wertz et al. 2013, Stoop et al. 2015). Contrary to the biological findings that suggest that oocytes should be cryopreserved before the age of 35 years, Mesen and coworkers (2015) concluded that 37 years is the most cost-effective age to take preventive action.

An electronic survey among women of reproductive age (21–40 years) has shown that 3.1% strongly consider preventive oocyte cryopreservation, while another 28.4% of young women are open to the idea (Stoop et al. 2011). Factors that would eventually convince them to embark on such treatment include the availability of more data about the effects of the procedure on their future fertility and more data on the neonatal outcome.

Follow-up studies have shown that women who have performed oocyte cryopreservation do not regret their actions, even though many may eventually not use or need their cryopreserved oocytes (Stoop et al. 2015). Centers offering the oocyte cryopreservation technique for non-medical reasons report increasing numbers of cycles (Cobo et al. 2016, Stoop et al 2015) and the growing awareness will undoubtedly further increase the number of women who opt for this treatment.

Individual women would benefit from assessing their personal risk of developing a future fertility problem. Studies by Devine et al. (2015) have indicated that the risk of future infertility largely influences the cost efficiency of preventive oocyte cryopreservation. Unfortunately, so far only limited data are available on the predictive value of several factors influencing fertility. Moreover, important factors such as the sperm quality of a future partner or the age at which women will start trying to conceive cannot be predicted. However, efforts are underway to collect these data in fertility assessment and counseling clinics (Hvidman et al. 2015).

Endometriosis, a fertility threatening disorder, is considered by some as an indication for preventive oocyte cryopreservation (see Chapter 7). This is particularly true for cases of bilateral nonoperated endometriosis or in women who have undergone unilateral excision of endometriosis with contralateral recurrence (Somigliana et al. 2015). Another nononcological medical indication that increases the risk for future infertility is a genetic predisposition for premature ovarian failure.

OOCYTE PRESERVATION: LABORATORY ASPECTS

Oocyte cryopreservation can be performed using slow freezing or vitrification methods. During slow freezing (equilibrium freezing), the oocytes are exposed to low concentrations of cryoprotective agents (CPAs) during a long exposure time. The oocytes are cooled in a slow controlled way, with the induction of extracellular ice (seeding) to prevent intracellular ice formation. This technique led to the first report of a baby born after oocyte cryopreservation in 1986 (Chen 1986).

By contrast, during vitrification (nonequilibrium freezing), oocytes are exposed to high concentrations of the CPAs with a shorter exposure time. By plunging the oocytes immediately into liquid nitrogen (LN2), there is not enough time for ice crystal formation and a vitreous state is obtained. The first report of a baby born after oocyte vitrification came more than a decade later (Kuleshova et al. 1999). Both methods are currently still applied; although the results obtained with vitrification appear to be superior to those obtained with slow freezing (Paramanantham et al. 2015).

Vitrification of oocytes

Procedures

Compared to embryos and blastocysts, oocytes have a specific structure to which particular attention should be devoted in order to obtain a high success rate after vitrification and warming. The mature oocyte, with a diameter of approximately 120 µm, is the largest cell in the human body and, because of the single cell structure, there is no back-up to regenerate after cell loss. Different oocytes from the same patient may react differently upon exposure to the hyperosmotic solutions, which may be attributed to the inherent biological variability between oocytes (Paynter 2005). The use of COS drugs might also influence this biological variability even more. It is therefore advisable for embryologists to follow the shrinking and swelling process of each individual oocyte microscopically.

Since the oocyte is a spherical cell with a large diameter and a very low surface-to-volume ratio, losing water and taking up the CPAs is less efficient when compared to embryos or blastocysts, which have a higher surface-to-volume ratio. Therefore, oocytes are more susceptible to cryodamage if the exposure to CPAs is not long enough. Besides, oocytes have an osmotically inactive volume of 20%, which is, together with the low surface-to-volume ratio, an important factor related to the formation of lethal intracellular ice during freezing.

Upon exposure to the hyperosmotic solutions during equilibration prior to vitrification, the oocyte will undergo a dramatic volume shrinkage that can be reduced by a gradual exposure, or stepwise addition of CPAs. The final exposure to the highly concentrated vitrification solution should be kept very short to allow the final removal of water from the oocyte and to minimize CPA-related toxicity.

When the oocytes are loaded on the vitrification device, it is important to apply the minimal volume cooling method which implies removal of all the excess vitrification solution from the device in order to increase the cooling rate even more. By contrast, upon warming, it is important to use a large volume (at least 200 µL) of preheated (37°C) thawing solution. To be able to obtain a very high warming rate, the step from LN2 to the thawing solution should be performed as fast as possible. Preheating of the initial thawing solution is also important to prevent over-swelling of the oocytes when they are placed in this hypo-osmotic solution. This then allows for a faster shift of the intracellular CPAs to the extracellular environment.

CRYOPRESERVATION TERMINOLOGY

Strictly speaking, when it comes to oocytes and embryos, the terms 'frozen' and 'thawing' should only be used in relation to the slow freezing technique. For vitrification, the terms 'cryopreserved / vitrified' and 'warming' should be used. A vitrified embryo cannot be thawed, as there are no ice crystals to thaw! However, to complicate matters, some commercial media manufacturers continue to label their warming solutions as 'thawing' solutions.

During the processes of vitrification and warming, different droplet volumes can be applied: the larger the droplets, the less disturbance of the composition and osmolarity during handling and, thus, the easier the use when compared to smaller droplet volumes. In order to prevent evaporation of the droplets during vitrification and warming procedures, it is advisable to switch off the laminar air flow and to use a lid to cover the dishes during incubation.

Subtle differences in oocyte vitrification procedures exist. Most commonly, oocyte vitrification is a two-step procedure involving an equilibration step and a vitrification step. Gradual equilibration is usually performed in three steps with a total equilibration time ranging from 12 to 15 minutes. The final vitrification step, including loading onto the vitrification device and plunging into LN2, should not exceed one minute. This vitrification step can be a two-step procedure in case smaller volumes are used or can be a one-step procedure in case of larger volumes (300 µL). In the latter case, the oocyte is subsequently replaced in different areas within the larger drop.

Most warming procedures are routinely performed in three steps including warming, dilution and washing. Warming is generally the only step performed at 37°C over a period of 1 minute only. This is then followed by a 3-minute dilution step and two washing steps, of which the first one takes 5 minutes and the second one is very short (only a few seconds). Commonly, manufacturers provide detailed instructions describing how to use vitrification devices and vitrification and warming media.

Devices

Different types of devices for oocyte vitrification are commercially available. They are mainly categorized as 'open' or 'closed', based on their direct contact with LN2 or not (Vajta et al. 2015).

Open devices allow a direct contact of the oocyte with LN2 and thereby generate very high cooling rates (≥20,000°C/min) and warming rates (~42,000°C/min). These devices are stored in unsealed protective straws or cryotubes which implies a theoretical risk of cross-contamination during handling and storage. Some open devices come with specially designed closed containers: after vitrification, the device is inserted in the precooled container and heat-sealed. By doing so, cross-contamination during storage is avoided.

Closed devices are sealed before any contact with LN2 during vitrification and thus offer the highest possible protection against cross-contamination. The major drawback of these devices is the impairment of the cooling rate (~2900°C/min) and to a lesser extent the warming rate (~25,000°C/min). Due to the lower cooling rate in the closed devices, there is more time for CPA uptake (and higher toxicity) in the final vitrification step; this is illustrated by a more extensive oocyte shrinking during dilution (**Figure 20.1**).

Examples of open and closed devices include the Cryotop device (Kitazato, Japan) and the CBSvit device (CryoBioSystems, France) respectively. However, there are other successful devices available in the market (Vajta et al. 2015) (**Table 20.1**).

To date, the highest reported fertilization and pregnancy rates have been obtained with open devices, with only limited published information available from the use of closed devices. Currently, only three reported studies have compared open and closed devices (De Munck et al. 2016, Paffoni et al. 2011, Papatheodorou et al. 2013).

Table 20.1 Open and closed vitrification devices currently used to vitrify oocytes

Tradename	Vitrification	Storage	Manufacturer
Cryotop	Open	Open	Kitazato, Japan
Cryotop SC	Open	Closed	Kitazato, Japan
Cryotop CS	Closed	Closed	Kitazato, Japan
Cryoleaf	Open	Open	Origio, Denmark
Cryoloop	Open	Open	Hampton Research, CA, USA
HSV straw	Closed	Closed	Cryo Bio Systems, France
Rapid-i	Closed	Closed	Vitrolife, Sweden
Cryotip	Closed	Closed	Irvine Scientific, CA, USA
Vitrisafe	Closed	Closed	Vitrimed, Germany

Interestingly, our group did not find a difference in oocyte survival rate following oocyte VIT-warming between open (Cryotop SC) and closed (CBSvit) devices (De Munck et al. 2016).

Cryoprotectants

For oocyte vitrification, it is generally accepted to use a combination of permeating and non-permeating CPAs. Permeating CPAs mainly protect the intracellular part of the oocyte by replacing a large proportion of water, whereas nonpermeating CPAs increase the viscosity of the solution and therefore reduce the amount of toxic permeating CPAs needed to obtain vitrification. By exerting an osmotic effect, CPAs reduce the time needed to dehydrate the oocyte before cooling and the time needed to restore the oocyte to an isoosmotic volume upon warming. Furthermore, they stabilize the cell membrane.

The permeating CPAs most commonly used are DMSO (dimethyl sulphoxide), EG (ethylene glycol) and PrOH (propanediol), whereas trehalose or sucrose are the most popular nonpermeating CPAs (Shaw and Jones 2003). Most protocols use 7.5% (v/v) DMSO and EG in the equilibration solution and 15.0% (v/v) DMSO and EG in the VIT solution. For closed devices, it has been proposed to use a three-step protocol, up to 20% (v/v), to obtain complete vitrification (Vanderzwalmen et al. 2009). The vitrification and warming protocol as used in our center is shown in **Figure 20.2**.

In vitro maturation of oocytes

Principle

In case of urgent FP for adult women or for prepubertal girls, the question raises whether to vitrify immature oocytes or vitrify mature oocytes obtained after IVM. In an immature oocyte at the germinal vesicle (GV) stage, chromatin is decondensed and protected by the nuclear envelop and the cytoskeleton is less specifically organized. Hence, vitrification of immature oocytes may theoretically bypass the problems encountered following mature oocyte vitrification, including disruption of the actin network, microtubule depolymerization, abnormal spindle configuration and chromosome scattering (Brambillasca et al. 2013). However, to ensure adequate maturation of GV oocytes in vitro, the bidirectional communication between the oocyte and the surrounding cumulus cells is imperative (Brambillasca et al. 2013). Clinically tested protocols for vitrification of cumulus oocyte complexes (COCs) maintaining this communication are not (yet) available. Therefore, it is currently recommended to mature obtained GV oocytes first and subsequently vitrify the mature oocytes, although robust data on efficiency, developmental capacity and safety of IVM vitrified-warmed oocytes are still lacking.

Unstimulated IVM can be challenging for the clinician performing the oocyte aspiration and for the embryologist searching for complexes

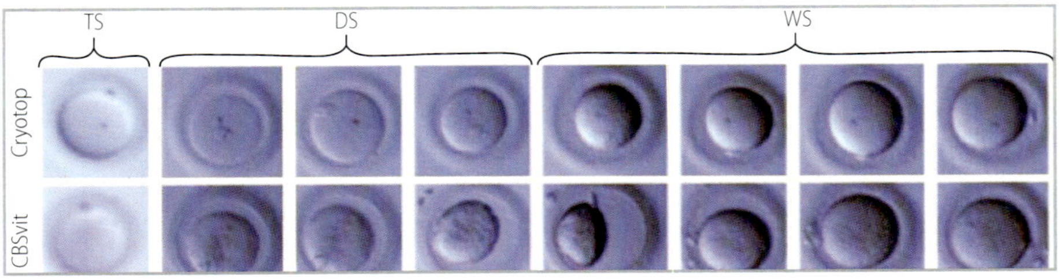

Figure 20.1 Oocyte dynamics after warming from the open or closed device. The shrinkage and re-expansion observed in both devices during warming was captured. The first picture was taken after 30 sec in thawing solution (TS), followed by pictures taken at time intervals of 1 minute in dilution solution (DS) and washing solution (WS). An oocyte vitrified with the CryotopSC device shows a less extensive shrinkage with the minimal oocyte volume mostly obtained in the last minute of exposure to the dilution solution. Once the oocyte is transferred to the first droplet of washing solution, the re-expansion starts and is mostly completed after 1.5 minutes. The oocyte vitrified with the CBSvit device shows a more pronounced shrinkage and its minimal shrinkage volume is obtained after 0.5 minute in the first droplet of warming solution and complete re-expansion is only obtained after 2.5 minutes in washing solution.

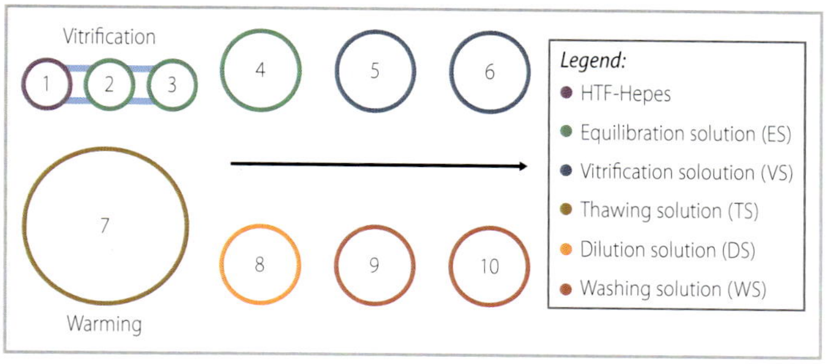

Figure 20.2 Flowchart of vitrification and warming in our center. *Vitrification*: oocytes are placed in 25 µL HTF-Hepes (1) and the droplet is immediately bridged with 25 µL ES (2). After 2 minutes, a second bridging with 25 µL ES is performed, again for 2 minutes (3). Bridging between the droplets is indicated in blue color lines. This is followed by 10 minutes equilibration in 50 µL ES (4). The final step in the vitrification has to be completed within 1 minute and comprises two washes in 50 µL VS (5 & 6), followed by loading and plunging into liquid nitrogen (LN2). All steps are performed at room temperature (RT). *Warming*: the straw containing the oocytes is opened and transfer to the preheated (37°C) 400 µL TS (7), is performed as fast as possible. Oocytes are kept here for 1 minute before they are placed in 50 µL dilution solution (DS) (8) at RT for 3 minutes. Afterwards, oocytes are washed in the first 50 µL (9) washing solution (WS) for 5 minutes followed by a short wash in the second 50 µL WS (10). Surviving oocytes are cultured in fertilization medium and injected within 1.5 hours after warming. Vitrification and warming procedures are indicated by the arrow.

in the follicular fluid. Unlike the large complexes of mucified, expanded cumulus cells (CC) surrounding in vivo matured oocytes, immature oocytes have only 2–5 layers of tightly packed cumulus cells, and complexes are therefore more difficult to identify, particularly if the follicular fluid is contaminated with blood. Filtering follicular fluid using a 70-µm mesh eliminates blood cells and concentrates the COCs to facilitate identification under a stereomicroscope. Since cumulus-enclosed oocytes have a significantly better developmental potential, 'naked' oocytes are excluded for IVM culture.

Procedures

Commercially available IVM culture media are usually based on basic cell culture media since they need to support both the gamete and the somatic cell compartment. Hence, IVM culture media differ from gamete and cleavage-stage media, e.g. in the glucose content. Investigational research in animal models revealed the benefits of further supplementing IVM media with a protein source (in human IVM this is autologous patient's serum or human serum albumin) and hormones (FSH and LH/hCG), with incubation in 5–6% CO_2 and 5% or 20% O_2.

Various IVM incubation periods have been reported (24–40 h). Furthermore, some laboratories check maturation at several time points during the maturation phase from 24 hours onwards, usually after cumulus cell (CC) removal. This practice allows insemination or vitrification shortly after polar body extrusion, but is labor-intense and implicates further incubation in vitro of immature oocytes which have been denuded of cumulus cells. On-site determination of the optimal IVM culture period in each specific clinical setting is vital, since increased maturation rates after increased incubation times may correlate with decreased developmental potential of resulting embryos (own observations).

Novel IVM systems are being developed to enhance further developmental potential of IVM oocytes, based on the use of meiotic inhibitors that allow a prolonged cytoplasmic maturation phase or based on the addition of (oocyte-secreted) growth factors, like *GDF9* and *BMP15*. These protocols are currently being tested in a preclinical phase (Coticchio et al. 2012, Smitz et al 2011).

Ovarian tissue cryopreservation

Ovarian cortex preparation

The ovary is a heterogeneous organ comprised of follicles at different stages of development, stromal tissue and blood vessels. Primordial resting follicles are packed in the dense cortical region of the ovary, while growing follicles are found near the medullar region, which is softer and contains more blood vessels.

Since primordial follicles represent the largest population of follicles and are able to withstand cryopreservation better than growing follicles, the ovarian cortex serves as a major contributor for the cryostorage of gametes. The ovarian cortex area of about 1-1.5 mm thick needs to be dissected from the ovary as depicted in **Figure 20.3**. With this technique, the cortex is dissected from the inside.

A different approach is dissecting cortex tissue from the outside, by 'peeling' the cortex with a blade from the medulla. This technique has been described in combination of vitrification since it creates slices of 0.7–1 mm thickness. Concerns have been raised, however, that reduced thickness will only preserve part of the primordial follicle pool and may result in a more pronounced 'burn out effect' upon transplantation.

Ovarian tissue freezing

Slow freezing versus vitrification

The procedure of OTC is increasingly applied to safeguard fertility in women facing POF due to gonadotoxic treatment. However, this technique is still considered experimental by the Practice Committee of the ASRM (2014), due to a lack of data to estimate the efficiency, safety and efficacy of ovarian tissue transplantation after cryopreservation. In this respect, the ASRM expert committee advises to use slow freezing (SF) protocols in the clinic, with more than 60 live births reported, rather than vitrification, with limited outcome data available (two live births). Research in animal models and human research material has shown that follicle survival and viability are comparable between both freezing strategies. The ultrastructure of the stromal tissue is better preserved after vitrification and warming, but this has not yet proven to result in increased live birth rates.

From a laboratory perspective, there are advantages and disadvantages with both protocols. Where vitrification requires highly skilled operators, expensive equipment for controlled freezing is necessary for the slow freezing procedure. Evidently, CPA concentrations are very high in VIT compared to SF, which imposes higher toxicity risks with increasing exposure time, although the level of toxicity is counterbalanced by reducing the size of the tissue pieces. Although VIT is a fast procedure (minutes), processing more and smaller tissue pieces will be more time consuming, compared to SF of large pieces in a single run of several hours (Amorim et al. 2011). These small vitrified tissue pieces may also require adapted transplantation techniques.

Cryoprotectants

A cryoprotectant solution for slow freezing is composed of a basic culture medium supplemented with permeable CPA and non-permeable CPA. In OTC, 1.5 M DMSO, 1.5 M EG or 1.5 M PROH are successfully used in combination with non-permeable CPA, a protein source (serum, a synthetic serum substitute or HSA, ranging from 10–20%) and often 0.1 M sucrose. These types of freezing solutions have been documented in literature and have resulted in the delivery of numerous healthy children (Dittrich 2015, Donnez and Dolmans 2015,

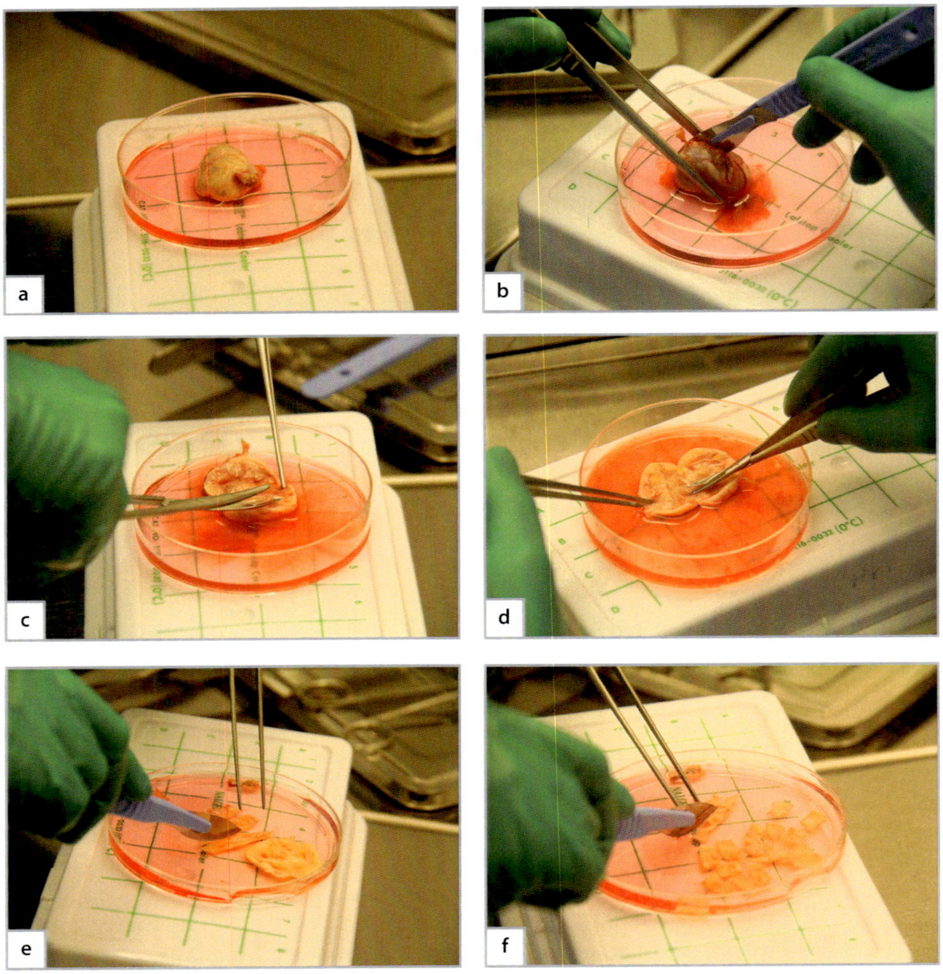

Figure 20.3 Ovarian cortex preparation. Upon arrival of the ovary in the lab, it is rinsed in ice cold medium on a cold working surface (a). The ovary is first cut into two halves (b). The difference in tissue density between the medullar tissue and the cortical tissue allows to trim medullar tissue apart with several sizes of scissors (c, d). As an alternative, the medullar tissue can also be scraped from the cortex with a scalpel (not shown). When the cortex is about 1–1.5 mm thick, the tissue is sliced in approximately 8 mm × 5 mm fragments (e, f) for slow freezing or in <5 mm^2 fragments for vitrification.

Stern et al. 2014). For CPA equilibration, a consensus 30-minute time period is used in the different cryobanking facilities. During controlled slow freezing of ovarian tissue, the used temperature curve is similar in most OTC facilities (**Figure 20.4**).

The OTC requires skilled personnel as well as stringent environmental conditions, which, in combination with the relatively rare application of OTC, promotes a centralization of the procedure in a limited number of specialized FP centers. This may entail transport of the tissue from the hospital where the patient has her ovarian tissue removed to the cryobanking facility. This transport must be as time-efficient as possible, whilst maintaining the integrity of the tissue (e.g. the temperature).

After laparoscopic removal of one ovary or several ovarian biopsies, the specimen can be transported. During transport, it has to be submerged completely in saline solution, basic cell culture or IVF media. In general, ovarian tissue is transported cold. Some centers allow transport on RT or 37°C if the cryobanking facility is on-site, only minutes away from the operation room. If ovarian tissue is to be sent to a remote cryobanking facility, it is kept on crushed ice or cold blocks to keep the tissue between 0°C and 4°C, to limit cellular activity and hence tissue damage in response to the cut off of blood supply. The birth of several babies from ovarian tissue transported cold for several hours and even overnight is reassuring (Dittrich et al. 2014).

Ex-vivo oocyte harvesting and IVM

All oocytes residing in follicles beyond the primordial and primary stage will not survive the freeze-thaw procedure and will be inevitably

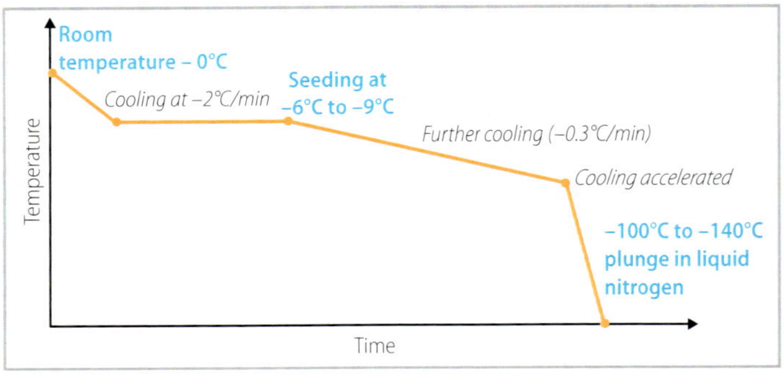

Figure 20.4 Starting at room temperature or 0°C–4°C at the moment of tissue preparation, cryovials containing freezing solution and cortical tissue fragments are first cooled up to –6°C to –9°C at a rate of 2°C/min, where a manual or automatic seeding step is performed. A further decline in temperature up to –30°C to –40°C is obtained at a rate of 0.3°C/min. Hereafter, cooling speed is accelerated to temperatures below –100°C and samples are transferred and stored into liquid nitrogen or stored in nitrogen vapor phase tanks.

lost. However, oocytes from antral follicles can be rescued by collecting them in the laboratory dish during tissue preparation. Before dissection of cortex tissue, follicular fluid can be aspirated from visible antral follicles appearing at the ovarian surface. Moreover, trimming of medulla tissue damages small antral follicles, releasing COC in the dissection medium. Filtration (**Figure 20.5**) and visual inspection of follicular fluid and dissection medium has been shown to lead to an average of 14.7 COCs harvested from one ovary (Segers et al. 2015). With an overall maturation rate of 39% if exposed to a

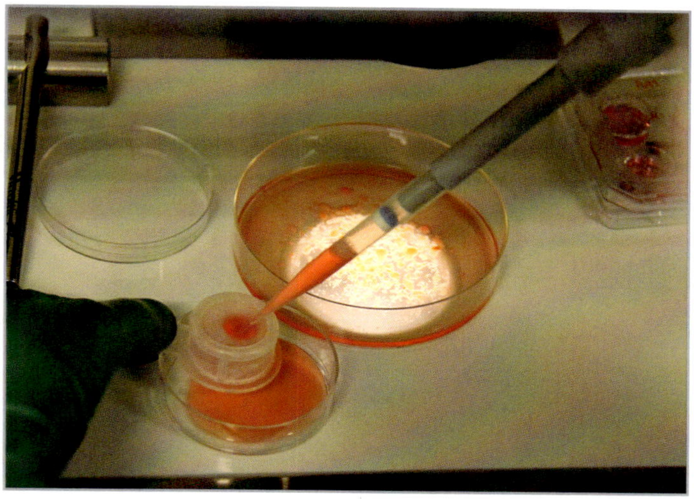

Figure 20.5 Filtration of medium after dissection of ovarian cortex. During tissue processing for ovarian tissue cryopreservation (OTC), medulla tissue is cut away with scissors, inevitably damaging the growing follicles present at the border of medulla and cortex tissue. Hereby, cumulus oocyte complexes (COC) are released in this 'waste material'. These COC can be visualized by filtering the medium in the dish and hence concentrating the COC and eliminating blood cells. Adding fresh medium to the remnant medulla pieces in the dish enhances visibility and allows further inspection of small COC in the dish.

standard IVM treatment, vitrification or insemination of these mature oocytes provides a valuable additional tool for FP.

Although the safety of this technique needs further investigation, three recent reports of deliveries of healthy children from IVM oocytes that had been harvested from extracorporeal tissue, followed by ICSI and embryo vitrification, should fuel the collection of these 'waste-material' oocytes (Prasath et al. 2014, Segers et al. 2015, Uzelac et al. 2015).

CONCLUSION

Oocyte vitrification can be considered as a major breakthrough in the field of FP for several indications, including oncofertility, disease-related and age-related fertility decline. Nevertheless, some controversies and uncertainties remain unsolved to date and need further investigation. The debate regarding the efficiency of open and closed devices for vitrification of oocytes is ongoing, and several studies are being performed to try to resolve this.

Furthermore, it is unclear which proportion of women will eventually use their stored oocytes or will request ovarian tissue transplantation, and how many vitrified oocytes will be needed in order to have a reasonable chance to deliver a child. Moreover, the safety of oocyte IVM is still an important topic of research. The overall efficiency and safety of ovarian tissue transplantation is still unknown since the reported data are scarce. Finally, the health of children born after long-term oocyte or OTC requires careful follow-up.

REFERENCES

Amorim CA, Curaba M, Van Langendonckt A, et al. Vitrification as an alternative means of cryopreserving ovarian tissue. Reprod Biomed Online 2011; 23:160–186.

Baart EB, Martini E, Eijkemans MJ, et al. Milder ovarian stimulation for in-vitro fertilization reduces aneuploidy in the human preimplantation embryo: a randomized controlled trial. Hum Reprod 2007; 22:980–988.

Baldwin K, Culley L, Hudson N, et al. Oocyte cryopreservation for social reasons: demographic profile and disposal intentions of UK users. Reprod Biomed Online 2015; 31:239–245.

Brambillasca F, Guglielmo MC, Coticchio G, et al. The current challenges to efficient immature oocyte cryopreservation. J Assist Reprod Genet 2013; 30:1531–1539.

Cakmak H, Katz A, Cedars MI, Rosen MP. Effective method for emergency fertility preservation: random-start controlled ovarian stimulation. Fertil Steril 2013; 100:1673–1680.

Chen C. Pregnancy after human oocyte cryopreservation. Lancet 1986; 1:884–886.

Cobo A, Garcia-Velasco JA, Coello A, et al. Oocyte vitrification as an efficient option for elective fertility preservation. Fertil Steril 2016; 105:755–758.

Coticchio G, Dal-Canto M, Guglielmo MC, et al. Human oocyte maturation in vitro. Int J Dev Biol 2012; 56:909–918.

De Munck N, Santos-Ribeiro S, Stoop D, et al. Open versus closed oocyte vitrification in an oocyte donation program: a prospective randomized sibling oocyte study. Human Reprod 2016; 31:377–384.

Demeestere I, Simon P, Dedeken L, et al. Live birth after autograft of ovarian tissue cryopreserved during childhood. Hum Reprod 2015; 30:2107–2109.

Devine K, Mumford SL, Goldman KN, et al. Baby budgeting: oocyte cryopreservation in women delaying reproduction can reduce cost per live birth. Fertil Steril 2015; 103:1446–1453.

Dittrich R, Hackl J, Lotz L, et al. Pregnancies and live births after 20 transplantations of cryopreserved ovarian tissue in a single center. Fertil Steril 2015; 103:462–468.

Donnez J, Martinez-Madrid B, Jadoul P, et al. Ovarian tissue cryopreservation and transplantation: a review. Hum Reprod Update 2006; 12:519–535.

Donnez J, Dolmans MM. Ovarian cortex transplantation: 60 reported live births brings the success and worldwide expansion of the technique towards routine clinical practice. J Assist Reprod Genet 2015; 32:1167–1170.

Donnez J, Dolmans MM, Díaz C, Pellicer A. Ovarian cortex transplantation: time to move on from experimental studies to open clinical application. Fertil Steril 2015; 104:1097–1098.

Fadini R, Mignini Renzini M, Guarnieri T, et al. Comparison of the obstetric and perinatal outcomes of children conceived from in vitro or in vivo matured oocytes in in vitro maturation treatments with births from conventional ICSI cycles. Hum Reprod 2012; 27:3601–3608.

Grynberg M, Poulain M, le Parco S, et al. Similar in vitro maturation rates of oocytes retrieved during the follicular or luteal phase offer flexible options for urgent fertility preservation in breast cancer patients. Hum Reprod 2016; 3´:623–629.

Guzman L, Ortega-Hrepich C, Polyzos N, et al. A prediction model to select PCOS patients suitable for IVM treatment based on anti-Mullerian hormone and antral follicle count. Hum Reprod 2013; 28:1261–1266.

Hodes-Wertz B, Druckenmiller S, Smith M, Noyes N. What do reproductive-age women who undergo oocyte cryopreservation think about the process as a means to preserve fertility? Fertil Steril 2013; 100:1343–1349.

Hvidman HW, Petersen KB, Larsen EC, et al. Individual fertility assessment and pro-fertility counselling; should this be offered to women and men of reproductive age? Hum Reprod 2015; 30:9–15.

Knopman JM, Noyes N, Grifo JA. Cryopreserved oocytes can serve as the treatment for secondary infertility: a novel model for egg donation. Fertil Steril 2010; 93:2413.e7–9.

Kuleshova L, Gianaroli L, Magli C, et al. Birth following vitrification of a small number of human oocytes: case report. Hum Reprod 1999; 14:3077–3079.

Lockwood G. Social Egg Freezing: the prospect of reproductive 'immortality' or a dangerous delusion? Reprod BioMed Online 2011; 23:334–340.

Mesen TB, Mersereau JE, Kane JB, Steiner AZ. Optimal timing for elective egg freezing. Fertil Steril 2015; 103:1551–1556.

Paffoni A, Guarneri C, Ferrari S, et al. Effects of two vitrification protocols on the developmental potential of human mature oocytes. Reprod Biomed Online 2011; 22:292–298.

Papatheodorou A, Vanderzwalmen P, Panagiotidis Y, et al. Open versus closed oocyte vitrification system: a prospective randomized sibling-oocyte study. Reprod Biomed Online 2013; 26:595–602.
Paramanantham J, Talmor A, Osianlis T, and Weston GC. Cryopreserved oocytes: update on clinical applications and success rates. Obstet Gynecol Surv 2015; 70:97–114.
Paynter SJ. A rational approach to oocyte cryopreservation. Reprod Biomed Online 2005; 10:578–586.
Prasath EB, Chan ML, Wong WH, et al. First pregnancy and live birth resulting from cryopreserved embryos obtained from in vitro matured oocytes after oophorectomy in an ovarian cancer patient. Hum Reprod 2014; 29:276–278.
Rosendahl M, Greve T, and Andersen CY. The safety of transplanting cryopreserved ovarian tissue in cancer patients: a review of the literature. J Assist Reprod Genet 2013; 30:11–24.
Segers I, Mateizel I, Van Moer E, et al. In vitro maturation (IVM) of oocytes recovered from ovariectomy specimens in the laboratory: a promising "ex vivo" method of oocyte cryopreservation resulting in the first report of an ongoing pregnancy in Europe. J Assist Reprod Genet 2015; 32:1221–1231.
Shaw JM, Jones GM. Terminology associated with vitrification and other cryopreservation procedures for oocytes and embryos. Hum Reprod Update 2003; 9:583–605.
Smitz JE, Thompson JG, Gilchrist RB. The promise of in vitro maturation in assisted reproduction and fertility preservation. Semin Reprod Med 2011; 29:24–37.
Somigliana E, Viganò P, Filippi F, et al. Fertility preservation in women with endometriosis: for all, for some, for none? Hum Reprod 2015; 30:1280–1286.
Sonigo C, Simon C, Boubaya M, et al. What threshold values of antral follicle count and serum AMH levels should be considered for oocyte cryopreservation after in vitro maturation? Hum Reprod 2016; 31:1493–1500.
Stern CJ, Gook D, Hale LG, et al. Delivery of twins following heterotopic grafting of frozen-thawed ovarian tissue. Hum Reprod 2014; 29:1828.
Stoop D, Maes E, Polyzos NP, et al. Does oocyte banking for anticipated gamete exhaustion influence future relational and reproductive choices? A follow-up of bankers and non-bankers. Hum Reprod 2015; 30:338–344.
Stoop D, Nekkebroeck J, Devroey P. A survey on the intentions and attitudes towards oocyte cryopreservation for non-medical reasons among women of reproductive age. Hum Reprod 2011; 26:655–661.
Stoop D, Van der Veen F, Deneyer M, et al. Oocyte banking for anticipated gamete exhaustion (AGE) is a preventive intervention, neither social nor nonmedical. Reprod Biomed Online 2014; 28:548–551.
The Practice Committee of the American Society for Reproductive Medicine. Fertility preservation in patients undergoing gonado-toxic therapy or gonadectomy: a committee opinion. Fertil Steril 2013; 100:1214–1223.
The Practice Committee of the American Society for Reproductive Medicine. Ovarian tissue cryopreservation: a committee opinion. Fertil Steril 2014; 101:1237–1243.
Turan V, Bedoschi G, Moy F, Oktay K. Safety and feasibility of performing two consecutive ovarian stimulation cycles with the use of letrozole-gonadotropin protocol for fertility preservation in breast cancer patients. Fertil Steril 2013; 100:1681–1685.
Uzelac PS, Delaney AA, Christensen GL, Bohler HC, Nakajima ST. Live birth following in vitro maturation of oocytes retrieved from extracorporeal ovarian tissue aspiration and embryo cryopreservation for 5 years. Fertil Steril 2015; 104:1258–1260.
Vajta G, Rienzi L, and Ubaldi FM. Open versus closed systems for vitrification of human oocytes and embryos. Reprod Biomed Online 2015; 30:325–333.
Van Loendersloot LL, Moolenaar LM, Mol BW, et al. Expanding reproductive lifespan: a cost-effectiveness study on oocyte freezing. Hum Reprod 2011; 26:3054–3060.
Vanderzwalmen P, Ectors F, Grobet L, et al. Aspectic vitrification of blastocysts from infertile patients, egg donors and after IVM. Reprod Biomed Online 2009; 19:700–707.
Walls ML, Hunter T, Ryan JP, et al. In vitro maturation as an alternative to standard in vitro fertilization for patients diagnosed with polycystic ovaries: a comparative analysis of fresh, frozen and cumulative cycle outcomes. Hum Reprod 2015; 30:88–96.
Zhang XY, Ata B, Son WY, et al. Chromosome abnormality rates in human embryos obtained from in-vitro maturation and IVF treatment cycles. Reprod Biomed Online 2010; 21:552–559.

Index

Note: Page numbers in **bold** or *italic* refer to tables or figures respectively.